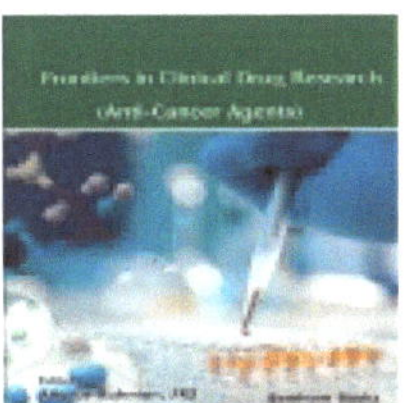

Frontiers in Clinical Drug Research
(Anti-Cancer Agents)
Bentham Books

AF407848

Table of Contents

Frontiers in Clinical Drug Research - Anti-Cancer Agents

(Volume 6)

Edited By

Atta-ur-Rahman, *FRS*
Kings College
University of Cambridge
Cambridge
UK

BENTHAM SCIENCE PUBLISHERS LTD.

End User License Agreement (for non-institutional, personal use)

This is an agreement between you and Bentham Science Publishers Ltd. Please read this License Agreement carefully before using the ebook/echapter/ejournal (**"Work"**). Your use of the Work constitutes your agreement to the terms and conditions set forth in this License Agreement. If you do not agree to these terms and conditions then you should not use the Work.

Bentham Science Publishers agrees to grant you a non-exclusive, non-transferable limited license to use the Work subject to and in accordance with the following terms and conditions. This License Agreement is for non-library, personal use only. For a library / institutional / multi user license in respect of the Work, please contact: permission@benthamscience.net.

Usage Rules:

misuse of the Work or any violation of this License Agreement, including any infringement by you of copyrights or proprietary rights.

Disclaimer:

Bentham Science Publishers does not guarantee that the information in the Work is error-free, or warrant that it will meet your requirements or that access to the Work will be uninterrupted or error-free. The Work is provided "as is" without warranty of any kind, either express or implied or statutory, including, without limitation, implied warranties of merchantability and fitness for a particular purpose. The entire risk as to the results and performance of the Work is assumed by you. No responsibility is assumed by Bentham Science Publishers, its staff, editors and/or authors for any injury and/or damage to persons or property as a matter of products liability, negligence or otherwise, or from any use or operation of any methods, products instruction, advertisements or ideas contained in the Work.

Limitation of Liability:

In no event will Bentham Science Publishers, its staff, editors and/or authors, be liable for any damages, including, without limitation, special, incidental and/or consequential damages and/or damages for lost data and/or profits arising out of (whether directly or indirectly) the use or inability to use the Work. The entire liability of Bentham Science Publishers shall be limited to the amount actually paid by you for the Work.

General:

1. Any dispute or claim arising out of or in connection with this License Agreement or the Work (including non-contractual disputes or claims) will be governed by and construed in accordance with the laws of Singapore. Each party agrees that the courts of the state of Singapore shall have exclusive jurisdiction to settle any dispute or claim arising out of or in connection with this License Agreement or the Work (including non-contractual disputes or claims).
2. Your rights under this License Agreement will automatically terminate without notice and without the need for a court order if at any point you breach any terms of this License Agreement. In no event will any delay or failure by Bentham Science Publishers in enforcing your compliance with this License Agreement constitute a waiver of any of its rights.
3. You acknowledge that you have read this License Agreement, and agree to be bound by its terms and conditions. To the extent that any other terms and conditions presented on any website of Bentham

Science Publishers conflict with, or are inconsistent with, the terms and conditions set out in this License Agreement, you acknowledge that the terms and conditions set out in this License Agreement shall prevail.

Bentham Science Publishers Pte. Ltd.
80 Robinson Road #02-00
Singapore 068898
Singapore
Email: subscriptions@benthamscience.net

PREFACE

Frontiers in Clinical Drug Research - Anti-Cancer Agents presents recent developments in various therapeutic approaches against different types of cancer. The book is a valuable resource for pharmaceutical scientists, postgraduate students, and researchers seeking updated and critical information for developing clinical trials and devising research plans in anti-cancer research.

The five chapters in this volume are written by eminent authorities in the field. Chapter 1 deals with the role of the PI3K/AKT/mTOR pathway in the survival of malignant cells as a potential target to combat relapse in AML patients. It also covers therapeutic agents involving a new class of inhibitors for plausible approaches to treat patients with relapsed or refractory AML diseases. Chapter 2 discusses the role of some natural products as potential novel anti-tumor agents treat CRPC patients. Chapter 3 presents an overview of key proteins and their coordinating and/or cooperating partner proteins in protein pathways which can be useful to design innovative chemotherapeutics. Chapter 4 deals with the effectiveness of Hepatic Arterial Infusion Chemotherapy (HAIC) for advanced hepatocellular carcinoma. Chapter 5 summarizes the current strategies and discusses lead molecules which have found their way to preclinical and clinical studies for targeting cancer stem cells.

I hope that the readers will find these reviews valuable and thought-provoking so that they may trigger further research in the quest for new and novel therapies against cancers.

I am grateful for the timely efforts made by the editorial personnel, especially Mr. Mahmood Alam (Director Publications) and Mrs. Salma Sarfaraz (Senior Manager Publications) at Bentham Science Publishers.

Atta-ur-Rahman, *FRS*
Kings College
University of Cambridge

Cambridge
UK

List of Contributors

Ademar A. da Silva Filho Faculty of Pharmacy, Department of Pharmaceutical Sciences, Federal University of Juiz de Fora, Juiz de Fora, Brazil

Aykut Özgür Tokat Gaziosmanpaşa University, Artova Vocational School, Department of Veterinary Medicine, Laboratory and Veterinary Health Program, Tokat, Turkey

Bilal Rah Immunology and Molecular Medicine, Sher-i-Kashmir Institute of Medical Sciences, Jammu and Kashmir, India

Danilo S. Costa Faculty of Pharmacy, Department of Pharmaceutical Sciences, Federal University of Juiz de Fora, Juiz de Fora, Brazil

Dil Afroze Adavnced Centre for Human Genetics, Sheri-Kashmir Institute of Medical Sciences, Jammu and Kashmir, India

Douglas C. Brandão Institute of Biotechnology, Federal University of Uberlandia, Uberlandia, Brazil

Ezgi Nurdan Yenilmez Tunoğlu Istanbul University, Aziz Sancar Institutes of Health, Division of Molecular Medicine, Istanbul, Turkey

Firdous A. Khanday Department of Biotechnology, University of Kashmir, Srinagar,, Jammu and Kashmir-190006, India

Gabriela S. Guimarães Institute of Biotechnology, Federal University of Uberlandia, Uberlandia, Brazil

Hilal Ahmad Mir Department of Biotechnology, University of Kashmir, Srinagar,, Jammu and Kashmir-190006, India

Hitoshi Yoshiji Department of Gastroenterology and Hepatology, Nara Medical University, Address: 840 Shijo-cho, Kashihara, Nara 634-8522, Japan

Igor M. Campos Faculty of Pharmacy, Department of Pharmaceutical Sciences, Federal University of Juiz de Fora, Juiz de Fora, Brazil

İrfan Koca Yozgat Bozok University, Faculty of Arts and Sciences, Department of Chemistry, Yozgat, Turkey

Javid Rasool	Department of Haematology, Sher-i-Kashmir Institute of Medical Sciences [SKIMS], Jammu and Kashmir, India
Kei Moriya	Department of Gastroenterology and Hepatology, Nara Medical University, Address: 840 Shijo-cho, Kashihara, Nara 634-8522, Japan
Khurshid I. Andrabi	Department of Biotechnology, University of Kashmir, Jammu and Kashmir, India
Lara Vecchi	Institute of Biotechnology, Federal University of Uberlandia, Uberlandia, Brazil
Lütfi Tutar	Ahi Evran University, Faculty of Science, Department of Molecular Biology and Genetics, Kırşehir, Turkey
Mariana A.P. Zóia	Institute of Biotechnology, Federal University of Uberlandia, Uberlandia, Brazil
Matheus A. Ribeiro	Institute of Biotechnology, Federal University of Uberlandia, Uberlandia, Brazil
Mehmet Gümüş	Yozgat Bozok University, Akdağmadeni Health College, Yozgat, Turkey
Paula M.A.P. Lima	Institute of Biotechnology, Federal University of Uberlandia, Uberlandia, Brazil
Rabia Hamid	Department of Nanotechnology, University of Kashmir, Srinagar, Jammu and Kashmir-190006, India
Roshia Ali	Department of Biochemistry, University of Kashmir, Srinagar,, Jammu and Kashmir-190006, India Department of Biotechnology, University of Kashmir, Srinagar,, Jammu and Kashmir-190006, India
Sahar Saleem Bhat	Division of Biotechnology, SKUAST-K, FVSc& AH, Shuhama, Srinagar, Jammu and Kashmir, India
Sara T.S. Mota	Institute of Biotechnology, Federal University of Uberlandia, Uberlandia, Brazil
Servet Tunoğlu	Istanbul University, Aziz Sancar Institutes of Health, Division of Molecular Medicine, Istanbul, Turkey
Shazia Ali	Adavnced Centre for Human Genetics, Sheri-Kashmir Institute of Medical Sciences, Jammu and Kashmir, India
Tadashi	Department of Gastroenterology and Hepatology, Nara Medical

Namisaki   University, Address: 840 Shijo-cho, Kashihara, Nara 634-8522, Japan

Thaise G. Araújo   Institute of Biotechnology, Federal University of Uberlandia, Uberlandia, Brazil

Yusuf Tutar   University of Health Sciences, Hamidiye Institute of Health Sciences, Division of Molecular Oncology, Istanbul, Turkey Hamidiye Faculty of Pharmacy, Department of Basic Pharmaceutical Sciences, Division of Biochemistry, Istanbul, Turkey

Immunomodulating Agents in the Treatment of Acute Myeloid Leukemia: A Combinatorial Immunotherapeutic Approach

Shazia Ali[1], Dil Afroze[1], [*], Javid Rasool[2], Bilal Rah[4], Khurshid I. Andrabi[3]

[1] Adavnced Centre for Human Genetics, Sheri-Kashmir Institute of Medical Sciences, Jammu and Kashmir, India

[2] Department of Haematology, Sher-i-Kashmir Institute of Medical Sciences [SKIMS], Jammu and Kashmir, India

[3] Department of Biotechnology, University of Kashmir, Jammu and Kashmir, India

[4] Immunology and Molecular Medicine, Sheri-Kashmir Institute of Medical Sciences, Jammu and Kashmir, India

Abstract

Regardless of the diverse modes of treatment, the prognosis and clinical response of AML (Acute myeloid leukemia) remain low as the conventional modes of treatment, including cytarabine and anthracycline have their limitations. Moreover, chemotherapy-induced cytotoxicity triggers the remission, thus most of AML patients succumb to relapse. The monotherapy is also not helping much due to the rapid growth of AML, while an insufficient period of time is a major barrier in immunotherapy. Therefore, the current focus has been on combination therapy, with different agents, possibly because chemotherapy for AML is associated with infection, inflammation and could be rather toxic when combined with immunotherapy. Thus, there is the utmost need for developing a new approach and treatment for AML. Recent therapies focus on various novel signaling pathways and proteins that promote the survival of cancer cells in AML patients. This single or combinatorial approach may be more effective with less harmful effects. In this context, here we are discussing the role of PI3K/AKT/mTOR pathway in the survival of malignant cells as a potential target to combat relapse in AML patients. Accordingly, the therapeutic agents with a new class of inhibitors for plausible approaches to treat the patients with relapsed or refractory AML diseases could be advocated.

Keywords: Acute myeloid leukemia, Inhibitors, Kinase, Rapamycin, Signaling, TORC1.

* **Corresponding author Dil Afroze:** Adavnced Centre for Human Genetics, Sheri-Kashmir Institute of Medical Sciences, Jammu and Kashmir, India;   E-mail: afrozedil@gmail.com

INTRODUCTION

Acute myeloid leukemia [AML] is a dysregulated proliferation of myeloid precursor cells leading to genomic instability. AML generally affects the people of older age and rarely occurs before the age of 45 and is thus a disease of later adulthood. 174,250 people were diagnosed with AML, in 2018, in the US alone. The overall incidence rate per 100,000 populations was reported in 2017 for leukemia based on age. 9.5 percent of the deaths was reported to be due to cancer in 2018, based on the predicted total of 609,640 cancer deaths [1, 2] The reckless progression of AML is fatal within a week or two if left untreated [3]. It is a multi-clonal disease involving the expansion of aberrant cells resulting in the impairment of the hematopoietic process, eventually leading to clinical relapse and death. The clonal heterogeneity in a large number of these patients intrigues different outcomes to chemotherapy in various individuals with AML.

Leukemogenesis is a multifactorial phenomenon involving genetic disposition, physical, chemical, or radiation exposure and chemotherapy. Many genetic aberrations have been associated with hyperproliferation and undifferentiated clonal populations in patients with AML. The distinct pattern of clonal cytogenetic abnormalities gives rise to acute myelogenous leukemia. Thus, the characterization of such clonal population and chromosomal aberrations will provide insights to understand the origin and development of leukemia. The mutations in epigenetic and transcriptional regulators represent one of the hallmarks of AML. There are numerous mutated genes present in AML, *e.g.*, FLT-3, fms-like tyrosine kinase-3, and IDH, isocitrate dehydrogenase associated with the sub-clonal population, which are difficult to analyze by an advanced technique like flow cytometry. It cannot be differentiated as to which sub-clone has refractory/ relapse properties. The mutations could be evaluated only after remission induction therapy in these patients for 5-7 days, which kills leukemic and normal blood marrow cells giving us an assessment of the improvement for the erased mutation after induction. Such trials can lead to identifying sub-clones having relapse markers by different techniques like cytogenetics, sequencing [4].

Chemotherapeutic Drugs Used in the Treatment of AML

Most of the patients can respond to the initial cytotoxic induction therapy; the common cause of death is the relapse of disease. The various chemotherapeutic regimes used for the treatment of AML are cytarabine, anthracycline, daunorubicin. Some of them are mentioned in Table 1. The other option for treatment is aggressive therapy to provide a path to an allogeneic hematopoietic stem cell transplant [alloHSCT], which is the promising option for patients with refractory or relapsed AML [RR-AML]. Patients should have at least a complete response before undergoing alloHSCT and fewer side effects with a suitable donor and in good health condition. The standard chemotherapy regimens do not help eliminate leukemia in patients showing relapse. It is due to the activation of various signaling cascades in leukemia stem cells and early leukemic precursors actively help in stimulating their survival. These signaling pathways are further targeted by several targeted agents. Some of the targeted agents are mentioned in Table 2, along with new combinational approaches of immunotherapeutic agents studied in clinical trials mentioned in Table 3. Such agents provide a potential therapeutic output and different signaling pathways like PI3K, mTOR can be targeted for the treatment of leukemia. New strategies and methods for treating AML individuals are being executed like a gene test variant of a patient, which helps in designing a drug and predicting the exact drug working for a specific patient [5].

The clinical relapse occurs due to three main sources; disease was chemosensitive with partial treatment and reoccurred with multiple mutations, a subclone originated from an initial clone at low frequency, but after treatment clone gets benefitted due to the decreased chemotherapy sensitiveness and a denovo generation of AML because of side effects from treatment. AML is treated with chemotherapy at the initial stage with an additional hematopoietic stem cell transplant depending on the patient's response [6].

AML Relapse

The relapse in AML occurs at any stage of the treatment or after completion of treatment. The standard recommendations by world health organization include monitoring blood counts for platelets every 1 to 3 months for the first two years and every 3 to 6 months thereafter for another three years [7]. The general practice of clinicians for treatment includes enrollment in a clinical trial, the reintroduction of a similar induction regimen if a relapse happens at a later stage [>12 months], or with a salvage regimen followed by allogeneic hematopoietic stem cell transplant. The relapse factor depends on age, pre-treatment cytogenetics, and chemotherapeutic drugs required for the first complete response. The prognosis factor is one of the important factors to be kept in mind at the time of relapse of disease. Relapse is one of the leading causes of death in such patients. The prognostic factor will help in facilitating appropriate chemotherapeutic agents for the successful treatment of disease [8, 9].

PI3K/mTOR Pathway

PI3K/mTOR, a mechanistic target of Rapamycin pathway is one of the main regulatory signaling cascades in mammals maintaining activities of a cellular system by regulating the transcription of genes encoding pro-oncogenic proteins which help in the survival of malignant cells. The growth-suppressive cytokines, for example, IFNs, help in activating the signaling cascades wherein a competition between growth factors and mitogenic factors occurs to regulate the mTOR pathway. Due to PTEN mutation, hyperactivation of PI3K leads to phosphorylation and activation of AKT on threonine 308, resulting in activation of downstream substrates and effectors promoting survival and proliferation in mammals. Extensive research and study are in progress to inhibit this pathway, which may pave the way for finding anti-tumorigenic therapy. The activation of this pathway also results in chemotherapy resistance. This makes the PI3K/AKT/mTOR signaling cascade pathway a major target for anticancer therapy in the treatment of AML and various other cancers. For the same reason, pharmacological inhibitors of the PI3K/AKT/mTOR pathway have been studied and are currently being evaluated in ongoing clinical trials. The first-generation mTOR inhibitors, including rapamycin, rapalogs, are in various phases of clinical trials. Two rapalogs, temsirolimus, and everolimus are approved by the FDA for treating renal cancer [10, 11]. The main pathway which is affected during AML is PI3K/mTOR signaling regulatory one. The study and elucidation of such pathways will pave the way to treat AML effectively.

Table 1 **Chemotherapy regimens in patients with relapsed or refractory acute myeloid leukemia [AML].**

Regimen	Agents	CR and Response Rate	TRM or 30-day Mortality	Reference	Overall Survival
HiDAC	Cytarabine	32-47%	12-15%	[12-15]	Overall response is 50%, Clinical remission is 30-40%
FLAG FLAG-IDA	Fludarabine Cytarabine	48-55%	10-11%	[16-18]	Overall and

	G-CSF				disease-free survivals were 19.3 and 11.3 months Overall CR rate for the salvage induction group was 73% Overall survival longer, superior disease-free survival [DFS at 5 years was 57% Vs 39%]
	Fludarabine Cytarabine Idarubicin	63%	17%	[19, 20]	
CLAG CLAG-M	Cladribine 5 mg/m^2 days 2-6 Cytarabine 2 g/m^2 days 2–6 G-CSF 300 mcg days 1–6	38-50%	0-17%	[21‑23]	Response rates and median overall survivals were 64% and 202 days
	Cladribine 5 mg/m^2 days 1–5 Cytarabine 2 g/m^2 days 1–5 G-CSF 300 mcg days 0–5 Mitoxantrone	50-58% [58% after first course]	0-7%		

MEC	Mitoxantrone 6 mg/m^2 days 1–6 Etoposide 80 mg/m^2 days 1–6 Cytarabine 1 g/m^2 days 1–6	59-66%	3-6%	[24⁻27]	Median overall survival [OS] was 6.8 months
MEC/Decitabine	Decitabine 20 mg/m^2 days 1–10 Mitoxantrone 8 mg/m^2 days 16–20 Etoposide 100 mg/m^2 days 16–20 Cytarabine 1 mg/m^2 days 16–20	30% [CR + CRp+CRi=50%]	20%	[27⁻29]	CR [30%], overall response rate was 50%, overall survival was longer [median of 211 days]
EMA-86	Mitoxantrone 12 mg/m^2 days 1–3 Cytarabine 500 mg/m^2 CI days 1–3 & 8–10 Etoposide 200 mg/m^2 CI days 8-10	60%	11%	[29]	60% CR, median survival was 7 months, 11% survival was 5 years
MAV	Mitomycin 10 mg/m^2 days 4–8 Cytarabine 100 mg/m^2 CI days 1–8 Etoposide 100–120	58%	11%	[30]	58.3% patients had complete remission

	mg/m^2 days 4–8					
FLAD	Fludarabine 30 mg/m^2 days 1–3 Cytarabine 2 g/m^2 days 1–3 Liposomal daunorubicin 100 mg/m^2 days 1–3	53%		7.5%	[31, 32]	Complete response rate was 44% and 56%, overall response rate of 52%. Median overall survival in AML patients was 9 months
GCLAC	Clofarabine 25 mg/m^2 days 1–5; Cytarabine 2 g/m^2 days 1–5; G-CSF 5 mcg/kg day 0 until ANC recovery	46%, [CR + CRp 61%]		13%	[33, 34]	Thirty-one patients, 52% had CR, an overall response rate of 60%. Among 35 patients older than 60 years of age, 20 patients [57%] achieved CR and 2 [6%] and OR of 63%.

complete response [CR], complete response with incomplete platelet recovery [CRP], complete response with incomplete blood count recovery [CRi], treatment-related mortality [TRM], High-dose arabinoside cytarabine

[HiDAC], granulocyte colony-stimulating factor [G-CSF], continuous infusion [CI], cyclin-dependent kinase [CDK].

Table 2 **Targeted agents in trials for the treatment of patients with relapsed/refractory AML [RR-AML].**

Agent	Mechanism of Action	Outcome	Overall Response	Complete Response	Reference
Quizartinib	FLT-3 inhibitor	It acts as a single agent against FLT3-ITD	61%-72%	44%-54%	[35]
Crenolanib	FLT-3 inhibitor	It inhibits signaling of wild-type and mutant isoforms of class III receptor *FLT3*, PDGFR α, and PDGFR β	234 days:238 days	39%	[36]
Rapamycin	mTOR inhibitor	It acts as a mTOR inhibitory agent	95%	95%	[37, 38]
Everolimus	mTOR inhibitor	It acts as a mTOR inhibitory agent	10.5-12 months	The objective response rate of 38%	[39]
Tosedostat	Aminopeptidase activity inhibitor CR 53%	It is an aminopeptidase inhibitor, has synergy with cytarabine and hypomethylating agents	CR/CR with incomplete count recovery [CRi] rate was 53%	Median survival was 11.5 months	[40-42]
Vorinostat	Histone deacetylase inhibitor	It is a cancer growth blocker, suberoylanilide hydroxamic acid, SAHA], a hydroxamic acid inhibitor of class I and class II HDAC	105-153 days overall maiden survival	complete remission rate was 4.5%	[43-45]

AG-120	IDH1 inhibitor	It acts as a single agent in R/R AML	Overall response rate 31%	Complete response 15%	NCT02074839
AG-221	IDH2 inhibitor	It acts as a single agent in R/R AML	ORR 41%	18%	[46]
Vosaroxin	Anticancer quinolone derivative	It intercalates DNA and inhibits topoisomerase II.	overall survival was 6.9 months	CR rate was 25%	[47, 48]
Pravastatin	HMG-CoA reductase inhibitor	It is a member of the drug class of statins	median overall survival was 12 months	response rate was 75%	[49]
Bortezomib	Proteasome inhibitor	It acts as a proteasome inhibitor	2-year overall survival [OS] was $39 \pm 15\%$	complete response [CR + CRp] rates were 29%	[50]
CPI-613	Lipoate derivative	It inhibits mitochondrial respiration in AML cells	Overall response rate was 48%	CR/CRi rate of 46%	[51]
ABT-199	BCL-2 inhibitor	It represents the first in class, selective, oral BCL-2 inhibitor sparing platelets	ORR was 15.5%	complete response [CR] of 23%	[52, 53]

Table 3 **Immunotherapeutic agents for the treatment of patients with relapsed/refractory AML.**

Agent	Overall Survival	Complete Response	Mechanism of Action	Reference
Gemtuzumab ozogamicin	Overall response rate 26%	Complete response [CR] rate was 16%	Conjugated Antibody targeting CD33	[54, 55]
SGN-CD33A	Overall survival 12.75	Complete response rate was 71 percent	Conjugated Antibody targeting	[56]

	months		CD33	
MGD006	phase 1 clinical trial, bispecific antibodies	MGD006 is a humanized, dual affinity retargeting, or DART, a molecule that recognizes both CD123 and CD3	Dual Affinity Re-Targeting Antibody targeting CD123 and CD3	[57]
CD16x33 BiKE		It activates NK cells at high potency against acute myelogenous leukemia [AML]	Bispecific Killer Cell Engager Antibody against CD16 and CD33	[58]
CART33		It is effective against long term myelosuppression and can be used alone or as part of a regimen before giving allogeneic transplantation in refractory AML.	Chimeric Antigen Receptor-Transduced T Cells targeting CD33	[59, 60]
CART123		It eliminates leukemia and leads to long term survival of AML	Chimeric Antigen Receptor-transduced T - cells targeting CD123	[61, 62]
WT1 peptide vaccine	It has relapse-free survival >1 year	It has long-lived [more than 8 years] remissions of disease	Vaccine targeting WT1	[63, 64]
WT1-specific CD8[+] T-cell infusion		WT1 with T-cells is safe and can lead to antileukemic activity	Adoptive Cell Transfer	[65, 66]
AlloHSCT	Leukemia-free survival, overall survival was improved	It reduced the risk of relapse for patients with AML	Adoptive Cell Transfer	[67, 68]
Donor lymphocyte infusion [post alloHCT]	Survival for all patients was 23% at 1-year post	CR rates of 29%	Adoptive Cell Transfer	[10, 62, 69-71]

| | relapse | | | |

mTOR Pathway in AML

The dis-functioning of pathways control both transcription and translation of genes encoding for oncogenic proteins. These emerge as the leading player's promotion and progression of AML disease. The PI3K/AKT/mTOR pathway is activated in AML. The activation of constitutive 3'K in AML is because of active PI3K p110δ isoform.

It has been found that AKT activation along with other cross-talk pathways like PKC-α and ERK leads to poor prognosis in AML. In recent years, proteomics study or single-cell network profiling with flow cytometry has been extensively used to check the chemotherapeutic response in AML patients. Their chemotherapy is highly ineffective in patients older than 60 years or secondary AML patients. Such AML ones are linked with increased phosphorylation of AKT, which is induced by FLT-3 ligand [72]. AML can be treated in a specific manner about identifying aberration in AKT/mTOR pathway. The use of mTOR inhibitor; Rapamycin has shown blast clearance in some patients of AML. The combinatorial approach of drugs like Rapamycin and etoposide has synergistic effects on AML cells *in vitro* and in AML mouse models under *in vivo* condition. The similar results of a combination of drugs in a chemotherapeutic regimen [mitoxanthrone, etoposide, and cytarbine] for the treatment of relapsed AML, but there weren't a similar response to AML patients. This gives an insight that the combinatorial approach of drugs can be successful for treatment. However, it needs to be extensively studied and practiced in clinical trials with the optimum dose and response of patients to the therapy before commercialization [73].

TORC1 Targeted Therapy in mTOR

Though there are various approaches to establish the dose and response of different rapalogs along with chemotherapy, the use of such agents is limited in the therapeutic aspect of the patient. To overcome such limitations, the agents are designed as inhibitors of multiple targeting pathways like mTORC1, mTORC2, and PI3K/AKT. For more effective treatment, dual TORC1, TORC2 inhibitors like PP242 or OSI-027 are being developed. These are very effective suppressors of TORC function in BCR-ABL transformed cells. These inhibitors showed anti-leukemic activity under *in vitro* and *in vivo* condition of CML cells, and on T3151 BCR-ABL mutated cells, which were resistant to such mTOR inhibitors are presently approved for CML and Ph+ ALL, for example, imatinib, mesylate, nilotinib, dasatinib. Such results lead to the possibility of using these agents in various other leukemias. The effects of dual TORC1/2 inhibition on different elements of the mTOR pathway in multiple AML cell lines and blasts of leukemia from AML patients were compared to mTOR inhibitor, rapamycin. The findings were that OSI-027 inhibited TORC2-specific cells of AML, leading to AKT phosphorylation on Ser473. In comparison to this finding, both OSI-027 and rapamycin were inhibiting activation of S6 kinase and its downstream target S6 ribosomal protein. There was an important finding that 4E-BP1 phosphorylation was inhibited by OSI-027 and not rapamycin stating that phosphorylation is a rapamycin-insensitive cell event in AML cells. The result is similar to other systems for rapamycin-insensitive TORC1-mediated signals. Some studies have established that OSI-027 is inhibiting primitive leukemic precursors from AML patients. Compared to rapamycin, OSI-021 was more inhibitory. It inhibited the effect of low dose cytarabine, stating that the combinatorial approach of dual TORC1/2 inhibitors with chemotherapy will provide an anti-leukemic response to chemotherapy [74].

In conclusion, clinical trials need to be done in more numbers for such dual TORC1/TORC2 inhibitors for AML. Apart from OSI-027, there are more TORC1/2 in clinical or pre-clinical development. Another approach is to block the mTOR pathway by inhibiting PI3K/AKT completely. The combined blockade of PI3K and mTOR has also been developed, for example, NVPBEZ235. This molecule has been effective, including rapamycin-insensitive TORC1 and 4E-BP1. The outcome was cell proliferation, and leukemic progenitor clonogenicity was decreased. This outcome makes this combinatorial approach as a progressive way for the treatment of AML [75].

Novel Therapies in the Treatment of AML

The overall survival rate in AML patients increases with the clinically active single agents like hypomethylating agents, and chemotherapies. The most effective response is a combination of such agents with chemotherapy or the dual approach of drugs. For example, the combination of FLT3, fms like tyrosine kinase-3, and IDH, isocitrate dehydrogenase inhibitors with chemotherapy, can be used. Targeted therapeutic agents and ADCs, antibody-drug conjugates in induction chemotherapy are another excellent combination and use, thereby it as maintenance therapy. The other combinational approach can be volasertib, guadecitabine, and SGN-CD33A along with targeted therapies, but such agents should be practiced in clinical trials [56, 72].

FLT3 Mutation in AML as a Therapeutic Target

FLT3, a cytokine receptor for FLT3 ligand, belongs to the class III family of tyrosine kinases [76]. Eventually expressed in myeloid series, FLT3 regulates the cell survival and proliferation of hematopoietic stem cells [77, 78]. It is commonly restricted in the region of juxtamembrane, FLT3 mutations are mostly seen in AML patients, contain 20% of mutations as internal tandem duplications, and 28-34% as CN-AML, however recent data suggest the association of the poor outcome with later mutation [79]. These constitutively active mutations activate the downstream cascade like RAS, MAPK, PI3K/Akt/mTOR, and STAT5 signaling pathways and accelerate immature blast count [80]. Various reports suggested that FLT3 mutations in AML patients are providing beneficial effects to allo-HSCT in CR1 [81]. Tyrosine kinase inhibitors [TKI] have been recently introduced in the therapeutics of an AML patient with FLT3 mutations alone or combinations with other chemotherapeutic drugs, thereby drastically reduces the blast count and increases overall survival time of AML patients [82].

Targeting Isocitrate Dehydrogenase [IDH] Mutations in AML

Isocitrate dehydrogenase [IDH] 1 and 2 genes encode vital physiological, metabolic enzymes that regulate the isocitrate and α-ketoglutarate metabolites [83]. In AML, the gain of function mutation of IDH1/2 is an oncogenic mutation in hematologic malignancies, increasing the oncometabolite's synthesis, the 2-hydroxyglutarate from the α-ketoglutarate [84]. The high production of 2-hydroxyglutarate inhibits TET enzymes, thus increases immature blast count [85]. The gain of function mutation in IDH1/2 accounts for approximately 15-20% of AML patients and 25-30% of CN-AML patients [86]. IDH1/2 mutations are afflicted with overall poor overall in CN-AML patients [87]. It is especially true for older patients. Recent findings revealed that many promising, selective, orally available inhibitors of mutant IDH1/2 are in clinical trials [phase I and II] for AML patients [Table 4], which might represent a novel class of drugs in targeted therapy [88⁻90].

Table 4 **Small molecule inhibitors and mutations in different malignancies as a therapeutic target in various clinical trials.**

Drug	Neoplasm/Cancer Studied	Clinical Trials	Mechanism/Target/Pathways	References
AG-120	Hematological malignancies	Phase I/II	IDH1 mutation	[89]
AG-120	Cholangiocarcinoma Chondrosarcoma Glioma Other advanced solid tumors	Phase I/II	IDH1 mutation	[89]
AG-221	Hematological	Phase I/II	IDH2 mutation	[89]

	malignancies			
AG-221	Solid tumor Glioma Angioimmunoblastic T-cell lymphoma Intrahepatic cholangiocarcinoma Chondrosarcoma	Phase I/II	IDH2 mutation	[89]
AG-221	Refractory or relapsed AML	Randomized Phase III: AG-221 vs physician's choice Patients ≥ 60 years of age after the second or third line of treatment	IDH2 mutation	[89]
AG-120 or AG-221	Newly diagnosed AML	Phase I	IDH1 mutation IDH2 mutation	[89]
AG-120 or AG-221	Newly diagnosed AML	Phase Ib/II	IDH1 mutation IDH2 mutation	[89]
In combination with subcutaneous azacitidine/In patients unfit for intensive chemotherapy				
AG-881	Advanced hematological malignancies	Phase I/II	IDH1 mutation IDH2 mutation	[89]
AG-881	Cholangiocarcinoma Chondrosarcoma Glioma	Phase I/II	IDH1 mutation IDH2 mutation	[89]
IDH305	Advanced haematological malignancies	Phase I/II	IDH1R132 mutation	[89]
IDH1 peptide vaccine	Grade III–IV gliomas	Phase I/II	IDH1R132H mutation	[89]
IDH1	Recurrent grade II	Phase I/II	IDH1 mutation	[89]

peptide vaccine	glioma			
FLT3 inhibitors as a single agent or in combination				
Midostaurin	Newly Diagnosed AML	Phase III	Protein Kinase C/another kinase inhibitor	[90]
Midostaurin	Newly diagnosed AML Elderly AML	Phase II	Protein Kinase C/another kinase inhibitor	[90]
Midostaurin	Newly diagnosed elderly MDS	Phase II	Protein Kinase C/another kinase inhibitor	[90]
Lestaurtinib	Newly diagnosed AML	Phase III	Janus kinase 2 [JAK2], tropomyosin receptor kinase A	[90]
Sorafenib	Newly diagnosed AML	Phase III	Pan-kinase inhibitor	[90]
Sorafenib	Newly diagnosed AML	Phase III	Pan-kinase inhibitor	[90]
Sorafenib	Maintenance after allogeneic transplantation of AML	Pilot Study	Pan-kinase inhibitor	[90]
Sorafenib	Maintenance after allogeneic transplantation of AML	Phase I/II	Pan-kinase inhibitor	[90]
Sunitinib	Newly diagnosed AML	Phase II	multi-kinase inhibitor/FLT3	[90]
Quizartinib	Relapsed/refractory AML	Phase II	c-KIT and another kinase inhibitor	[90]
Quizartinib	Newly diagnosed adults AML	Phase I	c-KIT and another kinase inhibitor	[90]
Quizartinib	Maintenance after allogeneic transplantation of AML	Phase I	c-KIT and another kinase inhibitor	[90]
Quizartinib	Newly diagnosed elderly AML	Phase II	c-KIT and another kinase inhibitor	[90]
Ponatinib	Relapsed/refractory AML	Phase I	BCR-ABL, FLT3, TKI-resistant CML/Ph+ ALL	[90]
Crenolanib	Relapsed/refractory AML	Phase I	PDGFR/FLT3 inhibitor	[90]
Gilteritinib		Phase III	FLT3/AXL inhibitoR	[97]

| | Relapsed/refractory AML | | | |

Immunologic Approaches for the Treatment of AML

There are various immunomodulating agents like lenalidomide, which are supposed to be effective in low proliferating diseases. The use of epigenetic modulators will be useful in relapsed patients. The same can be used in combination with other agents like tosedostat, midostaurin, or as a helping agent to allogeneic transplantation for unhealthy patients to reduce the intensity of drugs. Some of the agents which are used in AML patients like IDH1/2 mutations, FLT3-1TD, MLL-r are promising for molecularly defined groups [36, 46]. The poor prognosis factor in AML refractory/early relapse is the worrying aspect. To overcome such disadvantages, the use of next-generation sequencing is another way to see the genetic aberrations and design the drug according to the treatment of AML [93, 94].

The Use of Inhibitors in the Treatment of AML and Concluding Remarks

The inhibition of mTOR is one of the positive outcomes in the treatment of many malignancies, which selectively target agents like TORC1 [rapalogs] with limited activity and less impact in the clinical aspect. In this regard, selective ATP-catalytic inhibitors, which block both TORC1 and TORC2, are showing new ways to treat AML by targeting the mTOR pathway. Various approaches are going on, both *in vitro* and in clinical aspects, to overcome the negative issues of rapalogs and make them better inhibitors, for example, dual inhibitors like TORC1/2 or pan-PI3K-TORC1/2 are being developed and tested in clinical trials. The trials have to be optimized further by including a large number of patients and optimizing the dose and response of these inhibitors with minimal side effects and a major effect on the malignant part. The inclusion and exclusion criteria, while taking an inhibitor in trial and patient-specific inhibitors, are in the process of development. The dual inhibitors, apart from having an anti-leukemic effect, dual TORC1/2 catalytic inhibition also increases the effect of commonly used AML drug cytarabine on primitive leukemic precursor from AML patients. These studies will have a beneficial effect on AML patients. The combination of inhibitors and chemotherapeutic agents will provide a therapeutic approach to leukemic initiating stem cells and help to incur such patients. The revolution of newer techniques and low cost of next-generation sequencing of DNA, genetic mutation studies, to the pathogenesis of new cases of relapsed and refractory

AML. ChIP-seq has paved a way to understand genetic alterations present in leukemic disease [95, 96].

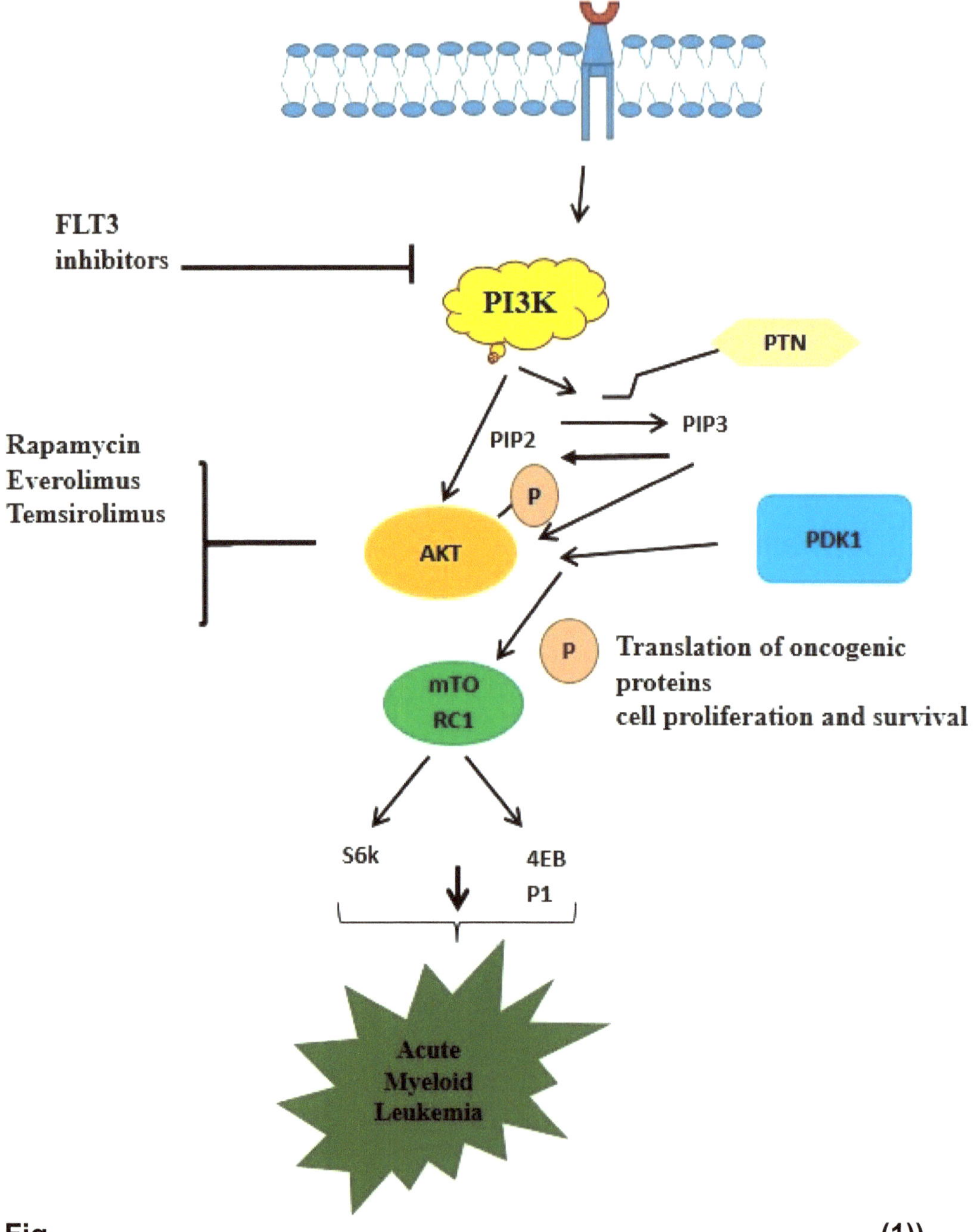

Fig. (1))

Direct mTOR inhibition by rapalogs (Rapamycin, Everolimus, Temsirolimus), inhibitors like FLT3 in AML.

Such genetic alterations can be studied using inhibitors like FLT3, NPM1, and CEBPA, which are in practice governed by world health organization guidelines for AML. Mutations in genes such as c-KIT, IDH1, IDH2, and FLT3 provide molecular aspects in AML that lead to an improvement in complete remission, disease-free survival, overall survival. Other inhibitors of proteins are also involved in clinical activity in phase 1 studies [7, 91, 92]. The newer approach is to translate preclinical data into the therapeutic regimen and in practice. The identification of a biomarker is another way to combine these agents with other drugs that show synergism. The pictorial representation of the mTOR inhibitors is shown in Fig. (1).

FUNDING

The funding body had no role in the writing of the review.

CONSENT FOR PUBLICATION

Not applicable.

CONFLICT OF INTEREST

The authors declare no conflict of interest, financial or otherwise.

ACKNOWLEDGEMENTS

This review was written by keeping in mind the relapse component in AML patients and data was compiled from the various studies to generate tables and figures accompanying this article. The article was critically reviewed and approved of its final version.

REFERENCES

[1]   Siegel RL, Miller KD, Jemal A. Cancer statistics, 2016. CA Cancer J Clin 2016; 66(1): 7-30.[http://dx.doi.org/10.3322/caac.21332] [PMID: 26742998]

[2]   Walter RB, Othus M, Burnett AK, et al. Resistance prediction in AML: analysis of 4601 patients from MRC/NCRI, HOVON/SAKK, SWOG and MD Anderson Cancer Center. Leukemia 2015; 29(2): 312-20.[http://dx.doi.org/10.1038/leu.2014.242] [PMID: 25113226]

[3]   Löwenberg B, Downing JR, Burnett A. Acute myeloid leukemia. N Engl J Med 1999; 341(14): 1051-62.[http://dx.doi.org/10.1056/NEJM199909303411407] [PMID: 10502596]

[4]   Ley TJ. Clonal Evolution and Relapse in Adult De Novo Acute Myeloid Leukemia. 2017.

[5]   Pemmaraju N, Kantarjian H, Garcia-Manero G, et al. Improving outcomes for patients with acute myeloid

leukemia in first relapse: a single center experience. Am J Hematol 2015; 90(1): 27-30.[http://dx.doi.org/10.1002/ajh.23858] [PMID: 25251041]

[6]   Ding L, Ley TJ, Larson DE, *et al.* Clonal evolution in relapsed acute myeloid leukaemia revealed by whole-genome sequencing. Nature 2012; 481(7382): 506-10.[http://dx.doi.org/10.1038/nature10738] [PMID: 22237025]

[7]   Breems DA, Van Putten WLJ, Huijgens PC, *et al.* Prognostic index for adult patients with acute myeloid leukemia in first relapse. J Clin Oncol 2005; 23(9): 1969-78.[http://dx.doi.org/10.1200/JCO.2005.06.027] [PMID: 15632409]

[8]   Kurosawa S, Yamaguchi T, Miyawaki S, *et al.* Prognostic factors and outcomes of adult patients with acute myeloid leukemia after first relapse. Haematologica 2010; 95(11): 1857-64.[http://dx.doi.org/10.3324/haematol.2010.027516] [PMID: 20634493]

[9]   Hourigan CS, Karp JE. New considerations in the design of clinical trials for the treatment of acute leukemia. Clin Investig (Lond) 2011; 1(4): 509-17.[http://dx.doi.org/10.4155/cli.11.24] [PMID: 23459118]

[10]   Meggendorfer M, Alpermann T, Perglerov K, Kern W, Schnittger S, Haferlach C. Genetic patterns of relapsed aml differ significantly from the first manifestation and are dependent on cytogenetic risk groups at diagnosis: Results in 175 patients with paired samples 2014.

[11]   Tian T, Li X, Zhang J. mTOR Signaling in Cancer and mTOR Inhibitors in Solid Tumor Targeting Therapy. Int J Mol Sci 2019; 20(3): 755.[http://dx.doi.org/10.3390/ijms20030755] [PMID: 30754640]

[12]   Karanes C, Kopecky KJ, Head DR, *et al.* A phase III comparison of high dose ARA-C (HIDAC) *versus* HIDAC plus mitoxantrone in the treatment of first relapsed or refractory acute myeloid leukemia Southwest Oncology Group Study. Leuk Res 1999; 23(9): 787-94.[http://dx.doi.org/10.1016/S0145-2126(99)00087-9] [PMID: 10475617]

[13]   Herzig RH, Lazarus HM, Wolff SN, Phillips GL, Herzig GP. High-dose cytosine arabinoside therapy with and without anthracycline antibiotics for remission reinduction of acute nonlymphoblastic leukemia. J Clin Oncol 1985; 3(7): 992-7.[http://dx.doi.org/10.1200/JCO.1985.3.7.992] [PMID: 3894588]

[14]   Montillo M, Mirto S, Petti MC, *et al.* Fludarabine, cytarabine, and G-CSF (FLAG) for the treatment of poor risk acute myeloid leukemia. Am J Hematol 1998; 58(2): 105-9.[http://dx.doi.org/10.1002/(SICI)1096-8652(199806)58:2<105::AID-AJH3>3.0.CO;2-W] [PMID: 9625576]

[15]   Virchis A, Koh M, Rankin P, *et al.* Fludarabine, cytosine arabinoside, granulocyte-colony stimulating factor with or without idarubicin in the treatment of high risk acute leukaemia or myelodysplastic syndromes. Br J Haematol 2004; 124(1): 26-32.[http://dx.doi.org/10.1046/j.1365-2141.2003.04728.x] [PMID: 14675405]

[16]   Martin MG, Welch JS, Augustin K, Hladnik L, DiPersio JF, Abboud CN. Cladribine in the treatment of acute myeloid leukemia: a single-institution experience. Clin Lymphoma Myeloma 2009; 9(4): 298-301.[http://dx.doi.org/10.3816/CLM.2009.n.058] [PMID: 19717379]

[17]   Wrzesień-Kuś A, Robak T, Lech-Marańda E, *et al.* A multicenter, open, non-comparative, phase II study of the combination of cladribine (2-chlorodeoxyadenosine), cytarabine, and G-CSF as induction therapy in refractory acute myeloid leukemia - a report of the Polish Adult Leukemia Group (PALG). Eur J Haematol 2003; 71(3): 155-62. [PALG].[http://dx.doi.org/10.1034/j.1600-0609.2003.00122.x] [PMID: 12930315]

[18]   Wrzesie Ku A, Robak T, Lecha araad E, Wierzbowski A, Dmoszyask A, Kowal M, et al.A multicenter, open, noncomparative, phase II study of the combination of cladribine [2-chlorodeoxyadenosine], cytarabine, and G-CSF as induction therapy in refractory acute myeloid leukemia a report of the Polish Adult Leukemia Group [PALG]. European journal of haematology 2003; 3: 155-62.

[19]   Lee SR, Yang DH, Ahn JS, *et al.* The clinical outcome of FLAG chemotherapy without idarubicin in patients with relapsed or refractory acute myeloid leukemia. J Korean Med Sci 2009; 24(3): 498-503.[http://dx.doi.org/10.3346/jkms.2009.24.3.498] [PMID: 19543516]

[20]   Bhella SD, Atenafu EG, Schuh AC, Minden MD, Schimmer AD, Gupta V. FLAG-IDA Has Significant Activity As Frontline Induction or Salvage Therapy for Patients with High Risk and/or Relapsed or Refractory Acute Myeloid Leukemia AML2014.[http://dx.doi.org/10.1182/blood.V124.21.5285.5285]

[21]   Price SL, Lancet JE, George TJ, *et al.* Salvage chemotherapy regimens for acute myeloid leukemia: Is one better? Efficacy comparison between CLAG and MEC regimens. Leuk Res 2011; 35(3): 301-4.[http://dx.doi.org/10.1016/j.leukres.2010.09.002] [PMID: 21109304]

[22]   Wierzbowska A, Robak T, Pluta A, *et al.* Cladribine combined with high doses of arabinoside cytosine, mitoxantrone, and G-CSF (CLAG-M) is a highly effective salvage regimen in patients with refractory and relapsed acute myeloid leukemia of the poor risk: a final report of the Polish Adult Leukemia Group. Eur J Haematol 2008; 80(2): 115-26.[http://dx.doi.org/10.1111/j.1600-0609.2007.00988.x] [PMID: 18076637]

[23]   Jaglal MV, Duong VH, Bello CM, *et al.* Cladribine, cytarabine, filgrastim, and mitoxantrone (CLAG-M)

compared to standard induction in acute myeloid leukemia from myelodysplastic syndrome after azanucleoside failure. Leuk Res 2014; 38(4): 443-6.[http://dx.doi.org/10.1016/j.leukres.2013.12.010] [PMID: 24439565]

[24] Trifilio SM, Rademaker AW, Newman D, *et al.* Mitoxantrone and etoposide with or without intermediate dose cytarabine for the treatment of primary induction failure or relapsed acute myeloid leukemia. Leuk Res 2012; 36(4): 394-6.[http://dx.doi.org/10.1016/j.leukres.2011.10.027] [PMID: 22172465]

[25] Greenberg PL, Lee SJ, Advani R, *et al.* Mitoxantrone, etoposide, and cytarabine with or without valspodar in patients with relapsed or refractory acute myeloid leukemia and high-risk myelodysplastic syndrome: a phase III trial (E2995). J Clin Oncol 2004; 22(6): 1078-86. [E2995].[http://dx.doi.org/10.1200/JCO.2004.07.048] [PMID: 15020609]

[26] Kohrt HE, Coutre SE. Optimizing therapy for acute myeloid leukemia. J Natl Compr Canc Netw 2008; 6(10): 1003-16.[http://dx.doi.org/10.6004/jnccn.2008.0076] [PMID: 19176198]

[27] Halpern AB, Estey EH, Othus M, Orlowski KF, Powell MA, Chen TL. Mitoxantrone, etoposide, and cytarabine [MEC] following epigenetic priming with decitabine in adults with relapsed/refractory acute myeloid leukemia [AML] or high-risk myelodysplastic syndrome [MDS]: A phase 1 study. Am Soc Hematology 2014.

[28] Kohrt HE, Patel S, Ho M, *et al.* Second-line mitoxantrone, etoposide, and cytarabine for acute myeloid leukemia: a single-center experience. Am J Hematol 2010; 85(11): 877-81.[http://dx.doi.org/10.1002/ajh.21857] [PMID: 20872554]

[29] Archimbaud E, Thomas X. Leblond Vr, Michallet M, Fenaux P, Dreyfus Fo, et al Sequential Chemotherapy with Mitoxantrone, Etoposide and Cytarabine for Previously Treated Acute Myeloid Leukemia: EMA 86 Regimen Acute Leukemias V 1996210-2.

[30] Link H, Freund M, Diedrich H, Wilke H, Austein J, Henke M. Mitoxantrone, cytosine arabinoside, and VP-16 in 36 patients with relapsed and refractory acute myeloid leukemia Acute Leukemias II 1990322-5.

[31] De Astis E, Clavio M, Raiola AM, *et al.* Liposomal daunorubicin, fludarabine, and cytarabine (FLAD) as bridge therapy to stem cell transplant in relapsed and refractory acute leukemia. Ann Hematol 2014; 93(12): 2011-8.[http://dx.doi.org/10.1007/s00277-014-2143-8] [PMID: 24989345]

[32] Camera A, Rinaldi CR, Palmieri S, *et al.* Sequential continuous infusion of fludarabine and cytarabine associated with liposomal daunorubicin (DaunoXome) (FLAD) in primary refractory or relapsed adult acute myeloid leukemia patients. Ann Hematol 2009; 88(2): 151-8.[http://dx.doi.org/10.1007/s00277-008-0571-z] [PMID: 18709502]

[33] Becker PS, Kantarjian HM, Appelbaum FR, *et al.* Clofarabine with high dose cytarabine and granulocyte colony-stimulating factor (G-CSF) priming for relapsed and refractory acute myeloid leukaemia. Br J Haematol 2011; 155(2): 182-9.[http://dx.doi.org/10.1111/j.1365-2141.2011.08831.x] [PMID: 21848522]

[34] Becker PS, Kantarjian HM, Appelbaum FR, *et al.* Retrospective comparison of clofarabine *versus* fludarabine in combination with high-dose cytarabine with or without granulocyte colony-stimulating factor as salvage therapies for acute myeloid leukemia. Haematologica 2013; 98(1): 114-8.[http://dx.doi.org/10.3324/haematol.2012.063438] [PMID: 22801963]

[35] Levis M. Quizartinib in acute myeloid leukemia. Clinical advances in hematology & oncology: H&O 2013; 11(9): 586.

[36] Cortes JE, Kantarjian HM, Kadia TM, Borthakur G, Konopleva M, Garcia-Manero G. Crenolanib besylate, a type I pan-FLT3 inhibitor, to demonstrate clinical activity in multiply relapsed FLT3-ITD and D835 AML 2016.[http://dx.doi.org/10.1200/JCO.2016.34.15_suppl.7008]

[37] RÃ©cher C, Beyne-Rauzy O, Demur Cc, Chicanne Gt, Dos Santos Cd, Mansat-De Mas Vr, et al.Antileukemic activity of rapamycin in acute myeloid leukemia. Blood 2005 2005; 105(6): 2527-34.

[38] Liesveld JL, O'Dwyer K, Walker A, *et al.* A phase I study of decitabine and rapamycin in relapsed/refractory AML. Leuk Res 2013; 37(12): 1622-7.[http://dx.doi.org/10.1016/j.leukres.2013.09.002] [PMID: 24138944]

[39] Park S, Chapuis N, Saint Marcoux F, *et al.* A phase Ib GOELAMS study of the mTOR inhibitor RAD001 in association with chemotherapy for AML patients in first relapse. Leukemia 2013; 27(7): 1479-86.[http://dx.doi.org/10.1038/leu.2013.17] [PMID: 23321953]

[40] Löwenberg B, Morgan G, Ossenkoppele GJ, *et al.* Phase I/II clinical study of Tosedostat, an inhibitor of aminopeptidases, in patients with acute myeloid leukemia and myelodysplasia. J Clin Oncol 2010; 28(28): 4333-8.[http://dx.doi.org/10.1200/JCO.2009.27.6295] [PMID: 20733120]

[41] Cortes J, Feldman E, Yee K, *et al.* Two dosing regimens of tosedostat in elderly patients with relapsed or refractory acute myeloid leukaemia (OPAL): a randomised open-label phase 2 study. Lancet Oncol 2013; 14(4): 354-62.[http://dx.doi.org/10.1016/S1470-2045(13)70037-8] [PMID: 23453583]

[42] Mawad R, Becker PS, Hendrie P, *et al.* Phase II study of tosedostat with cytarabine or decitabine in newly diagnosed older patients with acute myeloid leukaemia or high-risk MDS. Br J Haematol 2016; 172(2): 238-45.[http://dx.doi.org/10.1111/bjh.13829] [PMID: 26568032]

[43] Schaefer EW, Loaiza-Bonilla A, Juckett M, *et al.* A phase 2 study of vorinostat in acute myeloid leukemia. Haematologica 2009; 94(10): 1375-82.[http://dx.doi.org/10.3324/haematol.2009.009217] [PMID: 19794082]

[44] Walter RB, Medeiros BC, Gardner KM, Orlowski KF, Gallegos L, Scott BL. Gemtuzumab ozogamicin in combination with vorinostat and azacitidine in older patients with relapsed or refractory acute myeloid leukemia: a phase 1/2 study. Haematologica 2013: haematol 2013096545.

[45] Gojo I, Tan M, Fang H-B, *et al.* Translational phase I trial of vorinostat (suberoylanilide hydroxamic acid) combined with cytarabine and etoposide in patients with relapsed, refractory, or high-risk acute myeloid leukemia. Clin Cancer Res 2013; 19(7): 1838-51.[http://dx.doi.org/10.1158/1078-0432.CCR-12-3165] [PMID: 23403629]

[46] Stein E, Tallman M, Pollyea DA, Flinn IW, Fathi AT, Stone RM. Clinical safety and activity in phase I trial of AG-221, a first in class, a potent inhibitor of the IDH2-mutant protein, in patients with IDH2 mutant positive advanced hematologic malignancies. Proceedings of the 105th annual meeting of the American Association for Cancer Research 2014103.[http://dx.doi.org/10.1158/1538-7445.AM2014-CT103]

[47] Lancet JE, Roboz GJ, Cripe LD, Michelson GC, Fox JA, Leavitt RD. A phase 1b/2 study of combination vosaroxin and cytarabine in patients with relapsed or refractory acute myeloid leukemia. Haematologica 2014: haematol 2014114769.

[48] Roboz GJ, Rosenblat T, Arellano M, *et al.* International randomized phase III study of elacytarabine *versus* investigator choice in patients with relapsed/refractory acute myeloid leukemia. J Clin Oncol 2014; 32(18): 1919-26.[http://dx.doi.org/10.1200/JCO.2013.52.8562] [PMID: 24841975]

[49] Advani AS, McDonough S, Copelan E, *et al.* SWOG0919: a Phase 2 study of idarubicin and cytarabine in combination with pravastatin for relapsed acute myeloid leukaemia. Br J Haematol 2014; 167(2): 233-7.[http://dx.doi.org/10.1111/bjh.13035] [PMID: 25039477]

[50] Attar EC, Johnson JL, Amrein PC, *et al.* Bortezomib added to daunorubicin and cytarabine during induction therapy and to intermediate-dose cytarabine for consolidation in patients with previously untreated acute myeloid leukemia age 60 to 75 years: CALGB (Alliance) study 10502. J Clin Oncol 2013; 31(7): 923-9.[http://dx.doi.org/10.1200/JCO.2012.45.2177] [PMID: 23129738]

[51] Pardee TS, Stadelman K, Isom S, Ellis LR, Berenzon D, Hurd DD. Activity of the mitochondrial metabolism inhibitor cpi-613 in combination with high dose Ara-C [HDAC] and mitoxantrone in high risk relapsed or refractory acute myeloid leukemia [AML]. American Society of Clinical Oncology 2015.

[52] Cang S, Iragavarapu C, Savooji J, Song Y, Liu D. ABT-199 (venetoclax) and BCL-2 inhibitors in clinical development. J Hematol Oncol 2015; 8(1): 129.[http://dx.doi.org/10.1186/s13045-015-0224-3] [PMID: 26589495]

[53] Konopleva M, Pollyea DA, Potluri J, Chyla BJ, Busman T, McKeegan E. A phase 2 study of ABT-199 [GDC-0199] in patients with acute myelogenous leukemia [AML]. Am Soc Hematology 2014.

[54] Thol F, Schlenk RF. Gemtuzumab ozogamicin in acute myeloid leukemia revisited. Expert Opin Biol Ther 2014; 14(8): 1185-95.[http://dx.doi.org/10.1517/14712598.2014.922534] [PMID: 24865510]

[55] Pilorge S, Rigaudeau S, Rabian F, *et al.* Fractionated gemtuzumab ozogamicin and standard dose cytarabine produced prolonged second remissions in patients over the age of 55 years with acute myeloid leukemia in late first relapse. Am J Hematol 2014; 89(4): 399-403.[http://dx.doi.org/10.1002/ajh.23653] [PMID: 24375467]

[56] Stein EM, Stein A, Walter RB, Fathi AT, Lancet JE, Kovacsovics TJ. Interim analysis of a phase 1 trial of SGN-CD33A in patients with CD33-positive acute myeloid leukemia AML2014.[http://dx.doi.org/10.1182/blood.V124.21.623.623]

[57] Uy G, Stewart S, Baughman J, Rettig M, Chichili G, Bonvini E. A phase I trial of MGD006 in patients with relapsed acute myeloid leukemia. J Immunother Cancer 2014; 2(3): 87. [AML].[http://dx.doi.org/10.1186/2051-1426-2-S3-P87]

[58] Wiernik A, Foley B, Zhang B, *et al.* Targeting natural killer cells to acute myeloid leukemia *in vitro* with a CD16 x 33 bispecific killer cell engager and ADAM17 inhibition. Clin Cancer Res 2013; 19(14): 3844-55.[http://dx.doi.org/10.1158/1078-0432.CCR-13-0505] [PMID: 23690482]

[59] Wang QS, Wang Y, Lv HY, *et al.* Treatment of CD33-directed chimeric antigen receptor-modified T cells in one patient with relapsed and refractory acute myeloid leukemia. Mol Ther 2015; 23(1): 184-91.[http://dx.doi.org/10.1038/mt.2014.164] [PMID: 25174587]

[60] Kenderian SS, Ruella M, Shestova O, *et al.* CD33-specific chimeric antigen receptor T cells exhibit potent

preclinical activity against human acute myeloid leukemia. Leukemia 2015; 29(8): 1637-47.[http://dx.doi.org/10.1038/leu.2015.52] [PMID: 25721896]

[61] Gill S, Tasian SK, Ruella M, *et al.* Preclinical targeting of human acute myeloid leukemia and myeloablation using chimeric antigen receptor-modified T cells. Blood 2014; 123(15): 2343-54.[http://dx.doi.org/10.1182/blood-2013-09-529537] [PMID: 24596416]

[62] Pizzitola I, Anjos-Afonso F, Rouault-Pierre K, *et al.* Chimeric antigen receptors against CD33/CD123 antigens efficiently target primary acute myeloid leukemia cells *in vivo*. Leukemia 2014; 28(8): 1596-605.[http://dx.doi.org/10.1038/leu.2014.62] [PMID: 24504024]

[63] Berneman ZN, Van de Velde AL, Willemen Y, Anguille S, Saevels K, Germonpra P. Vaccination with WT1 mRNA-electroporated dendritic cells: report of clinical outcome in 66 cancer patients 2014.

[64] Di Stasi A, Jimenez AM, Minagawa K, Al-Obaidi M, Rezvani K. Review of the results of WT1 peptide vaccination strategies for myelodysplastic syndromes and acute myeloid leukemia from nine different studies. Front Immunol 2015; 6: 36.[http://dx.doi.org/10.3389/fimmu.2015.00036] [PMID: 25699052]

[65] Goswami M, Hensel N, Smith BD, *et al.* Expression of putative targets of immunotherapy in acute myeloid leukemia and healthy tissues. Leukemia 2014; 28(5): 1167-70.[http://dx.doi.org/10.1038/leu.2014.14] [PMID: 24472813]

[66] Chapuis AG, Ragnarsson GB, Nguyen HN, Chaney CN, Pufnock JS, Schmitt TM. Transferred WT1-reactive CD8+ T cells can mediate antileukemic activity and persist in post-transplant patients. Science translational medicine 2013; 5(174): 174ra127-.

[67] Sébert M, Porcher R, Robin M, *et al.* Equivalent outcomes using reduced intensity or conventional myeloablative conditioning transplantation for patients aged 35 years and over with AML. Bone Marrow Transplant 2015; 50(1): 74-81.[http://dx.doi.org/10.1038/bmt.2014.199] [PMID: 25243624]

[68] Grosicki S, Holowiecki J, Kuliczkowski K, *et al.* Assessing the efficacy of allogeneic hematopoietic stem cells transplantation (allo-HSCT) by analyzing survival end points in defined groups of acute myeloid leukemia patients: a retrospective, multicenter Polish Adult Leukemia Group study. Am J Hematol 2015; 90(10): 904-9.[http://dx.doi.org/10.1002/ajh.24113] [PMID: 26149802]

[69] Takami A, Yano S, Yokoyama H, *et al.* Donor lymphocyte infusion for the treatment of relapsed acute myeloid leukemia after allogeneic hematopoietic stem cell transplantation: a retrospective analysis by the Adult Acute Myeloid Leukemia Working Group of the Japan Society for Hematopoietic Cell Transplantation. Biol Blood Marrow Transplant 2014; 20(11): 1785-90.[http://dx.doi.org/10.1016/j.bbmt.2014.07.010] [PMID: 25034960]

[70] Weisdorf DJ, Wang H, Logan BR, Devine SM, de Lima M, Bunjes DW. Survival of AML patients relapsing after allogeneic stem cell transplantation: a center for international blood and marrow transplant research study 2015.

[71] Meggendorfer M, Alpermann T, Perglerov Ã. K, Kern W, Schnittger S, Haferlach C, et alGenetic patterns of relapsed aml differ significantly from the first manifestation and are dependent on cytogenetic risk groups at diagnosis: Results in 175 patients with paired samples 2014.

[72] Mirabilii S, Ricciardi MR, Piedimonte M, Gianfelici V, Bianchi MP, Tafuri A. Biological Aspects of mTOR in Leukemia. Int J Mol Sci 2018; 19(8): 2396.[http://dx.doi.org/10.3390/ijms19082396] [PMID: 30110936]

[73] Advani AS, Elson P, Kalaycio ME, Mukherjee S, Gerds AT, Hamilton BK. Bortezomib+ MEC [mitoxantrone, etoposide, cytarabine] for relapsed/refractory acute myeloid leukemia: Final results of an expanded phase 1 trial. Am Soc Hematology 2014.

[74] Récher C, Beyne-Rauzy O, Demur C, *et al.* Antileukemic activity of rapamycin in acute myeloid leukemia. Blood 2005; 105(6): 2527-34.[http://dx.doi.org/10.1182/blood-2004-06-2494] [PMID: 15550488]

[75] Kasner MT, Mick R, Jeschke GR, *et al.* Sirolimus enhances remission induction in patients with high risk acute myeloid leukemia and mTORC1 target inhibition. Invest New Drugs 2018; 36(4): 657-66.[http://dx.doi.org/10.1007/s10637-018-0585-x] [PMID: 29607465]

[76] Altman JK, Sassano A, Platanias LC. Targeting mTOR for the treatment of AML. New agents and new directions. Oncotarget 2011; 2(6): 510-7.[http://dx.doi.org/10.18632/oncotarget.290] [PMID: 21680954]

[77] Jessica K. Altman, Antonella Sassano, Surinder Kaur, Heather Glaser, Barbara Kroczynska, Amanda J. Redig, Suzanne Russo, Sharon Barr and Leonidas C. PlataniasDual mTORC2/mTORC1 Targeting Results in Potent Suppressive Effects on Acute Myeloid Leukemia [AML] Progenitors 2011 : July;10-2285.

[78] Julhash U. Kazi, Lars Rönnstrand. fms-like tyrosine kinase 3/FLT3. From Basic Science to Clinical Implications Physiol Rev 2019; 99: 1433-66.

[79] Yang J, Nie J, Ma X, Wei Y, Peng Y, Wei X. Targeting PI3K in cancer: mechanisms and advances in clinical trials. Mol Cancer 2019; 18(1): 26.[http://dx.doi.org/10.1186/s12943-019-0954-x] [PMID: 30782187]

[80]   Ramos NR, Mo CC, Karp JE, Hourigan CS. Current approaches in the treatment of relapsed and refractory acute myeloid leukemia. J Clin Med 2015; 4(4): 665-95.[http://dx.doi.org/10.3390/jcm4040665] [PMID: 25932335]

[81]   Meyer C, Drexler HG. FLT3 ligand inhibits apoptosis and promotes survival of myeloid leukemia cell lines. Leuk Lymphoma 1999; 32(5-6): 577-81.[http://dx.doi.org/10.3109/10428199909058416] [PMID: 10048431]

[82]   Montini E, Cesana D, Schmidt M, et al. Hematopoietic stem cell gene transfer in a tumor-prone mouse model uncovers low genotoxicity of lentiviral vector integration. Nat Biotechnol 2006; 24(6): 687-96.[http://dx.doi.org/10.1038/nbt1216] [PMID: 16732270]

[83]   Medinger M, Lengerke C, Passweg J. Novel therapeutic options in acute myeloid leukemia. Leuk Res Rep 2016; 6: 39-49.[http://dx.doi.org/10.1016/j.lrr.2016.09.001] [PMID: 27752467]

[84]   Dinner S, Platanias LC. Targeting the mTOR pathway in leukemia. J Cell Biochem 2016; 117(8): 1745-52.[http://dx.doi.org/10.1002/jcb.25559] [PMID: 27018341]

[85]   Schlenk RF, Kayser S, Bullinger L, Kobbe G, Casper J, Ringhoffer M. Differential impact of allelic ratio and insertion site in FLT3-ITD positive AML concerning allogeneic hematopoietic stem cell transplantation. Blood 2014. blood-2014-2005-578070.

[86]   Breitenbuecher F, Markova B, Kasper S, et al. A novel molecular mechanism of primary resistance to FLT3-kinase inhibitors in AML. Blood 2009; 113(17): 4063-73.[http://dx.doi.org/10.1182/blood-2007-11-126664] [PMID: 19144992]

[87]   Cairns RA, Harris IS, Mak TW. Regulation of cancer cell metabolism. Nat Rev Cancer 2011; 11(2): 85-95.[http://dx.doi.org/10.1038/nrc2981] [PMID: 21258394]

[88]   Yen KE, Bittinger MA, Su SM, Fantin VR. Cancer-associated IDH mutations: biomarker and therapeutic opportunities. Oncogene 2010; 29(49): 6409-17.[http://dx.doi.org/10.1038/onc.2010.444] [PMID: 20972461]

[89]   Wang F, Travins J, DeLaBarre B, et al. Targeted inhibition of mutant IDH2 in leukemia cells induces cellular differentiation. Science 2013; 340(6132): 622-6.[http://dx.doi.org/10.1126/science.1234769] [PMID: 23558173]

[90]   Tayyab M, Khan M, Iqbal Z, Altaf S, Noor Z, Noor N. Distinct gene mutations, their prognostic relevance, and molecularly targeted therapies in acute myeloid leukemia [AML] 2014.

[91]   Takahashi S. Current findings for recurring mutations in acute myeloid leukemia. J Hematol Oncol 2011; 4(1): 36.[http://dx.doi.org/10.1186/1756-8722-4-36] [PMID: 21917154]

[92]   Wouters BJ, Delwel R. Epigenetics and approaches to targeted epigenetic therapy in acute myeloid leukemia. Blood 2016; 127(1): 42-52.[http://dx.doi.org/10.1182/blood-2015-07-604512] [PMID: 26660432]

[93]   Wu Mei, Li Chuntuan, Zhu Xiongpeng. FLT3 inhibitors in acute myeloid leukemia. J Hematology & Oncology 2018; 11: Article number: 133.[http://dx.doi.org/10.1186/s13045-018-0675-4]

[94]   Keyur P. Patel, Farhad Ravandi, Deqin Ma, Abhaya Paladugu, Bedia A. Barkoh, L. Jeffrey Medeiros, Rajyalakshmi Luthra. Acute Myeloid Leukemia with IDH1 or IDH2 Mutations: Frequency and Clinicopathologic Features. Am J Clin Pathol 2011; 135(1): 35-45.[http://dx.doi.org/10.1309/AJCPD7NR2RMNQDVF] [PMID: 21173122]

[95]   Daver N, Cortes J. Molecular targeted therapy in acute myeloid leukemia. Hematology 2012; 17(sup1): s59-62.[http://dx.doi.org/10.1179/102453312X13336169155619]

[96]   Konopleva MY, Walter RB, Faderl SH, et al. Preclinical and early clinical evaluation of the oral AKT inhibitor, MK-2206, for the treatment of acute myelogenous leukemia. Clin Cancer Res 2014; 20(8): 2226-35.[http://dx.doi.org/10.1158/1078-0432.CCR-13-1978] [PMID: 24583795]

[97]   Iris Z. Uras, Barbara Maurer, Sofie Nebenfuehr, Markus Zojer, Peter Valent, Veronika Sexl Therapeutic Vulnerabilities in FLT3-Mutant AML Unmasked by Palbociclib. Int J Mol Sci 2018; 19(12): 3987.[http://dx.doi.org/10.3390/ijms19123987]

Potential Natural Products For Prostate Cancer Management: Prospects For Castration-Resistant Patients

Thaise G. Araújo[1],[*], Lara Vecchi[1], Danilo S. Costa[2], Sara T. S. Mota[1], Paula M. A. P. Lima[1], Igor M. Campos[2], Mariana A. P. Zóia[1], Douglas C. Brandão[1], Gabriela S. Guimarães[1], Matheus A. Ribeiro[1], Ademar A. da Silva Filho[2]

[1] Institute of Biotechnology, Federal University of Uberlandia, Uberlandia, Brazil

[2] Faculty of Pharmacy, Department of Pharmaceutical Sciences, Federal University of Juiz de Fora, Juiz de Fora, Brazil

Abstract

Prostate Cancer (PCa) is a major global health burden with alarming epidemiological indices. Research advances in this area have revealed complex molecular aspects associated with the disease, thus necessitating the novel development of diagnostic methods and therapeutic strategies. The main molecular target is the androgen receptor (AR), which is involved in both normal development and malignant transformation. However, many patients become resistant to conventional treatments, and the disease progresses to a castration-resistant stage (CRPC) in which tumor aggressiveness is driven by a constitutive activation of AR signaling. Tremendous effort has been made for elucidating CRPC and chemoresistance. In fact, multiple signaling pathways are related to the insurgence and maintenance of CRPC, highlighting the need for continuously updating such a complex scenario. Different drugs have been tested and used for CRPC treatment, facing unfavorable heterogeneity and leading to substantial morbidity and mortality. Thus, the clinical impact of advanced PCa with poorer outcomes still underscores the need for new compounds. The discovery and current use of natural products has given way to promising possibilities, offering alternative tools that aim to control the disease and to better manage patients. These natural products are versatile and effective molecules with different mechanisms of action and structures. In the present chapter, we explore the challenges of PCa and describe recent scientific contributions in this field, with special attention devoted to CRPC. We also discuss and suggest natural products as potential novel anti-tumor agents to overcome clinical limits and to treat and cure CRPC patients.

Keywords: Castration-Resistant, Chemotherapy, Phytochemicals, Prostate Cancer, Treatment.

---

* **Corresponding author Thaise Gonçalves Araújo**: Laboratory of Genetics and Biotechnology, Institute of Biotechnology, Federal University of Uberlandia, Rua Major Jerônimo, 566, Sala 604, 384700-128, Patos de Minas, MG, Brazil. Tel: +55 34 3814-2027; E-mail: tgaraujo@ufu.br

INTRODUCTION

Prostate cancer (PCa) is a hormonally-driven tumor that ranks fourth in incidence among human cancers and caused 358, 989 deaths worldwide in 2018 [1, 2]. When PCa is localized to the prostate and surrounding tissues, the overall survival (OS) rates are significantly high since these patients are efficiently treated with surgery and radiotherapy [3]. However, over 20% of patients evolve to a lethal treatment-refractory stage of the disease with OS ranging from 26% to 30% at 5 years [4].

Advanced PCa is treated with chemotherapy and, mainly, associated with androgen deprivation therapy (ADT) [5]. In chemotherapy, cytotoxic drugs are introduced to control or cure the disease, targeting circulating tumor cells. However, it also affects normal cells, which results in undesirable side effects [6]. In some PCa patients, it is not possible to reach a complete abrogation of the androgen receptor (AR)-mediated functions through ADT. Such a scenario is due to the ability of PCa cells to elicit aberrant AR signaling that sustains tumor progression towards castration-resistant PCa (CRPC) [7].

Current chemical therapies often fail to control PCa, especially CRPC [3]. Notably, the fact that Natural Products (NPs) present fewer side effects and greater efficacy, together with their ability to act on several cellular mechanisms, makes them particularly promising in the treatment of tumors. The ability of NPs to inhibit PCa has already been described and, owing to their low toxicity, they confer clear advantages over synthetic compounds used to control CRPC [6]. Herein, we discuss general aspects of PCa, focusing on CRPC. Considering that CRPC is characterized biochemically by increasing levels of AR-targeted genes, blocking the receptor-dependent transcriptional programmers is of particular interest. Hereafter, we describe the mechanisms of action of different NPs and their potential application for the management of advanced PCa, especially for modulating AR signaling.

OVERVIEW OF PROSTATE CANCER

Epidemiology and Etiopathology

The development of the human body is a complex and highly regulated process that needs a molecular equilibrium in order to carry out its essential functions [8]. Such an equilibrium is lost in the tumorigenesis process during which normal cells progressively evolve towards a neoplastic state. There are six hallmark traits that enable cells to become malignant, including sustained proliferative signaling, growth suppression evasion, cell death resistance, replicative immortality, sustained angiogenesis, and tissue invasion and metastasis. Such characteristics are also associated with genomic instability, reprogramming of energy metabolism, inflammation processes and evasion from immune destruction, which are responsible for the promotion and progression of cancer [9⁻11].

The progressive colonization of several sites of the body is the main cause of cancer-induced morbidity and relies on the capacity of cancer cells to invade tissues. During invasion, the extracellular matrix (ECM) is degraded and cancer cells survive in the lymphatic and vascular systems [12⁻15]. Epithelial-mesenchymal transition (EMT) is at the center of the metastatic process since it confers to cancer cells a more aggressive potential and allows the generation and accumulation of cancer stem cells (CSCs) in a highly dynamic and heterogeneous tumor microenvironment [14, 16].

Despite the notable advances in treatment methods and in detection of malignant neoplasms, cancer remains a major public health problem. Its epidemiological indexes are alarming, including its high incidence and mortality [17, 18]. The incidence of cancer in Brazil and in the world is growing at an accelerated pace, following the aging of the population (due to the increase in life expectancy) and the change in global lifestyles [19]. In 2017, according to the World Health Organization (WHO), there were 8.8

million cancer deaths worldwide with the vast majority in developing countries. About 12 million deaths are predicted by the year 2030 [17].

PCa, in absolute global values, is the fourth most common type and has the second highest incidence among men [17]. In 2018, 1.3 million new cases of PCa were registered worldwide with 358,989 deaths. The highest incidence of the disease was in Europe (449,761 - 35.2%), followed by Asia (297,215 - 23.3%), North America (234,278 - 18.4%), Latin America and the Caribbean (190,385 - 14.9%), Africa (80,971 - 6.3%) and Oceania (23,496 – 1.8%). Regarding the number of deaths, the continents were ranked as follows: Asia (118,427 - 33%), Europe (107,315 - 29.9%), Latin America and the Caribbean (53,798 - 15%), Africa (42,298 - 11.8%), North America (32,686 - 9.1%) and Oceania (4,465 - 1.2%) [2]. According to the American Cancer Society, 174,650 new cases of PCa were diagnosed in American men in 2019, with 31,620 deaths from the disease [17].

PCa is considered a malignant tumor of the elderly, since about three quarters of cases worldwide occur after age 65 [20]. In Brazil, according to the estimates of the National Cancer Institute (INCA), about 65,840 new cases will be identified in the 2020-2022 triennium. These values correspond to an estimated risk of 62.95 new cases per 100,000 men. Without considering non-melanoma skin tumors, PCa is the most prevalent among men in all regions from Brazil, with 72.35 / 100,000 in the Northeast; 65.29 / 100,000 in the Midwest; 63.94 / 100,000 in the Southeast; 62.00 / 100,000 in the South and 29.39 / 100,000 in the North [19, 21].

PCa is a multifactorial, heterogeneous and complex disease from the molecular and clinical points of view [22]. Prostate activity and the control of differentiation depend on a combination of different factors. Androgens are the main active hormones, maintaining homeostasis of the mature organ, guiding embryonic development and modulating the functional maturation by inducing epithelial proliferation, ductal ramification and differentiation of epithelial cells [23]. The hydroxylated form of testosterone, dihydrotestosterone (DHT), has the greatest action on the prostate, due to its high affinity for the AR. Other hormones, such as estrogens, glucocorticoids, prolactin and insulin, also control the organ's histopathology [24]. In addition, the prostatic microenvironment is characterized by the activation of several different pathways that, in order to modulate metabolism and gene expression, are linked together through the establishment of finely regulated networks [25, 26].

The human prostate is a pelvic gland located under the urinary bladder and in front of the rectum Fig. (1). This organ is traversed by the urethra [27]; for this reason, diseases related to prostate growths usually culminate in urinary symptoms [28]. A normal prostate measures 3 to 4 cm at the base, 4 to 6 cm in its cephalo-caudal dimension and 2 to 3 cm in its anteroposterior dimension with an approximate weight of 20 grams in adulthood. The prostate is subdivided into the following zones: peripheral, central, transitional and anterior (Fig. 1A) [29, 30]. Prostatic acini are composed of basal and luminal cells surrounded by the fibromuscular stroma. The epithelium is highly organized in a contiguous basal structure with three main cell subtypes: stem cells, transit-amplifying cells and committed basal cells (Fig. 1B) [31]. Columnar secretory luminal cells make up the rest of the epithelium. It has been shown that stromal cells can modulate the pattern of differentiation of normal epithelium and, therefore, are critical for prostate homeostasis [32].

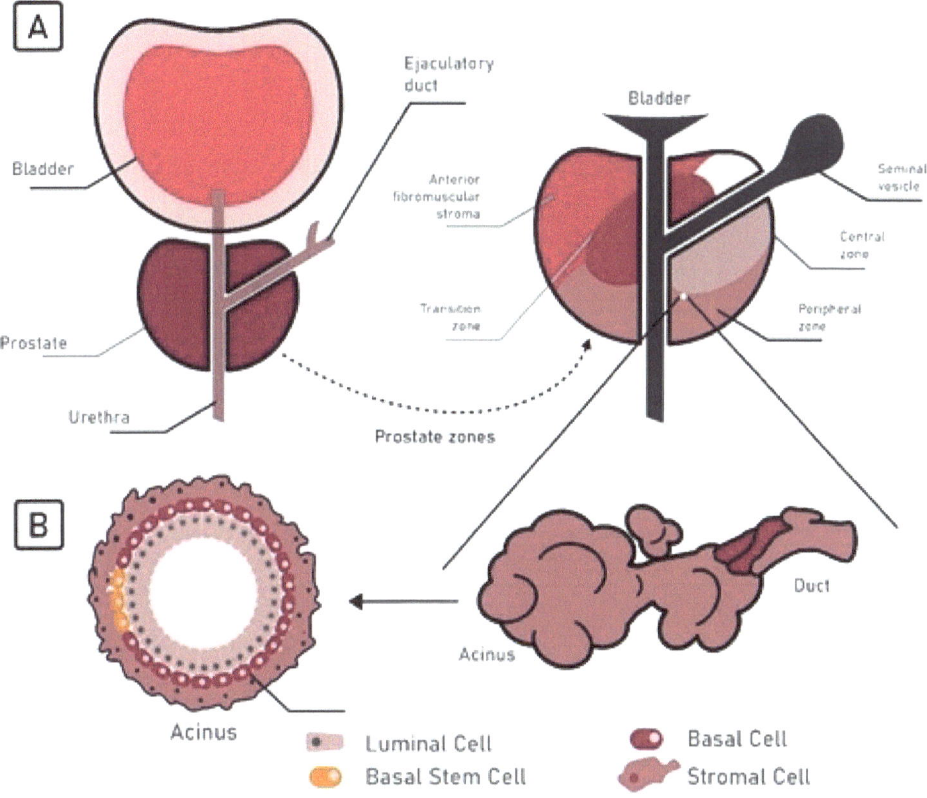

Fig. (1))

Representation of the prostate gland. **(A)** The prostate is located under the urinary bladder and in front of the rectum. It is subdivided into different zones. **(B)** Its acini are composed of a bilayer of basal and luminal epithelial cells surrounded by the fibromuscular stroma.

Benign Prostatic Hyperplasia (BPH) is a non-malignant enlargement of the stromal and epithelial compartments that occurs almost exclusively in the transition zone which is localized periurethrally in the central region of the gland. About 90% of men aged 70 to 80 years have histological evidence of this disease [33] that, when treated, is rarely fatal [34]. Clinical manifestations of BPH include lower urinary tract symptoms, insufficient emptying of the bladder, urinary retention, detrusor instability, urinary tract infection, hematuria and renal failure [35].

Changes in regulatory mechanisms of prostate growth, with a special emphasis on inflammatory processes, can lead to BPH. Stromal BPH nodules have infiltrates of B lymphocytes, T lymphocytes and macrophages that accumulate around the epithelial ducts and can disrupt the glandular epithelium [36]. Inflammation is also associated with the occurrence and progression of PCa. Tissue damage derived from an initial inflammatory injury leads to Proliferative Inflammatory Atrophy (PIA) [37, 38]. This is a focal hyperproliferative response of the epithelia. Highly proliferative epithelial cells of PIA lose their columnar structure, which leads to molecular and histological changes in secretory acini that meet with regions of the Prostate Intraepithelial Neoplasia (PIN) and PCa. PIN favors the development of malignant diseases [31] and is characterized by the appearance of enlarged nuclei of both ductal and acinar cells. PIN resemble prostate tumors from the biochemical, genetic and phenotypical points of view [38] and, for this reason, is considered a transition state between BPH and PCa [39].

Malignant neoplasm occurs mostly in the peripheral zone on the dorsal and dorsal-lateral side of the organ. Less than 30% of cancers progress in the transition zone [40⁻43]. Prostate tumors are predominantly luminal with disruption in the basal membrane. The etiology of PCa remains unknown, although some risk factors have already been described: advanced age, genetic predisposition, ethnicity, sexually transmitted infections, inflammatory atrophies, hormonal dysregulation and obesity [44⁻49]. The most well-established risk factor is age, since only 1% of diagnoses occur in men under 50 years of age. Therefore, it mainly affects men over 60 years of age [50⁻53]. Only 5% of PCa cases are attributed to heredity, which consists of at least three family members affected by the disease across 3 successive generations or at least two family members diagnosed before the age of 55 [49]. In addition, loci involved in susceptibility to PCa have already been described such as: 1q25.3, referring to the Ribonuclease L (*RNASEL*); 1q42.2-43 of the Predisposition to Prostate Cancer (*PCaP*) gene; Xq27-28, where the Hereditary Prostate Cancer, X-linked (*HPCX*) gene is located; 8p 22 of the Macrophage scavenger receptor 1 (*MSR1*) gene; 17p12 for the ElaC ribonuclease Z 2 (*ELAC2*) and 20q13 for Hereditary Prostate cancer, 3 (*HPC3*) [54]. Changes in these loci lead to the translation of proteins that act in several pathways such as angiogenesis, apoptosis, proliferation and cell differentiation [55]. Mutations in *BRCA1* (BRCA1, DNA repair associated) or *BRCA2* (BRCA2, DNA repair associated) genes can result in both breast and ovarian cancer, as well as in increased chances of developing PCa [56]. Ethnicity also influences PCa, which is more prevalent in African Americans. Genetic and hormonal variations are associated with these indexes [57].

About 95% of PCa cases are sporadic, resulting from mutations, chromosomal translocations, gene amplifications and epigenetic changes caused by carcinogenic agents. These include trans and saturated fats in the diet, smoking, obesity, pathogens (such as viruses and bacteria), radiation and environmental pollution [58]. Sexually transmitted diseases and prostatitis favor an inflammatory environment with high levels of cytokines, which regulate androgenic signaling and, therefore, lead to disease evolution [59]. Obesity is also considered a risk factor due to metabolic changes associated with oxidative stress and harmful levels of circulating insulin, which enhance cell growth [47]. Finally, personal habits [60], such as the high consumption of animal fat and sausages and the low intake of vitamin E, lycopene, selenium and isoflavonoids are also predictors of PCa [61].

Diagnosis Strategies and Current Treatments

In its initial phase, PCa has a silent evolution without defined symptoms or signs. These are similar to BPH, such as difficulty voiding and increased urinary frequency during the day and / or night [48, 62]. However, in advanced stages, the malignancy can be further characterized by hematuria, bone pain, generalized infections and / or renal failure [63].

Several tests are currently used for PCa diagnosis, even in asymptomatic cases. Prostate-Specific Antigen (PSA) is a glycoprotein identified in the seminal fluid, produced mainly by prostate tissue. PSA serum levels are routinely measured [64], and the detection of levels above normal values (2.5 ng / ml for men between 40 and 50 years old and up to 4.0 ng / ml between 50 and 60 years old) indicate possible changes in the prostate gland that can be either benign or malignant [65]. The isolated use of this procedure is not recommended, as 25% of patients with PCa have PSA levels less than 4 ng / ml and, on the other hand, hyperplasia is also responsible for raising these values [52, 66]. Therefore, the risk of unnecessary biopsy remains substantial. Considering that 80% of tumors are in the peripheral area of the prostate gland, digital rectal examination (DRE) remains a widely performed method by the medical community. It is an exam that allows the evaluation of different aspects of the prostate, such as size and shape, consistency and sensitivity (pain, discomfort or asymptomatic for finger pressure). At the normal or BPH stage, the organ has a fibroelastic aspect, yet when cancer develops, it becomes hardened or firm [66].

Additionally, the following tests are also performed: (1) measurement of serum acid phosphatase, an enzyme produced in the prostatic epithelium that is elevated in the bloodstream due to the development of cancer [66]; (2) transrectal ultrasound, capable of characterizing the size or volume of the tumor, its location, degree and pattern of growth, prostatic asymmetry and irregularity or capsular rupture; (3) magnetic resonance [66, 67]; (4) computed tomography, which allows for a better analysis of lymph node involvement [66, 67] and (5) abdominal or transrectal ultrasound to assess kidneys and the upper urinary tract (pelvis and ureters) [66].

After diagnosis, the tumor is clinically staged based on DRE, laboratory data, biopsy evaluation and image results. After surgical removal, the lesion is also pathologically staged, with microscopic analysis of the specimen [32, 68]. Pathological staging is based on the TNM system (Tumor, lymph Node and Metastasis) with: (T) the extension of the primary tumor; (N) the presence and number of compromised regional lymph nodes and; (M) the presence of metastasis. PSA levels at diagnosis and a Gleason score are also considered [69, 70]. This was introduced by Gleason et. al. in 1966, and has been utilized for half a century [71–74]. The Gleason score is internationally accepted [53, 75] to estimate cell differentiation in distinct patterns [76–78]. The last update was performed in 2014 by the International Society of Urological Pathology (ISUP) and five tier grades were established: (i) 1 to 5 as Gleason scores ≤6, (ii) 3 + 4 = 7, (iii) 4 + 3 = 7, (iv) 8 and (v) 9–10. This provides prognostic categories, and grade 4 was extensively discussed and considered critical for patients' outcomes [79].

Patients with low-risk and intermediate-risk PCa are those with organ-confined disease, displaying low PSA levels and Gleason ≤ 6. In the case of localized disease, the therapy consists of surgery or radiation therapy, associated with hormone therapy that blocks the production of male hormones [77]. Active surveillance is also an option for these cases, which consists of closer monitoring of the patient, with regular PSA tests and DRE (every six months). Biopsies are also performed to check the evolution of the disease. When the growth of the tumor or some critical alterations are observed, another treatment is initiated [80].

The objective of the above methods is to reduce the exposure of patients to the higher-risk therapies, including chemotherapy [78, 81]. The strategies vary according to the stage, presence of comorbidities and life expectancy of each man. In addition, possible side effects are also considered [82]. Radical prostatectomy is still commonly used [83], although about 20 to 40% of patients present cancer recurrence and progress to a metastatic condition [84]. In these cases, ADT is adopted, which includes androgen ablation by chemical or surgical castration [85]. Chemically, luteinizing hormone releasing hormone (LHRH) analogs, estrogens, pure or mixed antiandrogens such as flutamide, nilutamide, bicalutamide and cyproterone, and drugs that inhibit hormone production, such as abiraterone and enzalutamide, are used [86]. Bilateral orchiectomy is also an alternative in these cases [87]. Still, about 40% of cases are refractory to treatment, which defines CRPC. ADT is not effective in inhibiting CRPC progression, which is mainly reported by observing continuously rising PSA levels, a situation known as biochemical recurrence or relapse [88]. CRPC diagnosis is confirmed by the appearance of disease progression and metastasis despite ADT [89]. Chemotherapy, with the administration of cytotoxic chemical compounds such as Docetaxel, Cabazitaxel, Mitoxantrone and Estramustine, reaches circulating tumor cells, but also kills normal cells, which culminates in debilitating side effects. This treatment has evolved and has been used as a neoadjuvant, adjuvant, or for palliation, and mainly to improve OS [90].

Prostate-specific membrane antigen (PSMA) is upregulated during CRPC evolution, which makes it attractive as an indicator of PCa progression. In fact, this protein has been used in Positron Emission Tomography (PET) imaging, and the European Association of Urology (EAU) suggests the use of PSMA-PET/CT imaging in any case of biochemical recurrence. However, to avoid expensive and unnecessary technical procedures in low-risk patients, it is necessary to select the most suitable candidates for this procedure, considering ISUP grade, biochemical features and different clinical settings of PSA relapse [91, 92].

On the other hand, the disease can have a good prognosis when diagnosed early. In these cases, five-year survival ranges from 60% to 95% [93]. The rate can be improved by scientific-technological developments and through a better understanding of the molecular events involved in malignant transformation [94]. In this regard, the elucidation of the pathways associated with tumor suppressors and the activation of oncogenes can define better strategies for the diagnosis, surveillance and treatment of patients [95‑97]. Considering the physiological aspects, the development and physiology of the prostate are directly modulated by different hormones such as androgens, insulin, prolactin, growth hormone, retinoic acid and estrogen. The complexity of the molecular events involved in this modulation can evoke the insurgence of PCa [26, 98, 99].

Up to now, it is known that the putative target of PCa treatment is the AR, a protein that regulates prostate development and drives the expression of the main PCa biomarker: PSA [100, 101]. However, the complexity of PCa highlights the need to achieve a better understanding of this disease with the aim of improving patient management.

Biomarkers

The efficient and early detection of malignant changes is carried out by identifying and / or quantifying specific biomarkers, with a strong positive predictive value [102]. The term biomarker refers to a broad spectrum of molecular or physiological signals which are objectively measured. The quantification of a specific biomarker, besides indicating the presence or absence of a particular disease and its progression, can affect the therapeutic response and could predict which patients would benefit from a particular therapy [103]. Therefore, a biomarker must reflect the interaction between the organism's homeostasis and the disease. The measured response can be functional, physiological, biochemical and / or molecular [104, 105]. In the case of tumors, a biomarker consists of substances that can be produced either by the malignant cells or by normal tissues in response to the presence of the tumor. The concentration and nature of these substances may change with the occurrence, progression and treatment of cancer [106⁻108]. Body fluids, tissues and liquid biopsies are often used as biological samples [109].

Tumor biomarkers include gene mutations, transcripts, proteins, or metabolites, which demonstrate a correlation with malignant symptoms or phenotypes. They can be transcriptional activators, regulators, receptors, suppressors and oncogenes [110⁻115] capable of differentially modulating an individual molecular profile. The most commonly used biomarker in PCa is PSA, which helps in early diagnosis, and is associated with a decrease in the occurrence of aggressive cases [116].

However, due to the complexity of PCa, paradigm shifts are needed to better understand its molecular mechanisms. The advent of nanotechnology, genetic engineering, bioinformatics, molecular biology, and the reduction in the cost of next-generation sequencing technologies have enabled the scientific community to identify new biomarkers in a new era of molecular medicine. The initial effects of this change on oncology are beginning to impact patient care [51].

Prostate-Specific Antigen (PSA)

Kallikreins compose a subgroup of fifteen serine proteases that are involved in several physiological functions, including the regulation of blood pressure, peeling of the skin, liquefaction of the seminal clot, tissue remodeling and inflammatory signaling [117]. The kallikrein-related peptidase 3 gene (*KLK3*) is located in a 300kb cluster on chromosome 19. Its protein product is a protease present in seminal plasma. The quantification of its serum levels, in the clinical routine, helps in the screening, diagnosis, prognosis, monitoring of recurrence and evaluation of therapeutic efficacy [118-120].

PSA is synthesized by prostatic epithelial cells, either normal, hyperplastic or malignant [121]. PSA is produced in the ductal and acinar epithelium and is then secreted into the lumen. The main proteolytic function of PSA is the fragmentation of semenogelin I and II proteins of the seminal gel structure [122, 123]. The healthy prostate is surrounded by a continuous layer of basal cells and a basement membrane that prevent high concentrations of PSA from escaping into the blood [124].

There is a strong correlation between PSA levels and prostate volume [125]. Increase in serum PSA levels may represent abnormalities in gland architecture and vascularization [126]. Therefore, altered levels can suggest different alterations such as infections, chronic inflammation, BPH and / or PCa, since changes in the organization of the basement membrane culminate in the release of PSA into the bloodstream. Furthermore, it does not differentiate between indolent and aggressive tumors, which highlights the need for additional markers [118-120]. Since 1980 [127], PSA screening has significantly improved the management of patients with PCa [128, 129] and in 1994, together with DRE, it was approved by the Food Drug and Administration (FDA) [109] as a routine clinical test. Serum PSA values vary individually up to the upper limit of 4.0 ng / mL and, when elevated, additional tests are recommended, including biopsy of the gland [130]. Increased levels of this antigen are also indicative of PCa progression, since PSA regulates mechanisms involved in proliferation, angiogenesis and metastasis [116]. Therefore, it is also used in the monitoring of disease recurrence. In this context, the kinetics of the PSA or variations in its levels can also be measured over time, generating information related to the speed of the PSA (PSAV) [116] or PSA doubling-time (PSADT), which is defined as the time required for a 2-fold increase in PSA values [131].

PSA is found in the blood in its free form (fPSA) or in a complex with serum protease inhibitors [120]. Specifically, fPSA has no catalytic activity and does not form complexes [132]. fPSA levels can be detected and compared to the total PSA level in order to get the proportion of fPSA (% fPSA) [131]. fPSA corresponds to 5% to 35% of total PSA and encompasses three catalytically inactive molecular isoforms: pro-PSA, BPH-associated PSA (BPSA) and free intact PSA (iPSA) [133]. These isoforms occur in approximately equal proportions in the serum and are considered prostatic biomarkers [134].

Pro-PSA

Pro-PSA is an inactive pro-enzyme with a leading peptide of seven amino acids that is usually cleaved by human kallikrein enzymes to form PSA. In the prostate, peptidase 2 related to human kalicrein (hK2) cleaves pro-PSA and generates the enzymatically active mature form of PSA composed of 237 amino acids [135]. Several truncated pro-PSA isoforms have been found, which vary according to the number of amino acids of the leader peptide that remains bound to the PSA molecule [109, 136]. The most common are [-4] pro-PSA, [-5] pro-PSA and [-2] pro-PSA [137]. [-2] pro-PSA (p2PSA) has been described for being specific to PCa [138] and therefore, is a sensitive biomarker of the disease [139, 140].

The average percentage of prostate volume and the volume of the transition zone increase by approximately 2.2% and 3.5% per year [141]. Pro-PSA is generally higher in the peripheral region of prostatic tissues and undetectable in the transition region, with p2PSA being the most stable form [140, 142]. According to Mikolajczyk *et al.*, serum pro-PSA is clearly related to PCa and can be measured in addition to the PSA test, increasing the accuracy of the method [139].

BPH-related PSA (BPSA)

This isoform of fPSA is similar to total PSA, except for the internal cleavages between Lys 182 and Lys 145. In the tissue of the transition region its expression is generally limited, while it is highly expressed in BPH [134]. BPSA derives from a highly proteolytic environment, suggesting that the cleavage of PSA into BPSA is performed by specific proteases associated with nodular hyperplasia in patients with BPH [143].

Changes in BPSA levels are strongly associated with prostate volume [139], but it does not distinguish patients with PCa from healthy individuals [144]. However, Rhodes and collaborators (2012) reported high BPSA in groups with BPH and PCa compared to the general population [145]. Thus, BPSA is a useful and suggestive marker for benign prostate diseases, but it cannot reflect a full spectrum of malignant prostate disease [144].

Prostate Cancer Antigen 3 (PCA3)

PCA3 is a lncRNA whose expression is closely related to the prostate in malignant conditions, demonstrating its important role as a PCa-specific biomarker. It is located on the long arm of chromosome 9 and is characterized by a high density of stop codons and polyadenylation sites. The *PCA3* promoter region has a short repeat polymorphism (TAAA), identified as a risk marker for PCa [146]. In addition, new isoforms have also been described, which corroborates the molecular complexity of this lncRNA [147].

The *PCA3* gene plays essential roles in several cellular processes and biological functions. *PCA3* acts as a modulator of the transcriptional activity of the AR-target genes and controls the transcriptional levels of the tumor suppressor Prune homolog 2 with BCH domain (*PRUNE2*) [148]. In fact, *PCA3* is organized in an antisense orientation to intron 6 of the *PRUNE2* gene, modulating its expression. *PRUNE2* primary transcript anneals with *PCA3*, forming a double-stranded RNA, which becomes the target of adenosine deaminases (ADARs) that edit adenosine to inosine, suppressing *PRUNE2* expression. In this context, the overexpression of *PCA3* decreases the expression of *PRUNE2*, inducing the proliferation of malignant cells [149]. Moreover, it seems that *PCA3* can interfere with the expression of E-cadherin, a protein responsible for maintaining epithelial integrity and cell-cell interactions [146].

In angiogenesis, *PCA3* regulates the expression of Vascular endothelial growth factor A (VEGFA) and fibrillin-1 (FBN1). Regarding cell adhesion, it modulates MTSS I-BAR domain containing 1 (MTSS1) and Interferon beta 1 (IFNB1) and, in the signal transduction context, it modulates ERB-B2 receptor tyrosine kinase 2 (ERBB2), the Phosphoinositide-3-kinase regulatory subunit 1 (PIK3R1) and the Mitogen-activated protein kinase 1 (MAP2K1). It also influences apoptosis, regulating the Bcl-2- associated agonist of cell death (BAD), and Telomerase reverse transcriptase (TERT) activity [150].

Clinically, *PCA3* stands out as a diagnostic biomarker for PCa [151⁻154]. Studies have been conducted aiming at its quantitative detection by real-time PCR (qPCR) [154, 155] in body fluids like saliva [156, 157], blood [158, 159] and urine after DRE [160, 161]. The success regarding *PCA3* specificity culminated in its approval by the FDA as a diagnostic tool for PCa in urine samples from patients that underwent DRE [162]. Unlike PSA, *PCA3* expression levels are independent of the patient's age, presence of inflammation, trauma or previous biopsies [163]. Therefore, the quantification of *PCA3* by qPCR has been useful in guiding clinical practice, especially regarding the decision to perform or re-perform a biopsy in patients suspected of malignancy. The correct stratification of patients results from the combination of DRE, PSA and *PCA3* expression. However, the detection threshold for lncRNA remains controversial, especially considering the disease staging [132, 164]. It has been shown that *PCA3* levels in urine can be significantly affected when the patient underwent ADT [165, 166].

PCA3 has been described for being specific for PCa, since its expression is not altered by other clinical pathologies associated with the prostate, such as chronic prostatitis. Additionally, RT-PCR analysis did not detect *PCA3* in lung, esophageal, ileum, colon, pancreatic, testicular, breast, bladder and melanoma cancers [167]. However, it has been described in malignant and healthy ovarian tissues as well as in ovarian cancer cell lines. *PCA3* silencing in ovarian cancer cell lines has led to the suppression of cell migration, invasion and viability, in addition to inducing cell cycle arrest and apoptosis [168]. Recently, elevated transcriptional levels of *PCA3* have been identified in cerebrospinal fluid exosomes extracted from patients with Parkinson's and Alzheimer's diseases, suggesting their correlation with the pathogenesis of other chronic diseases [169].

TMPRSS2: ERG Fusion

Transcription factors have been reported as potential biomarkers for PCa diagnosis and prognosis [170] and are characterized by a diverse family of proteins that control gene expression through regulation of the transcription process. The ETS (erythroblast transformation-specific) family of transcription factors comprises different genes, *e.g.*, ETS transcription factor ERG (ERG), ETV1, ETV4, and ETV5, that mediate cellular processes such as angiogenesis, apoptosis, cell differentiation, oncogenic transformation and cancer progression [171].

In 2005, chromosomal rearrangements were identified in PCa [172], including fusions of ERG, ETV1, ETV4 and ETV5 genes with the TMPRSS2 (Transmembrane serine protease type 2) gene [172]. Interestingly, at the molecular level, TMPRSS2 and ERG are located on the same chromosome (21q), and the distance between them is short (3 Mb). Such vicinity contributes to the chromosomal rearrangement, upon which the TMPRSS2 allele loses its promoter while the ERG allele gains this promoter region [173, 174]. This event leads to TMPRSS2:ERG gene fusion, which is present in 50% [172] of PCa cases [171].

TMPRSS2 protein expression is regulated by androgens and characterized by a serine-linked transmembrane protease that is highly expressed on the membrane of the human prostate epithelial cells on the luminal surface. TMPRSS2 is found overexpressed in patients with PCa, which makes it a potential biomarker for the disease [175, 176]. On the other hand, ERG is a transcription factor that regulates many cellular functions such as proliferation, angiogenesis, apoptosis and oncogenic transformation. Scientific evidence indicates that ERG binds to AR-responsive genes, regulating androgen signaling, and, therefore, oncogenesis [177]. Moreover, cooperation between the AR and ERG favors the promotion of invasive adenocarcinomas.

TMPRSS2: ERG fusion may be a predictive biomarker in clinical practice for patients with PCa undergoing ADT [171, 177]. In fact, the presence of the TMPRSS2:ERG fusion-derived protein in PCa increases the risk of lymph node involvement, biochemical recurrence of PSA and disease relapse. Detection of this fusion also increases the mortality index and is correlated with phosphatase and tensin homolog (PTEN) loss [178] and phosphatisylinositol-3 kinase/protein kinase B (PI3K/Akt or PI3K/PKB) pathway activation [179]. Moreover, stromal alterations that favor the carcinogenic process have also been identified in patients with TMPRSS2:ERG [180].

Cells with TMPRSS2: ERG structural rearrangement overexpress the ERG transcription factor, activating the NOTCH signaling pathway and contributing to the invasion ability of PCa cells. Thus, the inhibition of NOTCH may be a viable alternative to antagonize the aggressive potential conferred by gene fusion on malignant prostate cells [171]. ERG overexpression also activates plasminogen, contributing to cellular invasion [181]. Since it can help PCa detection, TMPRSS2:ERG fusion has been used as biomarker for PCa in conjunction with other molecules such as *PCA3* [182]. These findings highlight the need for the discovery and analysis of multiple targets in order to unravel the molecular heterogeneity of PCa and develop more effective therapeutic strategies.

Urokinase-Type Plasminogen Activator (Upa) and its Receptor (Upar)

The coagulation process is essential for homeostasis by means of its action in preventing blood loss and in participating in tissue remodeling and healing processes [183]. The way by which the interaction between neoplastic cells and the coagulation system disrupts homeostasis is complex and not fully understood. So far, it is known that such a failure arises from the imbalance between procoagulant and anticoagulant factors [184, 185]. Urokinase-type plasminogen activator (uPA) and its receptor, uPAR, have stood out for acting in the proteolysis of the basement membrane and ECM components, promoting tumor invasion. uPa is a serine protease of approximately 50kDa synthesized by endothelial cells, muscle cells, epithelial cells, monocytes / macrophages, fibroblasts and tumor cells [183]. Its receptor is a glycoprotein rich in cysteines, composed of 283 amino acids [183, 184].

The uPA / uPAR interaction contributes to tumor growth through plasmin activation. Once connected, these two proteins catalyze the conversion of plasminogen to plasmin, with the cleavage of arginine-valine amino acids from plasminogen. Plasmin degrades laminin, collagen, vitronectin, fibronectin and fibrins and activates Matrix Metalloproteinases (MMPs), which are proteinases that causes the degradation of the basement membrane and ECM components. Plasmin is associated with increased levels of VEGF, fibroblast growth factor (FGF) and activation of transforming growth factor-β (TGF-β) [183, 186]. In addition, uPAR interacts with the epidermal growth factor receptor (EGFR), thereby activating the Extracellular signal Regulated Kinase / Mitogen Activated protein kinase (ERK / MAPK) pathway, triggering cell proliferation and tumor growth. The evaluation of uPA and uPAR in the prostate is centered on primary cancer and their location and expression are still controversial among researchers [184, 185].

Prostate-Specific Membrane Antigen (PSMA)

The PSMA is a transmembrane type II glycoprotein located on the surface of prostate epithelial cells. It consists of three regions: one cytoplasmic, composed of 19 amino acids, one transmembrane composed of 24 amino acids and an extracellular region of 707 amino acids. It is a folate hydrolase that was found to be significantly upregulated in PCa [187-189]. PSMA activity allows the release of free folate and, therefore, enables the participation of this molecule in the methylation of DNA and in the synthesis of polyamines. Therefore, PSMA is involved in PCa cells proliferation, contributing to the occurrence and progression of PCa [190, 191]. In addition, PSMA activates glutamate receptors and alters the membrane potential by modulating the function of the potassium / calcium channels supporting the influx of calcium into malignant cells [187, 192].

PSMA is promising as a target for imaging diagnosis and antineoplastic therapy because it is overexpressed in PCa. In addition, its expression in extra-prostatic tissues is highly restricted [188, 193]. Several studies have reported the importance of PSMA in clinical decisions regarding the treatment of patients, which can become a valuable method for imaging, even in cases of decreased PSA expression [194-196].

ANDROGEN RECEPTOR: FROM CURABLE TO LETHAL DISEASE

Androgen and ARs play important roles in the expression of the male phenotype since the binding of ARs to its ligands, DHT and testosterone, initiates male sexual development and differentiation. The AR is a type I nuclear receptor that functions as a transcriptional factor that controls the expression of specific genes. The AR gene is located on chromosome X, at the locus Xq11-Xq12, and is organized into 8 exons (2757 nucleotides). The AR is a protein of 110 kDa composed of 919 amino acids [197] with three major functional domains: the N-terminal domain (NTD) encoded by exon 1, the DNA-binding domain (DBD) encoded by exons 2 and 3, and the C-terminal ligand-binding domain (LBD) encoded by exons 4–8 [198].

The main natural androgen in males is testosterone, which enters prostate cells and, intracellularly, is converted by 5α reductase into DHT, a metabolite that promotes cell survival and growth Fig. (2). Meanwhile, in the absence of a ligand, the AR associates with heat shock proteins (HSP27 and HSP70) and other chaperones in the cytoplasm. Upon its binding to DHT, the AR changes its conformation, dimerizes, releases the chaperone molecules and binds to importin-α to translocate to the nucleus. In the nuclear compartment, the AR recognizes DNA sequences known as androgen-responsive elements (AREs), which are the promoter regions of target genes. By inducing the transcription of these genes, the AR promotes growth, survival, differentiation, proliferation, apoptosis and angiogenesis [199, 200]. AR activity is finely tuned by regulatory mechanisms that include the control of its protein levels within the cell, by the ubiquitin-proteasome system. The E3 ubiquitin ligase is encoded by *MDM2* and is responsible for AR ubiquitination, a process that is coupled to the proteasome-mediated degradation of this receptor [201].

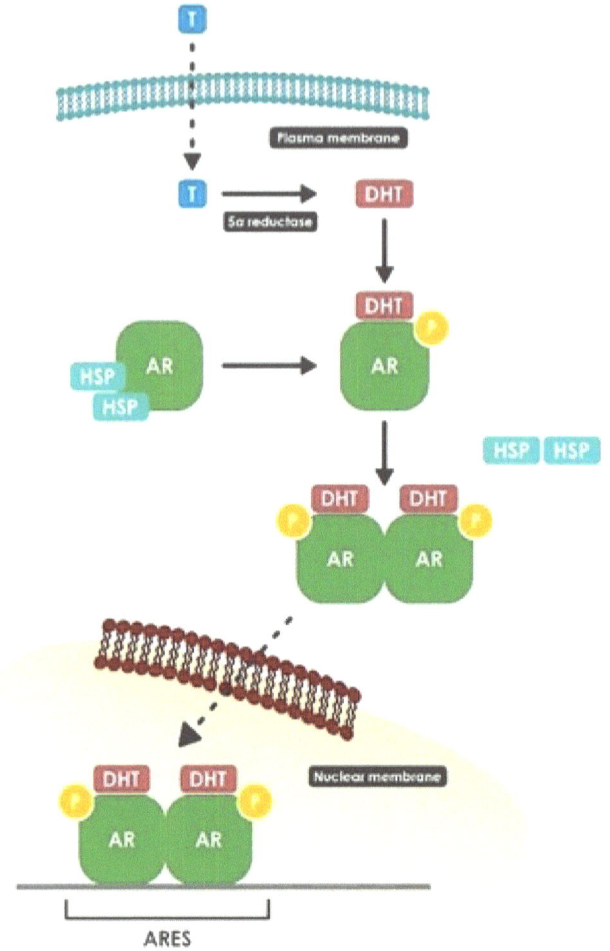

Fig.   **(2))**

Summary of the Androgen Receptor (AR) signaling pathway. Testosterone (T) is transported to the target tissues and is converted to dihydrotestosterone (DHT) by 5-α-reductase. DHT binds to the ligand-binding region of the AR, leading to the dissociation of heat-shock proteins (HSPs) from the receptor. The AR then is translocated into the nucleus, dimerizes and binds to the androgen response elements (AREs) in the promoter region of target genes. The AR orchestrates the cellular metabolism through regulation of the expression of genes that possess various functions such as growth stimulators, phosphatisylinositol-3 kinase (PI3K) modulation, metabolic enzymes, fusion genes, transcription factors and cell cycle regulators.

It is noteworthy that the AR orchestrates the cellular metabolism by regulating gene expression and, in this way, is able to modulate secreted proteins (KLK2 and KLK3), growth stimulators (APP and IGF1R), PI3K activation (FKBP5), metabolic enzyme function (CAMKK2), fusion genes (TMPRSS2:ERG), transcription factors (NKX3 and FOXP1) and cell cycle regulators (UBE2C and TACC2) [202]. In the context of a normal prostate, the AR acts to supply secretory proteins, such as PSA, to the prostate gland [203]. On the other hand, in PCa, the AR upregulates PSA expression, coordinates lipid metabolism, promotes cell growth and stimulates tumor aggressiveness [204].

AR activity is essential in PCa since prostatic cells depend on androgens to grow and survive. The development and progression of 80-90% of PCas encompass androgenic stimulation [205], and men with high transcriptional activity of AR display a higher risk of developing this type of cancer. Therefore, clinical practice uses ADT as the gold standard strategy to control PCa [206]. ADT is the first-line treatment for metastatic PCa and can be administered alone or in combination with chemotherapy. ADT provides favorable initial results with a reduction in disease progression and in the number of deaths. About 10-20% of patients treated with ADT progress to CRPC, with survival ranging from 9 to 78 months. Patients with CRPC do not derive substantial benefits from ADT and will display a continuous increase in PSA levels, an event that is defined as biochemical recurrence. The presence of biochemical recurrence and/or evidences of tumor progression and the formation of metastases, despite ADT, define CRPC. This is an aggressive and lethal disease in which AR signaling is constitutively activated [207-210]. In this context, contemporary research has demonstrated that progression to CRPC occurs from the alteration of the normal androgen axis through deregulation of AR activity through point mutations, amplification, changes in AR cofactors, changes of androgen biosynthesis, occurrence of AR variants, and activation of additional pathways [39, 211].

Hallmarks of CRPC

CRPC is characterized by an aberrant activation of the AR [212]. Mutations in the AR gene may contribute to the progression to CRPC since the receptor loses specificity for its agonist and the tumor becomes resistant to anti-androgens drugs such as enzalutamide and abiraterone. The most frequent mutation that occurs in CRPC is the AR T876A, which results in a promiscuous form of the AR that can be activated upon stimulation with progesterone, estradiol, androstenediol, dehydroepiandrosterone (DHEA), antiandrogens hydroxyflutamide (HF) and cyproterone acetate [213, 214]. AR gene amplification predominantly involves its wild-type sequence and results in the overexpression of the AR. Consequently, under ADT, tumor cells that can grow despite low concentrations of serum androgens are selected and pass through a clonal expansion process [215, 216].

An important CRPC feature is its resistance to therapies, which is favored by the existence of androgen receptor variants (AR-V) that originate from alternative splicing. In two decades, 20 variants of ARs have been described; most of them are characterized by truncations in the androgen-binding domain localized at the C terminal region and, for this reason, they confer to the AR the susceptibility to get activated even in the absence of androgens [211, 217ˉ 220]. In normal samples, AR variants are also found, but at a lower rate compared to full-length AR (AR-FL). Indeed, the expression of AR-V and AR-FL strongly correlate in normal samples while in CRPC models they are discrepant [219]. To clarify the functional relevance of these variants in cancer, the detection of specific protein products is important, and variant 7 (AR-V7, also known as AR3) is the only one that codifies for a protein product [221].

AR-V7 (Fig. 3) has been extensively studied and characterized for being involved in the regulation of AR-FL signaling, drug resistance, hormone-independent tumor growth, metastasis development and cell cycle control in PCa [220, 222ˉ224]. This variant can also repress tumor-suppressor genes [225]. Accordingly, AR-V7 expression in circulating tumor cells has been associated with a poor prognosis in patients treated with second- and third-line ADT therapies [224, 226].

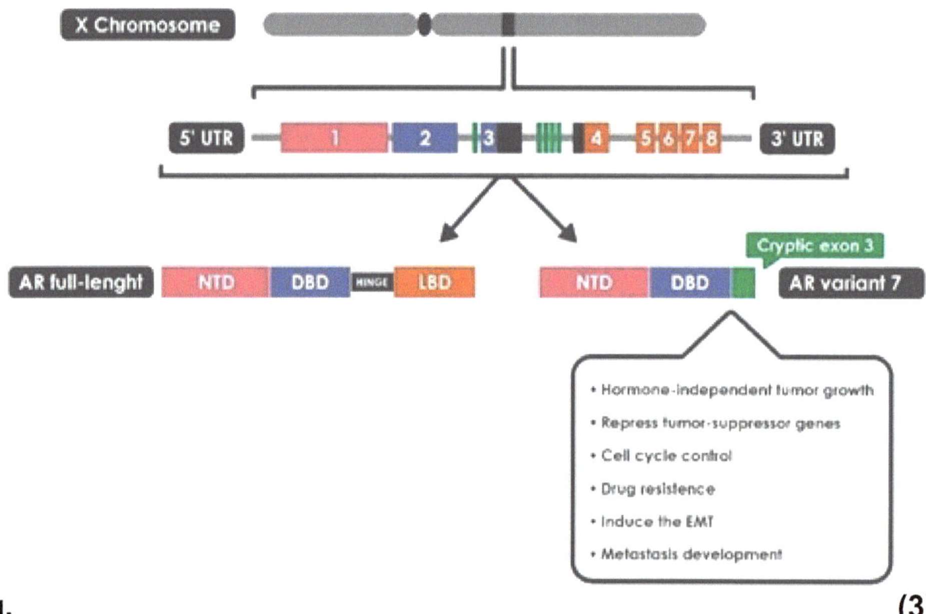

Fig. (3))
Schematic representation of the Androgen Receptor (AR) and AR variant 7 (AR-V7). The AR gene is composed of 8 exons. In the full-length AR, exon 1 encodes the amino-terminal domain (NTD), exons 2–3 encode the DNA-binding domain (DBD) and the 3′ region of exon 4 and exons 5–8 encode the ligand-binding domain (LBD). AR-V7 lacks the LBD and carries unique

amino acids from cryptic exon 3. AR-V7 is constitutively active, and thus involved in drug resistance, hormone-independent tumor growth, metastasis development, cell cycle control in prostate cancer, repression of tumor-suppressor genes and induction of the epithelial-mesenchymal transition (EMT).

CRPC cells also modulate the AR transcriptional activities using different AR co-regulators. Co-regulators are a group of proteins that interact with nuclear receptors or transcription factors in order to modulate gene expression. ARA55 inhibition, for example, hampers the transcriptional activity of AR and promotes anti-androgens to function as AR agonists instead of AR antagonists. For this reason, this AR co-regulator has been associated with a reduced PCa cell growth [227].

Forkhead box protein A1 (FOXA1), and GATA binding factor 2 (GATA2) are two other types of AR coactivators. FOXA1 is a member of the Forkhead family of DNA binding proteins and acts differentially between androgen-sensitive and CRPCs. Indeed, in CRPC, FOXA1 functions alone or together with the AR to promote the expression of genes involved in the progression of the cell cycle [228, 229]. GATA2 controls the expression of genes involved in cancer progression [230] and correlates with Gleason scores, tumor relapse and metastasis [231, 232]. GATA2 also regulates the activity of AR variants [233] and, therefore, contributes to the CRPC phenotype and resistance to chemotherapeutics [230].

Another class of co-activators is the steroid receptor co-activator family (SRC) that comprises several proteins that aid the transcription activity of progesterone, estrogen and androgen receptors [234]. SRC-1, SRC-2, and SRC-3 bind to the AR, open the chromatin structure at target sites, and, as a consequence, the transcriptional machinery is recruited. Scientific evidence demonstrated that suppression of SRC-1 reduces PCa cell growth [235]. SRC-2 is increased in metastatic prostate tumors and contributes to the increased expression of the AR [236]. In addition, SRC-3 is upregulated in aggressive PCa and is capable of activating Akt expression, which is necessary for CRPC development. Also, SRC-3 expression negatively correlates with the expression of the tumor suppressor protein PTEN and with recurrence-free survival of PCa patients [211, 216, 237].

Accordingly, an additional hallmark of CRPC is the inhibition of tumor-suppressor proteins and overexpression of oncogenes. PTEN is a lipid phosphatase that regulates different cellular signaling pathways, including the PI3K/Akt route. PI3K is responsible for the phosphorylation of phosphati-dylinositol bi-phosphate (PIP2) in order to generate the phosphatidylinositol tri-phosphate (PIP3) molecule. PIP3 activates the serine/threonine kinase Akt, which is involved in the promotion of cell proliferation and apoptosis inhibition. PTEN cleaves the phosphate group of PIP3 molecules and, therefore, prevents the activation of Akt [238, 239]. The tumor-suppressor p53 is also lost or mutated in CRPC. p53 is a transcription factor that regulates the cell cycle and promotes apoptosis [240]. Interestingly, in PCa a co-occurrence of *PTEN* and *P53* mutations can be frequently detected [241]. In CRPC, AR-V7 inhibits the expression of tumor-suppressor genes [225]. Tumor-suppressor genes, such as cyclin kinase inhibitors, also control cell cycles. It has been demonstrated that CRPC cells ensure their permanence into the cell cycle by shutting down the expression of two kinase inhibitors (p21 and p27), which is accompanied by the inhibition of the retinoblastoma protein (Rb), a critical regulator of cell division [242].

CRPC is further characterized by the ability to evade apoptosis, another hallmark of this disease. Apoptosis is programmed cell death, which is essential for the maintenance of homeostasis. One of the strategies developed by CRPC cells to inhibit apoptosis is the aberrant activation of members of the family of inhibitors of apoptosis proteins (IAPs). IAPs are well known for their role in preventing caspase activation and are involved in PCa progression. A member of the IAP family, baculoviral IAP repeat-containing 6 (BIRC6), has been described to be associated with a poor prognosis of cancer patients [243, 244]. Recently, it has been demonstrated that CRPC activates the PI3K/Akt pathway in response to enzalutamide and this activation leads to the inhibition of the pro-apoptotic protein, BAD, that culminates in apoptosis evasion [245].

Finally, EMT represents an essential hallmark for the acquisition of castration-resistance and tumor invasion properties [246]. EMT is a process through which an epithelial cell acquires an invasive mesenchymal phenotype and loses the ability to create cell-cell contacts. EMT occurs through the loss of expression of epithelial markers, such as E-Cadherin, and through the gain of expression of mesenchymal markers such as Vimentin, N-Cadherin, fibronectin and α-smooth muscle actin [247]. The mesenchymal phenotype plays a pivotal role in cancer progression and metastasis [246]. EMT is regulated by molecular mechanisms that include the signaling pathways of TGF-β and EGFR [248]. EMT occurs through the activation of several specific transcription factors such as Snail, Twist, Slug, E47, ZEB1 and ZEB2 that are able of increasing the expression of mesenchymal markers while decreasing the expression of epithelial markers [249]. In CRPC, AR-V7, induces the EMT process and leads to the expression of stem cell signature genes [250].

Signaling Pathways Involved in CRPC

The mechanisms associated with CRPC have been extensively investigated. Thus far, several pathways have been described to participate to the development of this aggressive phenotype (Fig. 4). All these pathways lead to aberrant AR activation that is responsible for an altered pattern of gene expression signatures [251, 252].

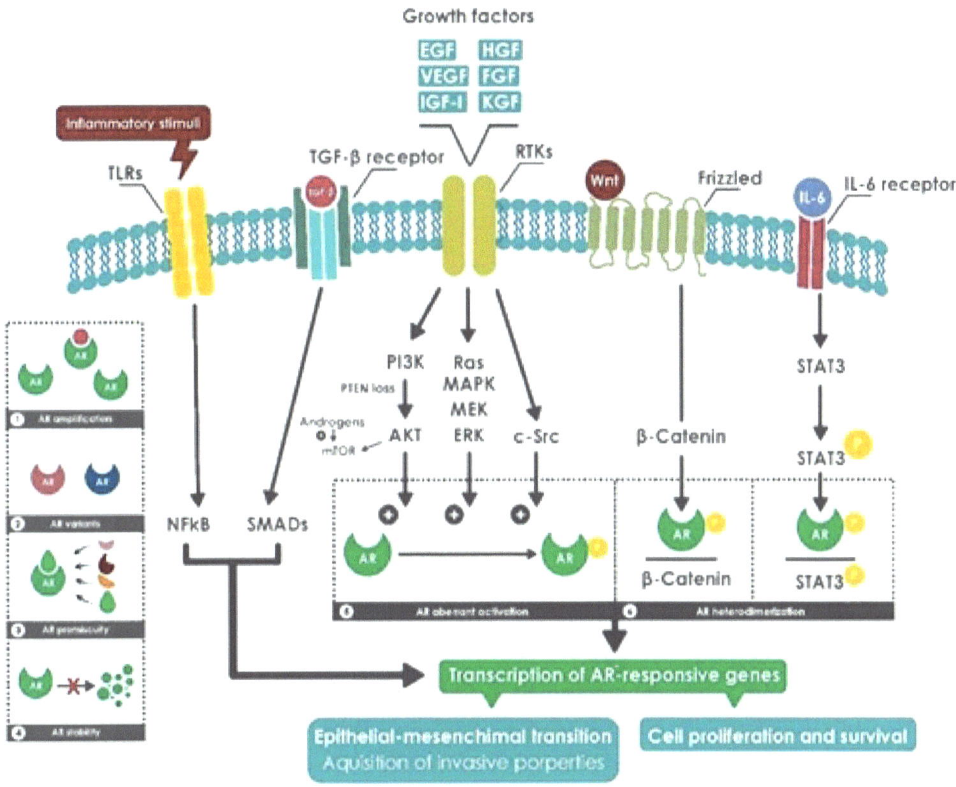

Fig. (4))

Scheme of molecules and cell signaling pathways involved in the occurrence and maintenance of castration-resistant Prostate Cancer (CRPC) phenotype. Regarding the Androgen Receptor (AR) pathway, several mechanisms used by CRPC cells to support AR signaling are represented in the image, even in the absence of androgens. These strategies rely on: (i) AR gene amplification that allows a higher expression of this receptor; (ii) the expression of AR variants, with the acquired ability of the AR to become activated by non-androgens ligands (AR promiscuity); and (iii) AR protein stability, which implies a lower degradation rate of the AR though ubiquitin-proteasome system. The image also shows signaling pathways that communicate, either directly or indirectly, with the AR pathway in order to activate the transcription of AR-responsive genes. Thus, these routes promote cell survival and proliferation and sustain cell invasion by stimulating the epithelial-mesenchymal transition (EMT) process. Cellular response can be mediated by growth factors that interact with tyrosine kinase receptors (RTKs) by transforming growth factor-β (TGF-β) and interleukin-6 (IL-6), upon their binding to their specific receptors and through the interaction between Wnt ligands and Frizzled and by Toll-like receptor

(TLR) activation by inflammatory stimuli. Nuclear Factor Kappa light chain enhancer of activated B cells (NFkB) and TGF-β signaling are directly implicated in the increase of transcriptional activity of the AR. The RTK signaling pathway activates (+) several molecules including protein kinase B (Akt), the Mitogen Activated protein kinase (MAPK) that culminates in the activation of Extracellular signal Regulated Kinase (ERK) and in the activation of the cytoplasmic kinase c-Src. Akt, ERK and c-Src enhance AR signaling by stimulating its phosphorylation and thus leading to aberrant AR activation. By binding to their receptor, Frizzled, Wnt ligands activate β-catenin that interact directly with the AR, forming a transcriptional active heterodimer. The IL-6 signaling pathway promotes the phosphorylation and activation of Signal Transducer and Activator of Transcription 3 (STAT3). Phospho-STAT3 (pSTAT3), in turn, binds to the AR, forming a transcriptional active heterodimer.

The clinical significance of these mechanisms is actively researched, mainly because the molecular alterations are not punctual and much remains to be learned regarding multiple unknown CRPC drivers [253].

EGF: Epidermal growth factor; FGF: Fibroblast growth factor 2; HGF: Hepatocyte growth factor; IGF-1: Insulin-like growth factor 1; KGF: Keratinocyte growth factor; MEK: Mitogen activated protein kinase kinase; ERK: extracellular signal regulated kinase; mTOR: Mammalian Target of Rapamycin; PI3K: Phosphatisylinositol-3 kinase; PTEN: Phosphatase and Tensin Homolog; SMAD: Small Mothers Against Decapentaplegic; VEGF: Vascular endothelial growth factor.

TGF-β

One of the main pathways that promotes and sustains the CRPC phenotype is the signaling mediated by a multifunctional cytokine called TGF-β. The TGF-β signaling pathway regulates several cellular processes including proliferation, apoptosis and EMT [254]. TGF-β signaling is mediated by two types of serine/threonine receptors: TFG-β RII, which binds directly to the TGF-β, and TGF-β RI. TGF-β RI and TGF-β RII form a heterodimer once the binding to TGF-β has occurred, and subsequently TGF-β RI is phosphorylated, leading to the activation of SMAD family member 2 and 3 (Smad2 and 3) [254]. Afterwards, Smad2 and 3 bind to Smad4 forming a complex that migrates to nuclei where it induces the transcription of specific genes involved in the control of cell proliferation, apoptosis, angiogenesis and EMT [255, 256]. In addition to the Smad-dependent pathway, Smad-independent pathways, involving the activation of MAPK, Mammalian Target of Rapamycin (mTOR), c-Src and PI3K/Akt downstream of the TGF-β receptor, have been described [257]. Nevertheless, Smad-independent pathways, which do not directly involve TGF-β receptor activation, have also been reported and described for driving the expression of growth factors, such as epidermal growth factor (EGF) [258]. TGF-β enhances the progression of cancer by means of its de-differentiation activity in tumor cells, immune system suppression and angiogenesis process promotion [259]. Moreover, TGF- β signaling regulates the expression of the MMP-2 and MMP-9, which are endopeptidases that are directly implicated in cancer cell invasion and formation of metastases, due to their property of degrading ECM components [256, 260].

The TGF-β/Smad pathway plays an essential role in CSC proliferation and, consequently, its up-regulation associates with chemoresistance [261]. It has been demonstrated that TGF-β expression is increased in PCa when compared to BPH and PIN [262]. Interestingly, TGF-β displays a dichotomist behavior in PCa; while it inhibits proliferation at early stages of the disease, it promotes PCa growth at advanced stages of the disease [256]. It has been shown that the TGF-β signaling pathway is able to activate the transcriptional activity of the AR. The molecule responsible for this action is Smad3, which binds directly to the AR at the DBD and LBD and acts as AR co-activator. Indeed, the binding of Smad3 to the AR has been linked to increased PSA expression levels [263, 264]. On the other hand, it has been reported that the high expression of the AR in the presence of another AR co-activator, ARA55, inhibits the TGF-β pathway. When bound to ARA55, the AR inhibits TGF-β up-regulation of Smad transcriptional activity [265]. Those findings highlight the essential role played by AR co-activators in the development and progression of PCa. Previous reports demonstrated that the activation of the Smad proteins, elicited by the TGF-β signaling, induces the expression of ZEB, SNAIL and TWIST which are transcriptional repressors of the epithelial marker, E-Cadherin [266]. Finally, the AR can induce EMT [267] by virtue of its ability to suppress the expression of E-Cadherin [268].

Tyrosine Kinase Receptors

Tyrosine kinase receptors (RTKs) constitute a family of receptors that are usually activated by growth factors. These receptors elicit a signal cascade that lead to activation of molecules involved in cell growth and cell survival. The main pathways activated during RTK stimulation comprise the PI3K/Akt or PI3K/PKB, the janus kinase (JAK)/ signal transducer and activator of transcription proteins (STATs) and the MAPK [269]. EGFR signaling is frequently up regulated in PCa thus promoting cancer progression towards the CRPC phenotype, drug resistance and metastasis formation [270]. Interestingly, androgens downregulate EGFR in normal prostate cells but not in PCa cells. Therefore, the lack of regulation in EGFR expression seems to be responsible for the high rate of proliferation and for the progression toward the CRPC phenotype [271]. Consistently, a strong correlation has been shown between EGFR expression and the CRPC phenotype [272]. In PCa cells, EGFR activates the AR in an androgen-independent manner, thus contributing to the progression of PCa in low androgen conditions [273]. The EGFR-downstream signaling molecules, such as STATs and Akt activate the AR by enhancing its phosphorylation in the absence of androgens [274, 275].

The insulin-like growth factor receptor (IGF-1R) seems to be involved in the development and progression of PCa. PCa cells frequently express both insulin-like growth factor-1 (IGF-1) and IGF-1R and the expression of these molecules is increased in CRPC [276⁻278]. IGF-1 regulates the expression of the EMT transcription factor ZEB1 in PCa. ZEB1, in turns, represses the expression of E-Cadherin [279]. It has also been demonstrated that the AR upregulates ZEB1 [280], presenting a paramount role in inducing EMT and, therefore, in promoting PCa progression towards CRPC [246]. In this scenario, since a crosstalk between the AR and IGF-IR has been described, the expression of ZEB1 [281] could result from the IGF-1R-dependent activation of the AR.

VEGF plays a crucial role in promoting the angiogenesis process by eliciting a signaling pathway through its tyrosine kinase receptor, VEGFR. Angiogenesis is essential for sustaining tumor growth since the new vessels formed supply nutrients and oxygen to tumor cells [282]. VEGF expression is higher in PCa metastatic disease *versus* non-metastatic disease and is increased in CRPC [283]. It has also been shown that the AR regulates the expression of VEGF [284, 285]. The angiogenesis process is also promoted by the signaling of the hepatocyte growth factor (HGF) mediated by its receptor c-MET [286]. Previous findings also correlated the c-MET expression with the CRPC phenotype [287].

One of the main signaling pathways triggered by RTKs is the MAPK and ERK1 and 2, which plays a crucial role in cell proliferation, cancer progression and EMT [288]. A constitutive activation of MAPK has been associated with PCa progression to CRPC [289]. In PCa, a crosstalk between the AR and MAPK has been reported and described for being responsible for the ligand-independent activation of the AR [290]. Another RTK downstream signaling pathway that has been described for being involved in a functional interaction with the androgenic route is the PI3K/Akt pathway [291]. Reports showed that Akt, by means of its activity of phosphorylating the AR, inhibits the pro-apoptotic functions of this receptor [292].

An additional molecule which is activated by RTKs and that is frequently over activated in mCRPC is mTOR [293]. mTOR is a serine/threonine protein kinase that regulates cell proliferation, migration, protein synthesis, transcription and autophagy [294]. It has been demonstrated that the cytoplasmic fraction of mTOR can be activated by androgens [295], which results in its migration to the nucleus, where it regulates AR-dependent transcription [296]. Finally, a non-receptor tyrosine kinase, which is also a downstream effector of RTKs, is c-Src. When cells receive the proper stimuli, c-Src gets activated and displays its tyrosine kinase activity, which is involved in both physiological and pathological processes. Indeed, c-Src promotes the activation of several effectors of cell function and thus modulates processes such as proliferation, cell cycle progression, cell migration and differentiation [297]. It has been shown that c-Src is highly expressed in PCa and over-activated in CRPC [298]. A cross-activation between c-Src and the AR has also been reported [299].

Il-6 Signaling

The inflammatory cytokine IL-6 has also been associated with the EMT process. IL-6 elicits a signaling pathway upon binding to the IL-6 receptor (gp130). Once activated by IL-6, gp130 dimerizes and activates the JAK/STAT pathway. The IL-6 pathway triggers the activation of JAK, which is responsible for the phosphorylation of tyrosine residues within the cytoplasmic tail of the IL-6 receptor. Signal transducer and activator of transcription 3 (STAT3) is therefore recruited at the phospho-tyrosine residues of IL-6 receptor and is phosphorylated by JAK. Once phosphorylated, STAT3 dimerizes and migrates to the nucleus where it regulates gene transcription [300].

It has been reported that in PCa cells, both IL-6 and gp130 are expressed [301], and in CRPC cells, IL-6 elicits an autocrine loop that promotes their aggressive phenotype [302]. In PCa cells, the IL-6 autocrine loop increases the AR nuclear localization and transcriptional activity [303⁻307]. In fact, IL-6 promotes PCa progression and androgen-independency [308] and induces EMT through the activation of STAT3 [309]. In addition, STAT3 has been described to promote resistance towards chemotherapies [310].

Wnt/frizzled/β-Catenin

One of the signaling pathways that have been associated with the CRPC phenotype is Wnt/Frizzled/β-catenin. β-catenin promotes cell adhesion when localized at the cell membrane through its interaction with E-Cadherin and α-catenin. On the other hand, the cytoplasmic fraction of β-catenin is sequestered in a protein complex that promotes its phosphorylation. Once phosphorylated, β-catenin is ubiquitinated and directed to proteasomal degradation. This type of fine regulation occurs in the absence of signaling mediated by Wnt ligands and is essential in order to maintain the tissue's homeostasis [311].

The class of Wnt ligands comprises several secreted glycoproteins that have been deeply studied for their role in the control of the morphogenesis processes [311]. The signaling pathway elicited by Wnt ligands aims to activate the transcriptional activities of β-catenin. In order to do that, Wnt ligands activate Frizzled, a G-protein-coupled receptor, leading to an inhibition of proteasomal degradation of β-catenin that therefore starts to accumulate in the cytoplasm. In this situation β-catenin can migrate to the nucleus where it binds to transcription factors and lead to the expression of genes involved in cell proliferation [312, 313].

It has been shown that the Wnt/Frizzled/β-catenin pathway is frequently mutated in CRPC [241] and in aggressive cells there is an increased co-localization of the AR and β-catenin at the nuclear level [314]. Indeed, a crosstalk between the AR and the Wnt pathway has been already described and can occur through an interaction between β-catenin and the AR or through the transactivation of the AR by Wnt ligands. It is also possible that the AR is responsible for an increase in β-catenin activation levels, thus leading to EMT [314]. Reports also described that the Wnt/Frizzled/β-catenin axis significantly contributes to treatment resistance [315] and to EMT [316].

NFkB

NFkB (nuclear factor kappa light chain enhancer of activated B cells) is a protein complex that controls, through gene transcription modulation, the cell response to various stimuli, including inflammation and stress. NFkB is composed by RelA (p65), RelB, c-Rel and p50/150 subunits [317]. P50 and p65 forms a heterodimer that is sequestered in the cytoplasm in an inactive form by the regulatory protein, IkB. IkB masks the nuclear localization signal (NLS) present in the p50/p65 complex thus impeding its nuclear transport. In order to get activated, the complex p50/p65 must uncouple from IkB. Upon receiving the proper stimuli, cells activate the IkB kinases enzyme complex (IKK) that promotes the phosphorylation and the subsequent proteasomal degradation of IkB, resulting in the activation of the p50/p65 complex [318].

NFkB expression correlates with PCa progression, chemoresistance and metastasis and is up regulated in CRPC [319, 320]. NFkB induces IL-6 expression and promotes the hormone-independent growth of PCa cells [321]. Cancer cells can display a constitutive activation of a specific IKK subunit, the IKKε, which is responsible for the constitutive activation of NFkB. IKK induces the NFkB-dependent expression of IL-6 [322, 323]. Moreover, IKKε phosphorylates and subsequently promotes the degradation of tumor suppressors proteins thus contributing to the escape from cell cycle check-points [324]. The over-activation of the NFkB pathway seems to be responsible for the increased transcription of AR variants, thus promoting the progression towards the CRPC phenotype [325].

Approved Treatments for CRPC

According to Scher and his collaborators (2016), CRPC patients are divided into non-metastatic (nmCRPC) and metastatic (mCRPC) cases [326]. In nmCRPC there is biochemical recurrence with increasing PSA levels but no evidence of metastasis in conventional scans. Initially, ADT is performed, which results in reduced PSA levels and in a decrease risk of metastasis. Eventually, many of these patients refract and develop metastasis within 19 months, progressing to mCRPC [207, 327, 328].

The treatment of CRPC focuses on the androgenic axis and consists in blocking its biosynthesis, inhibiting its ligands, interrupting its interaction with co-activators and preventing its nuclear translocation [210, 329, 330]. First-generation antiandrogens have been used to block AR signaling in PCa cells, inhibiting the binding of the AR to its target, and so, preventing disease progression. Flutamide, bicalutamide and nilutamide are included in this class of drugs [331]. However, resistance to these inhibitors and the presence of notable side effects have led to the approval of second-generation compounds [332]. Second-generation antiandrogens act on different mechanisms on the androgenic axis, with advantages when compared to the first generation, including a higher affinity for the AR without agonistic properties [333].

Docetaxel is the current first-line treatment for CRPC patients. This chemotherapeutic compound works by binding to microtubules and prevents the depolymerization required for mitosis. Consequently, the cell cycle is compromised, and apoptosis is activated. Particularly in CRPC, docetaxel induces Bcl-2 (B-cell lymphoma 2) phosphorylation, which leads to caspase activation and finally apoptosis. In addition, AR expression is decreased in docetaxel-treated CRPC cells, since the receptor traffic depends on the microtubules machinery. Therefore, AR nuclear localization is reduced and, consequently, its transcriptional effects are inhibited [207, 208, 329].

Cabazitaxel is indicated for second-line treatment of docetaxel-resistant CRPC patients. This is a semisynthetic taxane with less affinity for drug efflux proteins, such as the P-glycoprotein efflux pump, which is responsible for constitutive and acquired resistance to taxanes [207, 332, 334]. In addition, treatment with cabazitaxel associated with prednisone has demonstrated significant antitumor activity and improved overall survival in patients with CRPC [335].

CRPC cells produce DHT from steroids of adrenal origin through the 5 α-dione pathways, without depending on testosterone directly. The enzyme CYP17A1 (cytochrome P450 family 17 subfamily A member 1) is involved in this mechanism for androgen synthesis. Abiratone acetate is a potent and irreversible inhibitor of CYP17A1 activity, leading to loss of CYP17A1 activity and, consequently, causing a significant loss of androgen production in the peripheral organs, especially from adrenals [336–339]

Enzalutamide, apalutamide and darolutamide are AR antagonist and therefore prevent testosterone binding to the AR, AR nuclear translocation, the AR binding to DNA, and AR co-activators recruitment. Enzalutamide and apalutamide are used in treatments of men with nmCRPC who are at high risk of metastases. These drugs are able to balance the risk of disease progression with collateral effects [328, 338, 340, 341].

Radio dichloride 223 (Radium-223 / RA-223) is an FDA approved therapy for mCRPC that have been shown to improve overall patient survival. RA-223 is an alpha-emitting radiopharmaceutical that delivers high energy, short range irradiation, inducing irreversible DNA double-strand breaks and consequently tumor cell death. RA-223 is a calcium mimetic agent that is incorporated in the bone matrix at sites of active mineralization *via* osteoblasts. Therefore, RA-223 specifically targets bone metastases [342–344]. Lutetium-177 PSMA (Theranos-tic) is a targeted radionuclide therapy that has been used to treat advanced PCa. Low toxicity and tolerance by men with end stage metastatic disease have been demonstrated in different trials [345]. Since PSMA expression is correlated with androgen independence, this strategy is promising for CRPC treatment.

Sipuleucel-T is an autologous cellular immunotherapy for CRPC and is the first therapeutic cancer vaccine approved by the FDA with improvement in overall survival. Sipuleucel-T is a dendritic cell vaccine. Dendritic cells from PCa patients are harvested from peripheral-blood and cocultured with recombinant prostatic acid phosphatase fusion protein and then infused back into the patient. Through this therapy, host antigen-specific T cells are activated in order to kill tumoral cells [207, 346–348].

Research targeting the variant forms of the AR have been carried out and have been revealed to be very promising [349–352]. For all approaches, the clarification of the mechanism by which PCa evolves to the castration-resistant phenotype and acquires resistance to drugs already used is essential for success in treating CRPC. AR activation can occur regardless of ligands, which is known as aberrant activation. In this case, androgen signaling activation is mediated by growth factors, such as EGF, IGF-1 and keratinocyte growth factor (KGF), in addition to cytokines such as IL-6 [208, 210].

Although current strategies against CRPC improve overall survival and quality of life of PCa patients, the disease still progresses. Therefore, new therapies are needed, and inhibiting a single target is not enough to suppress the tumor. The PCa complex must be addressed, especially considering the AR signaling pathway. In this context, NPs emerge as promising compounds, with multi-targeting properties and relatively lower systemic toxicity, which must be explored and better understood.

CHALLENGES AND THE WAY FORWARD TO TREAT CRPC: NATURAL PRODUCTS AS ANTICANCER AGENTS

The first records of the medicinal use of plant species date back to 2600 BC. Documents describe the historical use of about 1000 different herbal preparations in the composition of tea, tinctures, plasters and other formulations [353]. However, its applicability in medicine is not restricted to ancient times and different species continue to be studied in the care of patients affected by different diseases [354, 355].

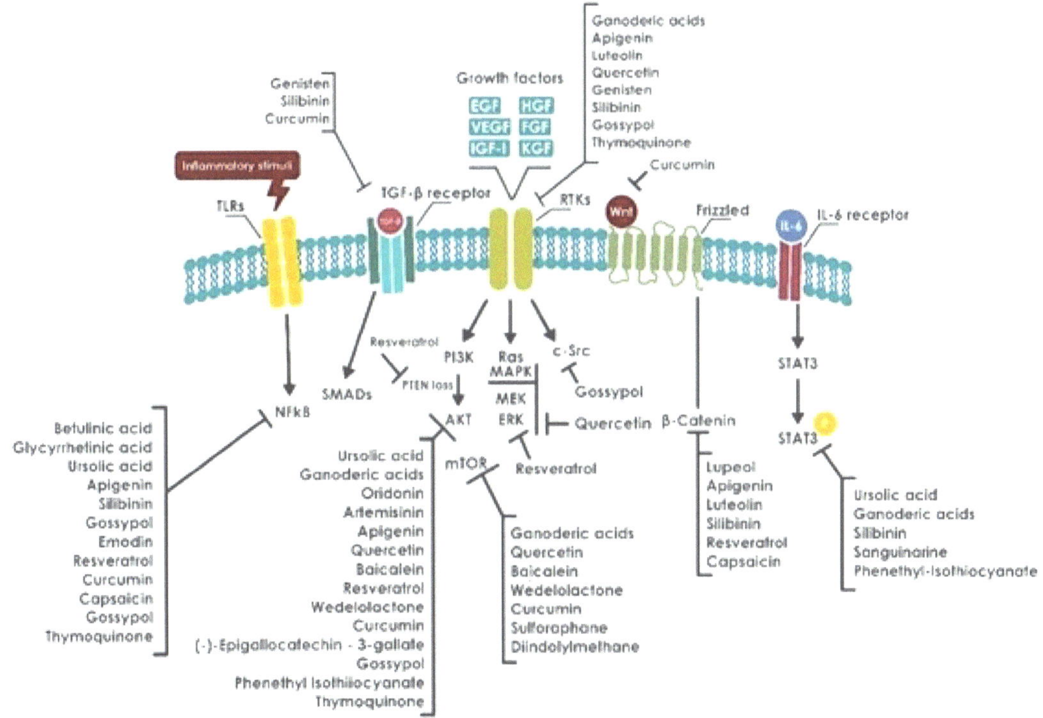

Fig. **(5))**

Scheme of Natural Products (NPs) acting on cell signaling pathways that are involved in the occurrence and maintenance of the castration-resistant Prostate Cancer (CRPC) phenotype. The image indicates NPs that are inhibitors (—|) of the signaling pathways elicited by transforming growth factor-β (TGF-β), growth factors (GFs) and Wnt ligands. NPs specifically inhibit (—|) the following signaling molecules: Nuclear Factor Kappa light chain enhancer of activated B cells (NFkB), protein kinase B (Akt), Mammalian Target of Rapamycin (mTOR), Extracellular signal Regulated Kinase (ERK), β -catenin, c-Src and Transducer and Activator of Transcription 3 (STAT3). Quercetin acts as a broad-spectrum inhibitor of Mitogen Activated protein kinas (MAPK) pathway and Resveratrol has been associated with the re-acquisition of Phosphatase and Tensin Homolog (PTEN) expression that is responsible for a reduced Akt activation.

NPs are compounds produced by living systems, including plants, microorganisms or animals [356]. They offer several advantages since their action has been reported to be highly effective without leading to toxicity or to relevant side effects [18, 354]. Additionally, they have a broader range of targets, which makes them particularly attractive for the treatment of complex diseases like cancer [3]. The therapeutic action of plants is mediated by mainly their secondary metabolites, and great efforts have been undertaken in order to study the activities of these compounds. Secondary metabolites play a relevant adaptive role during a plant's life, being classified by their chemical structure and biosynthesized from essential pathways, such as chiquimic acid and mevalonate [357].

There are different groups of secondary metabolites, such as: terpenes, flavonoids, alkaloids and others [356]. The first alkaloid to be isolated was morphine, by Serturner in 1804 [358]. Since then, secondary metabolites have been attracting pharmacological interest over the years because of their biologic activities, revolutionizing the treatment of different diseases, including cancer [353].

Research on NPs offers numerous possibilities for innovation in the oncology field. In fact, secondary metabolites from NPs are excellent candidates for drug development because they modulate intracellular signaling pathways related to oxidative stress, inflammation, proliferation, apoptosis, angiogenesis and invasion of neoplastic cells. About 25 thousand phytochemicals have already been identified in plants and their anti-cancer properties have been demonstrated [359]. Here we describe some bioactive compounds for the treatment of PCa (Fig. 5), highlighting those that are promising for the treatment of CRPC. The therapeutic landscape of PCa has been transformed and NPs may bring the benefit of survival for those patients with a serious and lethal disease.

EGF: Epidermal growth factor; FGF: Fibroblast growth factor 2; HGF: Hepatocyte growth factor; IGF-1: Insulin-like growth factor 1; KGF: Keratinocyte growth factor; MEK: Mitogen activated protein kinase kinase; ERK: extracellular signal regulated kinase; PI3K: Phosphatisylinositol-3 kinase; PTEN: Phosphatase and Tensin Homolog; RTKs: tyrosine kinase receptors; SMAD: Small Mothers Against Decapentaplegic; TLRs: Toll-like receptors; VEGF: Vascular endothelial growth factor.

Terpenes

Betulinic Acid

Fig. (6))
Betulinic Acid.

Betulinic acid (BA) (Fig. 6) is a natural pentacyclic lupane-type triterpenoid present in many plant species, including *Syzygium* spp. (Myrtaceae), *Ziziphus* spp. (Rhamnaceae), and particularly in *Betula* species, such as the White birch (Betula *pubescens* Ehrh., Betulaceae) [6, 360]. BA possesses anti-inflammatory properties and was initially known for its high cytotoxicity against human melanoma cancer cells. Later studies also suggested that this compound is a broad inhibitor of other tumors, including breast cancer [361].

BA induces apoptosis in tumor cells without affecting normal cells. A synergy in controlling cancer was observed when BA was used in combination with the apoptosis-inducing ligand related to tumor necrosis factor α (TNF- α), or with ionizing radiation. In CRPC, BA sensitizes PC-3 cells to TNF-α-induced apoptosis by suppressing NFκB [362]. BA also increases degradation of the AR in PCa cell lines, LNCaP and PC-3, but not in normal cells. This effect is possibly attributed to the inhibition of deubiquitinase activity, which is crucial for the regulation of the ubiquitin-proteasome system-mediated protein degradation [3]. In addition, BA acts on the regulation of the cell cycle and the angiogenic pathway *via* specific protein (Sp) transcription factors, and through the inhibition of cyclin D1 and EGFR, causing cell cycle arrest. In addition, by inhibiting the expression of Sp1, Sp2 and Sp4 through the microRNA (miR)-27a-ZBTB10-Sp1 axis, BA impairs tumor cell aggressiveness [363].

Glycyrrhetinic Acid

Fig. (7))
Glycyrrhetinic Acid.

18β-Glycyrrhetinic acid (GRA) (Fig. 7) is a pentacyclic oleane triterpenoid found mainly in the roots of Licorice (*Glycyrrhiza glabra*, Fabaceae), a plant which has been extensively used in traditional medicines. Evidence has demonstrated the anti-leishmanial, anti-ulcerative, anti-tumor and antiviral effects of GRA. Anti-tumor properties include inhibition of proliferation and induction of apoptosis [364].

GRA can modulate the activity of cellular enzymes in the normal prostate such as 17, 20 lyase and 17b-hydroxysteroid dehydrogenase, which catalyze the conversion of 17-hydroxyprogesterone into androstenedione and androstenedione to testosterone. GRA is also a potent inhibitor of cytosolic 5α-reductase [365]. Studies suggest that GRA modulates androgen-dependent PCa growth through inhibition of cell proliferation and down-regulation of PSA production [6, 365]. In CRPC cells, DU145, GRA suppresses proliferation, induces apoptosis and downregulates the expression of NFκB (p65), VEGF and MMP-9, impairing aggressiveness [6, 366].

Ursolic Acid

Fig. (8))
Ursolic acid.

Ursolic acid (UA) (Fig. 8) is a pentacyclic triterpenoid found in fruits, vegetables and medicinal plant species, such as *Cornus officinalis* (Cornaceae). This compound exhibits pharmacological activities and, by means of its ability of modulating several signaling pathways, it prevents the development of chronic diseases. Moreover, UA has demonstrated significant anticancer activities against CRPC cells (DU145, and PC-3) and LNCaP cells *in vitro* [367].

In PC-3 cells, UA induces apoptosis by extrinsic and intrinsic mechanisms, while limiting cell invasion by inhibiting Akt and MMP-9. Furthermore, UA suppresses NFκB and STAT3, as well as reduces serum levels of TNF-α and IL-6, modulating proliferation, survival, angiogenesis and apoptosis of PCa cell lines (DU145 and LNCaP). Additionally, UA controls metastasis by suppressing CXCR4 expression in PCa, both *in vitro* (PC-3, DU145 and LNCaP cell lines) and *in vivo* models [6].

Ganoderic Acids

Fig. (9))
Ganoderic acid A.

Ganoderic acids, a group of oxygenated lanostane-type triterpenoids, are the major bioactive compounds produced by the well-known medicinal macro fungus Ganoderma lucidum. More than 150 ganoderic acids have been identified, and the genome of G. lucidum was recently sequenced. However, the biosynthetic pathways of ganoderic acids have not yet been elucidated [368].

Ganoderic acid isoforms induce apoptosis, through intrinsic and extrinsic pathways and regulate proteins and adaptor molecules involved in cancer signaling pathways. Specifically, ganoderic acid A (Fig. 9) modulates NFκB, PI3K / Akt / mTOR pathway in the CRPC cell line, PC-3 [369]. Ganoderic acid A inhibits the proliferation, viability and Reactive oxygen species (ROS) index, modulating the expression of superoxide dismutase SOD1, SOD2, SOD3 and STAT3 in CRPC in a dose-dependent manner [370]. Johnson *et al.* have also shown that this compound controls the conversion of testosterone to DHT and prevent DHT binding to the AR through competitive inhibition [77].

Lupeol

Fig.   **(10))**
Lupeol.

Lupeol (Fig. 10) is a pentacyclic lupane-type triterpene compound found in edible vegetables and fruits, such as cabbage and carrots, as well as in medicinal plants, such as licorice, *Tamarindus indica* and *Celastrus paniculatus* [371]. Over the last decade several studies have revealed important pharmacological activities of lupeol, such as anti-inflammatory, anti-microbial and anti-proliferative [371⁻373].

Lupeol inhibits the tumorigenicity of androgen-independent 22Rn1 PCa cells under *in vivo* conditions. Additionally, lupeol demonstrated a significant anti-proliferative effect on PC-3 cells, not only exerting its pro-apoptotic activity against cancer cells but also working synergistically with natural DNA-damaging compounds to increase cell cytotoxicity through disruption of DNA repair systems [374].

Lupeol deregulates the function of β-catenin signaling during the G2 / M phase and sensitizes CRPC cells to cytotoxic stress. Lupeol can also compete antagonistically with androgen for binding to the AR, can block the binding of the AR to AR-responsive genes including PSA, TCDD inducible poly(ADP-ribose) polymerase (TIPARP), Serum/glucocorticoid regulated kinase 1 (SGK) and IL-6, by inhibiting the recruitment of RNA Pol II to target genes and finally sensitize CRPC cells to anti-hormone therapy [371]. According to the literature, lupeol is a potential chemopreventive agent against CRPC [374].

Oridonin

Fig. (11))
Oridonin.

Oridonin Fig. (11) is a kaurene diterpenoid isolated from herb *Rabdosia rubescens* (Lamiaceae), which has been widely used for thousands of years in traditional Chinese medicine for the treatment of different types of tumors. In PCa, this compound exerts anti-proliferative and pro-apoptotic activities, including in CRPC cells (PC-3 and DU145).

Oridonin stimulates caspase-3 activation [16], probably through ROS generation [375]. In addition, oridonin has been found to elicit G0/G1 cell cycle arrest and apoptosis of LNCaP cells through the upregulation of p53 and Bax and through the downregulation of Bcl-2 in a dose-dependent manner. This compound has also been shown to trigger G2/M cell cycle arrest, autophagy and apoptosis in LNCaP and PC-3 cells by upregulating the expression of p21 [6]. Oridonin downregulates the AR and PSA expression and is a potent inhibitor of NFkB transcriptional activity, also inhibiting the Akt pathway [6, 16, 376].

Although here we are focusing on PCa, it is important to mention that Oridonin is a potential inhibitor of ovarian cancer by blocking the mTOR signaling pathway [377] and it induces apoptosis in cervical carcinoma by suppressing PI3K/Akt genes [378].

Artemisinin

Fig. (12))
Artemisinin.

Artemisinin Fig. (**12**) is a sesquiterpene lactone and a naturally occurring antimalarial substance of *Artemisia annua* (Asteraceae) that presents anti-proliferative effects on a number of human cancer cell lines, such as those of lung, breast, ovarian and prostate [379]. In addition, this compound induces the ubiquitin-proteasome-mediated degradation of the AR in LNCaP and PC-3 cells thus decreasing androgen responsiveness. In addition, it was demonstrated that Akt signaling plays a pivotal role in Artemisin-induced degradation of AR protein in PCa cells [380].

In LNCaP cells, artemisinin treatment triggered G1 cell cycle arrest due to the downregulation of Cyclin-dependent kinase 4 (CDK4) expression [6]. Regarding derivatives, several cancer cells, such as breast, prostate, ovarian, colon, kidney, central nervous system and melanoma cells demonstrated susceptibility to artesunate [379]. Dihydroartemisinin (DHA), reduced viability of LNCaP, DU145 and PC-3 cells, by activating caspases 8 and 9, thus suggesting that DHA activates apoptosis through extrinsic and intrinsic pathways [6].

Lycopene

Fig. (13))
Lycopene.

Lycopene (a ψ,ψ-carotene) Fig. (**13**) is a naturally tetraterpenoid carotene found mainly in tomato (*Solanum lycopersicum*; Solanaceae) [381] that has been identified as an antioxidant with antitumoral properties without any relevant side effects [382]. This compound has demonstrated antiproliferative effects against PCa and suppressed migration and invasion of LNCaP and PC-3 cells [6].

The relation between lycopene and PCa risk have been investigated, including in clinical trials. In fact, lycopene also exerts chemopreventive action and there is evidence for a positive association between its dairy intake and overall PCa risk. In 2013, a 24-year follow-up study in the US suggested a reduced risk of developing PCa in patients with higher lycopene intake, when compared to those with a lower intake [383]. Moreover, evidence showed that high lycopene intake can suppress the angiogenesis within the tumor [384], both *in vitro* and *in vivo*. This effect may involve the inhibition of MMP-2 that has the ability to degrade type IV collagen and is directly associated with endothelial cell migration during the angiogenesis process [385].

In addition, the evidence suggests that Lycopene intake decreased the expression of genes involved in androgen signaling/metabolism such as Srd5a1, Srd5a2 and Srebf1 [386]. Finally, this compound is a powerful antioxidant agent that inhibits IGF-1 [382]. Overall, there is consistent evidence showing that lycopene is associated with a lower risk of advanced or fatal PCa, such as CRPC [387].

Physachenolide D

Fig. (14))
Physachenolide D.

Physachenolide D Fig. (14) is a withasteroid, a group of natural steroids with an intact or modified ergostane skeleton and a C_{28} lactone structure that exhibits various biological activities [388]. Some withanolides, such as Physachenolide D, act as potential activators of quinone reductase or selective inhibitors of the COX-2 enzyme, exhibiting cytotoxic or cell differentiation inducing activities. The proposed mechanism of action, based on the results of bioassay evaluation in withanolides, relies on the α, β-unsaturated ketone unit in ring A and group 5β, 6β-epoxy in ring B [389].

Several withanolides present selective toxicity for LNCaP and PC-3 cell lines [390]. 17β-hydroxywithanolides is as a new class of potent anti-androgenic molecules capable of inhibiting PSA expression and displaying selectivity for LNCaP and PC-3 cell lines. Preliminary structure-activity relationships identified physacenolide D as a 17β-hydroxywitanolide with promising antitumor activity in xenograft mice implanted with LNCaP and PC-3 cells [389, 391].

Flavonoids

Luteolin

Fig. (15))

Luteolin.

Luteolin Fig. (15), a 3',4',5,6-tetrahydroxyflavone, is a common dietary flavonoid found in a large variety of fruits, vegetables and plants, such as celery, *Chrysanthemum* flowers, sweet bell peppers, carrots, onion leaves and broccoli. Luteolin displays multiple biological activities, such as anti-inflammatory and anti-allergy with both antioxidant and pro-oxidant properties [392]. Moreover, luteolin is as a flavonoid compound that possesses anticancer activity against various types of human malignancies such as lung, breast, prostate, and colon tumors [392].

Some studies have proposed that luteolin has an antiangiogenic effect [393]. This compound controls PCa growth and blocks EMT and NFkB pathways [394]. In addition, the evidence suggests that luteolin is a negative regulator of VEGF-2R in PC-3 cells and decreases the expression of the AR and PSA in PCa cells. In PC-3 cells, luteolin acts as a ligand for the type II nuclear estradiol binding site [(3) H], modulating genes involved in the cell cycle [6].

Luteolin inhibits *in vitro* proliferation and induces apoptosis in both PC-3 and LNCaP cells through downregulation of miR-301, which triggers Death effector domain containing 2 (DEDD2) silence, a proapoptotic factor that plays important role in Luteolin's effect on PCa cells [395]. In addition, another mechanism underlying luteonin-induced inhibition of PCa stemness is the suppression of Wnt signaling *via* the upregulation of frizzled class receptor 6 (FZD6), a negative regulator of β-catenin transcriptional activity [396].

Apigenin

Fig. **(16))**

Apigenin.

Apigenin Fig. (16) is one of the most widespread flavonoids in plants and formally belongs to the flavone subclass. Plants of Asteraceae family, such as those of *Artemisia, Achillea, Matricaria*, and *Tanacetum* genera, are the main source of this compound [397].

Apigenin has been shown to suppress cytokine-induced NFkB activation by blocking IKKβ activity [398]. It was demonstrated that apigenin inhibits constitutive and TNFα-induced NFkB activation in PC-3 and 22Rv1 cells. Moreover, apigenin intake by transgenic adenocarcinoma of the mouse prostate (TRAMP) mice inhibited prostatic carcinogenesis and completely blocked tumor metastasis by increasing E-cadherin expression, inhibiting nuclear translocation of β-catenin and decreasing c-myc and cyclin D1 levels [399]. Treatment of CRPC cells (PC-3 and DU145) with apigenin resulted in a significant decrease in Akt phosphorylation in its Serine 473. *In vivo* analyses showed that apigenin compromised tumor cell survival, induced apoptosis [400] and suppressed tumor growth through IGF-IR inactivation and dephosphorylation of Akt in PC-3 xenografts [401].

Wedelia chinensis (WCE) is rich in apigenin and others compounds that act synergistically to suppress AR activity in PCa [402]. Oral administration of WCE significantly inhibited angiogenesis, tumor growth and metastasis in orthotopic PC-3 and DU145 xenografts. In addition, when WCE was combined with docetaxel, docetaxel-induced NFκB signaling was significantly suppressed, boosting the therapeutic effect of this drug with reduced toxicity [403].

Quercetin

Fig. (17))

Quercetin.

Among the various flavonoids present in food and plants, quercetin Fig. (17) is one of the most scientifically explored [404]. Quercetin is found in many foods, plants, vegetables and in their fruit juices. Sources of this compound include apples, berries, broccoli, black tea, green tea, pepper, red wine, tomatoes and especially grapes (*V. vinifera*, Vitaceae) [404-406].

Quercetin was found to reduce cell proliferation and induce apoptosis in various cancer cell lines, such as bladder, breast, colon, and prostate. This compound suppresses tumor growth in PC-3, LNCaP, and DU145 PCa cells. In LNCaP, quercetin elicits G2/M cycle arrest due to p21 upregulation and cyclin B suppression. Studies in PC-3 cells suggested that antitumor activities were caused by decreasing phosphorylation of RTKs, c-Raf, MAPK kinase 1/2 (MEK1/2) and Akt. *In vitro* and *in vivo* studies in prostate xenograft mouse models depicted quercetin's antiangiogenetic effects as it interacts with the VEGF-R2-regulated autophagic pathway (Akt/mTOR/P70S6K) when administered at a dose of 20 mg/kg/day [6, 407].

Quercetin modulates c-Jun and Sp1 pathways, also decreasing AR expression. Tummala and co-authors demonstrated that quercetin antagonizes AR signaling by reducing the expression of hnRNPA1 and, consequently, the expression of AR-V7. In this sense, quercetin was able to restore sensitiveness to enzalutamide treatment in mice bearing enzalutamide-resistant PCa [401. In addition, this flavonoid triggers apoptosis in PCa cell lines through caspase activation, inhibition of fatty acid synthase and downregulation of HSP 90 [408, 409].

Genistein and other Soy Isoflavones

Fig. **(18))**
Genistein.

Genistein Fig. (18) is the most abundant isoflavone compound of soybeans and the suggested active agent underlying the putative anticancer effect of soy. The mechanisms by which genistein inhibits growth are not entirely understood. However, it is becoming clear that genistein exerts multiple effects on prostate tumorigenesis [410].

Previous studies have reported that genistein inhibited angiogenesis, protein tyrosine kinases and topoisomerase II activities, oncogene expression and prostaglandin synthesis [411-413]. According with Basak and co-authors, genistein modulated the HDAC6–HSP90 chaperone function, which has been shown to cause a down-regulation and degradation of the AR in PCa [414]. In addition, genistein treatment increased the expression of the pro-apoptotic protein Bax, activated apoptotic signals and enhanced the response to cabazitaxel treatment in mCRPC cell lines C4-2, ARCaPM and PC-3. In a PC-3-luciferase xenograft model, the combined treatment with genistein and cabazitaxel significantly retarded the growth of mCRPC when compared to vehicle control, cabazitaxel or genistein [415].

Genistein inhibits the proliferation of VCaP CRPC cells by eliciting cell cycle arrest in G2/M phase, decreasing the expression of PSA, Cyclin D1 and PCNA and upregulating p53 [416]. In a PC-3 cell line, genistein led to a significant increase in apoptosis and to cell migration inhibition. At low physiological concentrations (≤10 µM) genistein induced CDKs, and MAPKs activation, while high concentrations (>10 µM) down-regulated TGF-β signaling [417].

Silibinin

Fig. (19))

Silibinin.

Silibinin or silybin Fig. (19) is a flavolignan isolated from the fruits of *Silybum marianum* (Asteraceae). Silibinin has been described as causing G1 cell cycle arrest and decreasing both intracellular and secreted forms of PSA in LNCaP cells, through downregulation of AR coactivators and the epithelium-derived Ets transcription factor (PDEF). This flavolignan also modulates retinoblastoma protein (Rb) levels and its phosphorylation status decreasing CDKs activities [6, 418].

Silibinin was shown to suppress global protein translation that leads to a decreased activity of Hypoxia inducible factor 1 (HIF-1) alpha and telomerase. Furthermore, for being a lipophilic compound, silibinin seems to compete in the EGF-ERBB1 interaction and to modulate the proliferation signaling and DNA synthesis in LNCaP and DU145 cells. Silibinin also restrains Wnt pathway signaling by inhibiting the Wnt co-receptor, LRp6, and induces apoptosis through the inhibition of STAT3 while it sensitizes cells to TNFα-induced apoptosis, through constitutive NFkB inactivation. Previous studies demonstrated that silibinin prevents migratory and invasive potential of PC-3, PC-3MM2, C4-2B LNCaP and DU145 cells. In general, this compound inhibits EMT of PCa cells through inhibition of the NFkB pathway. Such inhibition downregulates the EMT transcription factors ZEB1 and SLUG, and therefore culminates in a decreased expression of Vimentin and MMP2 [6, 419], increased levels of E-cadherin, suppression of Akt phosphorylation at the Ser-473 site and inhibition of β-catenin expression [420]. In CRPC cell lines, silibinin inhibits osteoclastogenesis, reducing the expression of osteomimicry biomarkers (RANKL, Runx2, osteocalcin, and PTHrP) and decreasing the level of several cytokines that promote osteoclastogenesis including IGF-1, TGF-β, TNF-α, HGF, TARC and IL-17 [421].

Baicalin and Baicalein

Fig. (20))

Baicalin **(a)** and Baicalein **(b)**.

Baicalin (**a**) and its aglycone, baicalein (**b**) Fig. ([20](#)) are the major flavonoid constituents in the plants of genus *Scutellaria* (Lamiaceae), including *S. baicalensis* Georgi, *S. lateflora* L., *S. galericulata*, and *S. rivularia* Wall. Both baicalin and baicalein have been found to exhibit several pharmacological activities, including antioxidant, anti-inflammatory, anticancer, anticardiovascular, antidiabetic, hepatoprotective, antiviral, anti-ulcerative, antithrombotic, eye protective and neuroprotective [422, 423].

In vivo, baicalin is converted to baicalein. Baicalin inhibits cell proliferation of various cancer cell lines, including bladder, bone, breast, colon, liver, and prostate. A previous study in LNCaP cells revealed that baicalin increased the expression of CDK inhibitors and caused G1 cell cycle arrest. Similar results were found for baicalein. Baicalin also induced G1 arrest and apoptosis in DU145 cells, through the inhibition of Bcl-2, loss of Bax and upregulation of Fas. In PC-3 cells, baicalein was able to overcome TRAIL resistance by upregulating DR5. Both baicalin and baicalein prevented angiogenesis and reduced tumor volume in xenograft models [6, 423].

In CRPC cells, baicalein inhibits AR dimerization and AR-coactivators interaction [424]. However, cell growth inhibition by baicalin and its metabolite, baicalein, is independent of AR status. In LNCaP cells this compound blocked AR transactivation and AR-mediated PCa cell growth, suppressing AR target genes (PSA, TMPRSS2 and TMEPA1) expression. In both models, androgen-dependent and androgen-independent cells, baicalein causes an apparent accumulation of cells in G1 phase, induced apoptosis at higher concentrations and, in LNCaP cells, decreased expression of the AR [425]. Additionally, baicalein induces apoptosis and controlled metastasis in CRPC cells lines through inhibition of the caveolin-1/Akt/mTOR pathway [426].

Alkaloids and Anthraquinones

Sanguinarine

Fig. (21))
Sanguinarine.

Sanguinarine Fig. (21) is a benzophenanthridine alkaloid derived from the roots of *Sanguinaria canadensis* (Papaveraceae) (known as the bloodroot plant). In LNCaP and DU145 PCa cells, sanguinarine elicits G0/G1 cell cycle arrest in a dose-dependent manner by modulating the expression of p21/WAF1 and p27/KIP1 (cyclin kinase inhibitors), cyclin E, D1, and D2 and CDKs 2, 4, and 6 [427, 428].

Sanguinarine has also been shown to control PCa cells growth and induce apoptosis by suppressing the expression of Survivin and STAT3 proteins. Inactivation of STAT3, by sanguinarine, occurs by inhibiting phosphorylation of JAK2 and c-Src. In DU145 cell xenografts, the administration of sanguinarine reduced tumor weight and volume after 31 days [6, 427].

Emodin

Fig. (22))
Emodin.

Emodin Fig. (22) is an anthraquinone isolated from many plants, including *Rheum palmatum* (Polygonaceae), *Polygonum cuspidatum* (Polygonaceae), *Polygonum multiforum* (Polygonaceae), and *Cassia obtusifolia* (Fabaceae). Emodin exhibits remarkable biological effects, such as anti-inflammatory, antioxidant and preventive of DNA damage and intrahepatic fat accumulation. Emodin can attenuate numerous cancers, including those affecting the nasopharyngeal, gall bladder, lung, colorectal, oral, ovarian, bladder, prostate and breast tissues, mainly through the inhibition of cell proliferation and growth, metastasis, angiogenesis and induction of apoptosis [429].

Emodin could be qualified as endogenous ROS generators because of its property of transferring electrons. Emodin's mechanism of action in inhibiting the development of cancer remains barely elucidated [430]. Against PCa, emodin has been shown to be more potent than the compounds curcumin or genistein. Also, investigators have shown that emodin induces dissociation of the AR from HSP90 and increases its interaction with the E3 ligase MDM2, thus promoting the proteasome-mediated degradation of the AR in LNCaP cells. In this context, emodin inhibits nuclear translocation of the AR and, consequently, hampers its transcriptional activity downregulating AR-targeting genes, including PSA [431].

Importantly, emodin also promoted AR degradation in tumor tissues and suppressed tumor growth in C3(1)/SV40 transgenic mice with no effect on body weight and physical activity [432]. In CRPC cells emodin suppressed NFkB activation, which probably triggers the downregulation of the CSC markers [433].

Other Phenolic and Miscellaneous Compounds

Resveratrol

Fig. (23))
Resveratrol.

Resveratrol Fig. (23) is a plant–derived stilbene phenolic and phytoalexin compound that is produced in response to environmental stress, such as vicissitudes in climate and infection by pathogenic microorganisms. Resveratrol is primarily found in the skin of grapes, as well as in other fruits and plants, such as raspberries, blueberries, mulberries, and knotweed [434].

Resveratrol exerts anticancer activity on PCa cells PC-3, DU145 and LNCaP-FGC, at least in part, through epigenetic mechanisms, including post-translational modification and reactivation of PTEN tumor suppressor. Resveratrol promotes acetylation and reactivation of PTEN *via* inhibition of the metastasis-associated protein 1 (MTA1)/HDAC complex, hampering the Akt pathway. These findings highlight the importance of resveratrol and other MTA1/HDAC inhibitors for PCa chemoprevention and treatment [435].

In LNCaP cells, resveratrol significantly reduced DHT-induced cell viability, inhibiting the EMT process with increased expression of E-cadherin and downregulation of N-cadherin, Vimentin and the AR [436]. In DU145 and LNCaP cells, resveratrol increased expression of the suppressor tumor programmed cell death protein 4 (PDCD4) and of the LncRNA prostate associated transcript (PCAT29), through modulation of IL-6 / STAT3 / miR-21 signaling [437]. In CRPC lineages, different concentrations of resveratrol have been found to hamper the activation of NFkB by impeding the nuclear translocation of its component, p65 [438].

In addition, it was described that resveratrol activates autophagy-mediated cell death in CRPC cells, PC-3 and DU145, through regulation of sore-operated calcium entry (SOCE) mechanisms that involve downregulation of stromal interaction molecule 1 (STIM1) expression and activation of endoplasmic reticulum (ER) stress, by depleting the ER calcium pool [435, 439, 440]. When TRAMP mice were fed with resveratrol, the progression of the lesions was reduced. It was also possible to observe an inhibition of ERK 1 and 2 activation [441].

Honokiol

Fig. (24))

Honokinol.

Honokiol Fig. (24) is a biphenolic natural neolignan compound, found mainly in the bark of *Magnolia officinalis* (Magnoliaceae) and reported to be efficient in preventing several tumors, such as those involving the brain, breast, cervix, colon, liver, lung and prostate [442, 443]. Honokiol is a small molecule with relevant cytotoxicity against a variety of human cancer cells, including PCa. Activation of caspases-3, -8 and -9 and enhanced cleavage of poly (ADP-ribose) polymerase (PARP) is responsible for its cytotoxic effects, through apoptosis induction [405, 443-445].

In LNCaP cells, honokiol downregulated AR expression, suppressed its nuclear translocation and altered the regulatory functions of this receptor in a p53 independent manner. Also, this compound promoted the proteasome-mediated degradation of the AR [446]. Considering the DU145 cell line, honokiol downregulated mRNA levels of FOXM1 and Aurora B kinase, controlling the aggressiveness of CRPC [447].

Curcumin

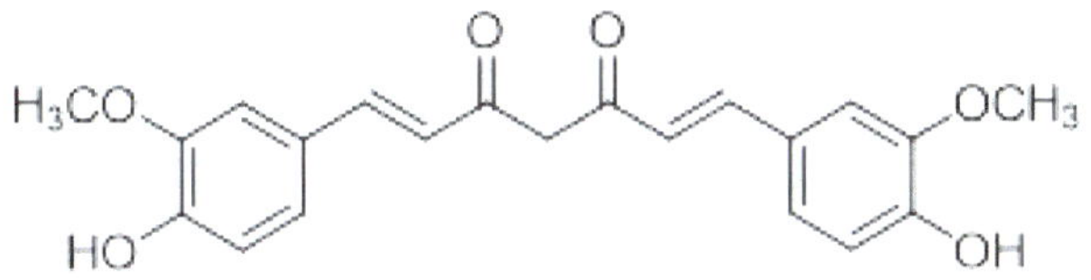

Fig. **(25))**

Curcumin

Curcumin Fig. (25) is a diarylheptanoid natural compound and the most important component of the rhizomes of *Curcuma longa L.* (turmeric) (Zingiberaceae). Curcumin and its derivatives have received immense attention in the past two decades due to their pharmacological properties, such as anti-tumor, antioxidant, and anti-inflammatory activities [448]. After treatment of LNCaP cells with curcumin, the TGF-β, Wnt, NFkB, and PI3K/Akt/mTOR signaling pathways were downregulated [449]. AR expression was also suppressed, followed by inhibition of β-catenin expression, repression of Akt and GSK-3β phosphorylation and degradation of cyclin D1 and c-myc [450].

Curcumins is described to inhibit the growth of mCRPC. In PC-3 cells, curcumin shows its anti-cancer effects by inducing apoptosis and eliciting G2/M cell cycle arrest [451]. The mechanism relies on the upregulation of p21 and suppression of TNF-α-mediated NFkB pathway [452].

Capsaicin and Derivatives

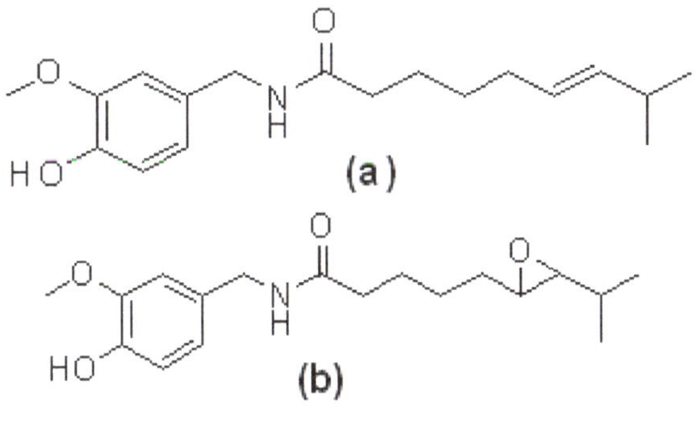

Fig. **(26))**

Capsaicin **(a)** capsaicin epoxide **(b)**.

Capsaicin (Fig. 26a) is a natural pungent amide constituent of hot chili peppers (*Capsicum frutescence L.*) or hot red peppers (*Capsicum annum L.*). The anticancer effects of capsaicin are partly mediated through the inhibition of cancer cell proliferation. In LNCaP cells capsaicin was shown to exert a dual effect, while it induces AR expression and proliferation at lower doses, it triggers apoptosis and hampers AR expression at 200 µM [432, 453, 454]. In these cases, the compound inhibited the AR-mediated expression of PSA and increased p53, p21 and Bax [432].

Experiments in CRPC cells, DU145 and PC-3, previously demonstrated that capsaicin downregulated the expression of CD133, CD44, ALDH1A1, OCT-4, Nanog and Sox-2. PC-3 and DU145 tumorspheres were also treated with the compound, which downregulated Wnt/β-catenin pathway and leads to c-myc and cyclin D1 expression suppression [455]. In another study, capsaicin inhibited TNF-α degradation of IkBa in the cytoplasm, blocking the nuclear translocation and, hence, the transcriptional activities of NFkB [453].

Regarding its derivatives, the growth-inhibitory activity of capsaicin epoxide Fig. (26b) was found to be better than capsaicin in PCa, breast cancer, cervical cancer and renal cancer cell lines [456]. The human breast cancer cell line, MCF-7, was found to be the most responsive to capsaicin epoxide-induced cell death. Capsaicin epoxide was shown to trigger robust apoptosis in these cell lines by inducing oxidative stress [457].

Wedelolactone

Fig. (27))
Wedelolactone.

Wedelolactone Fig. (27) is a coumestane-type and plant-derived natural compound found in species of the Asteraceae family. A major source of wedelolactone are plants of the genus *Eclipta* sp. Wedelolactone inhibits breast cancer-induced osteoclastogenesis by inhibiting the Akt/mTOR signaling while in PCa cells it has been shown to induce caspase-dependent apoptosis [458, 459] through a novel mechanism involving inhibition of protein kinase Cε (PKCε) but without suppressing Akt. These results suggest that wedelolactone should be further tested as a novel candidate for PCa treatment [460].

(-)-Epigallocatechin- 3-Gallate and other Polyphenols Form Green Tea

Fig. (28))

Epigallocatechin 3-gallate.

Epigallocatechin-3-gallate (EGCG) Fig. (28) is a catechin derived natural compound found mainly in green tea (*Camellia sinensis*, Theaceae). Among the four major types of catechins derived from the tea, (EGCG, epigallocatechin, epicatechin-3-gallate and epicatechin), EGCG is recognized as the most potent catechin that inhibits carcinogenesis. This compound can specifically control the growth of LNCaP cells and reduce androgen actions. In LNCaP and DU145 cells, EGCG elicited G0/G1 cell cycle arrest regardless of the p53 status of the cells [6, 461]. EGCG markedly suppresses the expression of Vimentin through inhibition of Akt in PC-3 cells [462]. In DU145 cells, apoptosis was activated by lyophilized EGCG though increased levels of Bax / Bcl-2 ratio, cytochrome c release and caspase cleavage [463]. Finally, chitosan nanoparticles encapsulating EGCG inhibited tumor growth in mice models and decreased PSA levels [6, 461, 464].

Gossypol

Fig. (29))

Gossypol.

Gossypol Fig. (29) is a polyphenolic aldehyde present in cottonseed (*Gossypium hirsutum*, Malvaceae), which has been shown to exert antiproliferative and cytotoxic effects in PCa cell lines [465]. This compound has demonstrated antitumor effects through induction of G0/G1 cell cycle arrest and autophagy in CRPC cells with high levels of Bcl-2 [466]. Gossypol also controls tumor aggressiveness, suppressing migration, invasion and angiogenesis. In PC-3 cells, this compound inhibited NFkB pathway, hampering the secretion of the urokinase plasminogen activator and VEGF, even in PC-3 xenografts. In these experiments, gossypol caused the subsequent suppression of phosphorylation of focal adhesion kinase, Akt, and key intracellular proangiogenic kinases such as those belonging to the Src family [6, 467]. Finally, nanoparticles of (-) - gossypol loaded with mPEG-Mal demonstrated favorable antitumor activity and no toxicity. The ability of these nanoparticles to induce apoptosis of PCa cells highlights its potential use as anticancer nanodrug [468].

Phenethyl-Isothiocyanate

$$\text{N=C=S}$$

Fig.   **(30))**
Phenethyl-isothiocyanate.

Phenethyl-isothiocyanate (PEITC) Fig. (30) is one of the most extensively studied isothiocyanates that is found in cruciferous vegetables, such as broccoli (*Brassica oleracea*) and watercress (*Nasturtium officinale*) of the *Brassicaceae* family. In DU145 cells, PEITC (1–20 μM) suppressed cell proliferation and elicited cell cycle arrest in the G2/M phase, inducing apoptosis in a dose-dependent manner. The mechanism of PEITC action suggests that it increases p53 expression, while it reduces the expression of cell division cycle 25C (CDC25C), blocks the JAK-STAT3 signal cascade and modulates the activation of the caspase's pathway [469]. PEITC has also been described to suppress the expression of α- and β-tubulin proteins in LNCaP, DU145, PC-3 and C4-2B cells through ROS generation and protein degradation. In addition, PEITC downregulated AR expression by inhibiting Sp1-mediated transcription, thus promoting growth arrest both in androgen-dependent and CRPC cells. It is noteworthy that PEITC triggers both apoptotic and autophagic cell death in PC-3 and LNCaP cells through the Atg5 protein. Exposure of LNCaP and 22Rv1 (CRPC cell line) to PEITC resulted in the suppression of expression and transcriptional activity of c-myc. Furthermore, PEITC was shown to restrain migration of PC-3 and LNCaP cells by inactivating Akt with a subsequent suppression of VEGF [470].

In an LNCaP xenograft model, PEITC controlled tumor growth by downregulating the expression of the platelet/endothelial cell adhesion molecule (PECAM1-CD31) and by suppressing angiogenesis. When mice bearing PCa xenografts were fed with 3 μmol PEITC/g for 19 weeks it was possible to observe an inhibition in tumor growth rates, which was accompanied by a restoration of E-cadherin expression and autophagy-regulated pathways [469].

Ellagic Acid

Fig. (31))
Ellagic acid.

Ellagic acid Fig. (31) (EA) is a polyphenolic compound found in various plants and fruits, including blackberries (*Rubus sp.*, Rosaceae), cranberries (*Vaccinium sp.*, Ericaceae) and pomegranates. In LNCaP cells, EA causes DNA damage and leads to a cooccurring downregulation of antiapoptotic proteins (such as silent information regulator 1-SIRT1), upregulation of p21 and modulation of the expression of AIF, resulting in ROS-mediated and caspase-mediated apoptosis [471]. The antiangiogenetic effects of EA were reported in LNCaP cells. In CRPC cells, DU145 and PC-3, EA elicits cell cycle arrest in the S phase and induces apoptosis through caspase-dependent pathways, which was associated with decreased levels of cyclin B1 and cyclin D1. Finally, EA controls the invasive potential of PC-3 by decreasing the secretion of MMP-2 [6, 472].

Thymoquinone

Fig. (32))
Thymoquinone.

Thymoquinone Fig. (32) is a natural quinone found mainly in *Nigella sativa* (Ranunculaceae). This compound reduces cell growth both in androgen-dependent (LNCaP, C4-B) and CRPC (DU145, PC-3) PCa cell lines.

Biological effects are associated with downregulation of the AR, E2F-1 and E2F-1 expression. In PC-3 and C4-B cells, thymoquinone induces apoptosis through an increase in ROS generation and decreased GSH levels. In PC-3 thymoquinone also inhibits cell proliferation by suppressing the Akt pathway and prevents tumor angiogenesis by repressing VEGF [6].

In addition, when thymoquinone was combined with Docetaxel, the PI3K / Akt pathway was inhibited and an increased expression of pro-apoptotic markers (BAX, BID, caspase-3) and a downregulation of the Bcl-2 family was detected [473]. Thymoquinone also suppressed the phosphorylation of NFkB and IKKα / β, reducing metastasis [474].

Atraric Acid

Fig. (33))
Atraric acid.

Atraric acid (AA) Fig. (33), a natural benzoic acid derivative, occurs in lichens and has also been isolated from higher plants, like *Newbouldia laevis* (Bignoniaceae), *Alseodaphne andersonii* (Lauraceae) and *Frullania brasiliensis* (Frullaniaceae) [475]. *In vitro* studies have shown that AA presents antiandrogenic activity, controlling PCa cells proliferation when they express the AR, suggesting an AR-dependent growth inhibitory mechanism. In this sense, AA represses the androgen AR-mediated transactivation by about 90% when this compound is used at higher concentrations. Additionally, AA inhibits the cellular invasion of PCa, suggesting its important role in control aggressiveness. Finally, AA leads to senescence associated with beta-galactosidase activity. Therefore, the ability of AA to suppress the AR and decrease PCa cells proliferation can be potentially employed in the chemoprevention and chemotherapy [476].

Diindolylmethane

Fig. (34))
Diindolylmethane.

The diindolylmethane Fig. (**34**), is a dimeric product of indole-3-carbinol, which is mainly found from naturally occurring glucosinolates that exist in vegetables, including members of the family Cruciferae, and particularly members of the genus *Brassica* [477]. Anticancer bisindole derivatives of diindolylmethane have been developed by different research groups. Diindolylmethane was reported as a strong mitochondrial Hþ-aTPase inhibitor and stimulated mitochondrial ROS production [478]. Also, diindolylmethane blocks multiple pro-oncogenic molecular pathways in tumors derived from different organs and tissues. In PCa, diindolylmethane inhibits tumor growth in TRAMP mice through inhibition of CDK and induction of p27 and Bax expression. A formulated compound of diindolylmethane, with greater bioavailability (B-DIM), suppressed critical survival signaling pathways and enhanced the efficacy of radiation treatment in a murine PCa xenograft model [479].

Sulforaphane

Fig. (35))

Sulforaphane.

Sulforaphane Fig. (**35**) is a natural isothiocyanate found in many cruciferous vegetables, first isolated from broccoli (*Brassica oleracea*, Brassicaceae). Sulforaphane elicits cell cycle arrest and apoptosis in androgen-dependent and CRPC PCa cell lines. The antiproliferative effects of SFN involve modulation of methyltransferase expression, which inhibited phosphorylation of mTOR substrates in PC-3 cells [6, 480]. Sulforaphane also decreases the transcription-mediated by NFkB, the expression of cyclin D2, and upregulates Nrf2. Additionally, the sulforaphane - induction of the ubiquitination and proteasome activity observed in CRPC 22Rv1 cells, led to an enhancement of AR degradation and hence, to a reduction in AR functions [481].

CONCLUDING REMARKS

PCa depends on androgen for growth and progression and, accordingly, ADT is effective for the treatment of non-metastatic lesions. However, tumors evolve to a resistant phenotype and keep the AR axis continually activated. In this state patients are more likely to die since current treatments are no longer effective. We presented promising bioactive NPs and their respective mechanisms of action, principally focusing on AR signaling and its interaction with other signaling pathways. Indeed, NPs interfere in different cancer hallmarks without eliciting severe side effects. Therefore, the use of NPs in combination with other current therapies can potentially offer greater anti-tumor efficacy, especially if we consider that the complexity of CRPC pathways demands a broad-spectrum clinical approach Fig. (36). Despite AR antagonists, different NPs act at the nuclear level, inhibiting AR transcriptional activity such as Lupeol, AA, GRA, Physachenolide D, Luteolin, Genistein, Emodin, and EGCG. These NPs can be effective for CRPC control, especially in combined therapies with synergistic effects. Furthermore, NPs also trigger AR-independent mechanisms such as upregulation of apoptosis, reactivation of PTEN (Resveratrol) and modulation of EMT (Apigenin, Silibinin, Resveratrol, and PEITC).

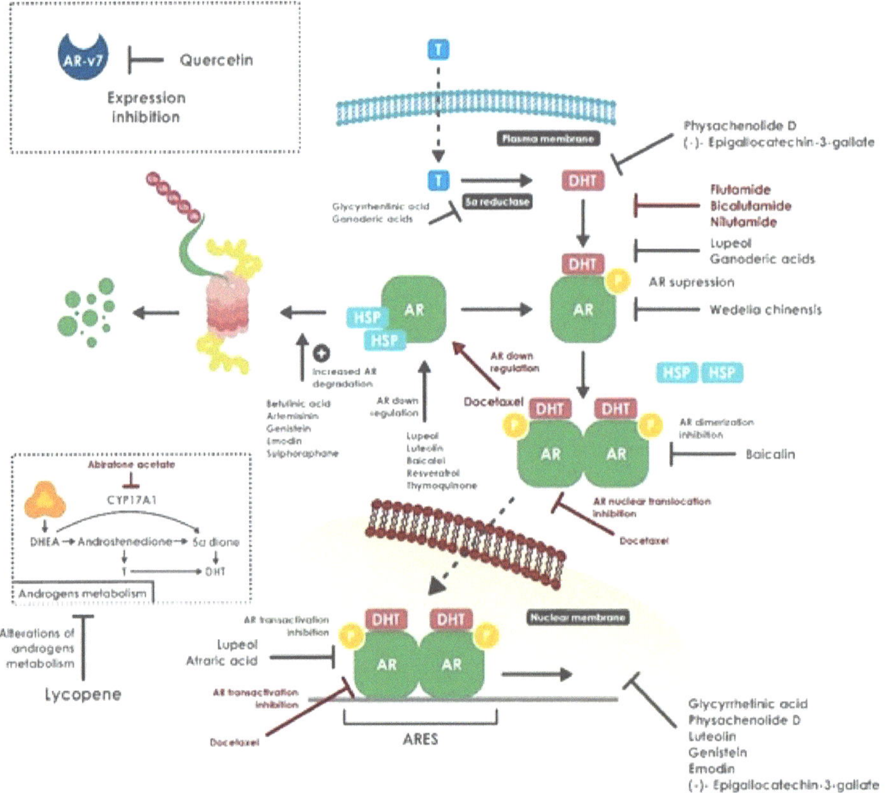

Fig.   **(36))**

Scheme showing both conventional drugs and Natural Products (NPs) acting on androgen metabolism, and Androgen Receptor (AR) activation / signaling pathway. The image shows drugs and NPs that act inhibiting (—|) the conversion of testosterone (T) to Dihydrotestosterone (DHT), inhibiting DHT action and / or inhibiting AR activation, either by blocking the AR binding to

DHT or by suppressing AR dimerization. The image also shows drugs and NPs that downregulate AR expression or that promote (+) the AR degradation through the ubiquitin-proteasome pathway. In addition, drugs and NPs that inhibit the transactivation of the AR and that therefore control the transcription of AR–responsive genes (AREs), such as Prostate-Specific Antigen (PSA), are shown. In dotted upper box Quercetin is depicted as specific inhibitor of AR variant 7 (AR-V7) expression. In dotted bottom box it is represented the androgen metabolic pathway that starts from the production of dehydroepiandrosterone (DHEA) from adrenal glands. Regarding this pathway, Lycopene has been indicated as a general inhibitor of androgen metabolism while the conventional drug, Abiratone acetate, is a specific inhibitor of the cytochrome P450 family 17 subfamily A member 1 (CYP17A1) that converts DHEA into DHT without the need of passing through the step of production of T. HSP: heat shock proteins; Ub: ubiquitin.

Coordinated actions are needed to unravel the molecular mechanisms that are still obscure in CRPC. A better understanding of the pathways that lead to aberrant AR activation may contribute to the development of novel inhibitors. All new knowledge is crucial for the development of strategies to prevent and control this aggressive disease. In this context, therapeutic compounds, including NPs, may be effectively contributing to overcome the therapeutic challenges of CRPC. However, further modifications, including nanoformulations, and *in vivo* studies should be performed in order to clarify whether these NPs can exert their effects in physiologic concentrations alone or need to be combined with conventional therapies.

CONSENT FOR PUBLICATION

Not applicable.

CONFLICT OF INTEREST

The authors declare no conflict of interest, financial or otherwise.

ACKNOWLEDGEMENTS

Declared none.

REFERENCES

[1]   Rawla P. Epidemiology of Prostate Cancer. World J Oncol 2019; 10(2): 63-89.[http://dx.doi.org/10.14740/wjon1191] [PMID: 31068988]

[2]   Bray F, Ferlay J, Soerjomataram I, Siegel RL, Torre LA, Jemal A. Global cancer statistics 2018: GLOBOCAN estimates of incidence and mortality worldwide for 36 cancers in 185 countries. CA Cancer J Clin 2018; 68(6): 394-424.[http://dx.doi.org/10.3322/caac.21492] [PMID: 30207593]

[3]   Kallifatidis G, Hoy JJ, Lokeshwar BL. Bioactive natural products for chemoprevention and treatment of castration-resistant prostate cancer. Semin Cancer Biol 2016; 40-41: 160-9.[http://dx.doi.org/10.1016/j.semcancer.2016.06.003] [PMID: 27370570]

[4]   Steele CB, Li J, Huang B, Weir HK. Prostate cancer survival in the United States by race and stage (2001-2009): Findings from the CONCORD-2 study. Cancer 2017; 123 (Suppl. 24): 5160-77.[http://dx.doi.org/10.1002/cncr.31026] [PMID: 29205313]

[5]   Dai C, Heemers H, Sharifi N. Androgen Signaling in Prostate Cancer. Cold Spring Harb Perspect Med 2017; 7(9): 7.[http://dx.doi.org/10.1101/cshperspect.a030452] [PMID: 28389515]

[6]   Gioti K, Tenta R. Bioactive natural products against prostate cancer: mechanism of action and autophagic/apoptotic molecular pathways. Planta Med 2015; 81(7): 543-62.[http://dx.doi.org/10.1055/s-0035-1545845] [PMID: 25875508]

[7]   Liu VWS, Yau WL, Tam CW, Yao KM, Shiu SYW. Melatonin inhibits androgen receptor splice variant-7 (ar-v7)-induced nuclear factor-kappa B (NF-κB) activation and NF-κB activator-induced AR-V7 expression in prostate cancer cells: potential implications for the use of melatonin in castration-resistant prostate cancer (CRPC) therapy. Int J Mol Sci 2017; 18(6): 18.[http://dx.doi.org/10.3390/ijms18061130] [PMID: 28561752]

[8]   Redzović A, Dintinjana RD, Nacinović AD. R. DOBRILA DINTINJANA, A. DULETIĆ NAČINOVIĆ, Indicators of cellular and developmental disorders in multiple primary cancers. Coll Antropol 2016; 40(1): 59-62.[PMID: 27301239]

[9]   Hanahan D, Weinberg RA. Hallmarks of cancer: the next generation cell 2011; 1442011: 646-74.

[10]   Hagan I, Sharrocks AD. Understanding cancer: from the gene to the organism. Conference on genes and cancer. EMBO Rep 2002; 3(5): 415-9.[http://dx.doi.org/10.1093/embo-reports/kvf100] [PMID: 11991945]

[11]   Menyhárt O, Harami-Papp H, Sukumar S, *et al.* Guidelines for the selection of functional assays to evaluate the hallmarks of cancer. Biochim Biophys Acta 2016; 1866(2): 300-19.[PMID: 27742530]

[12]   Massagué J, Obenauf AC. Metastatic colonization by circulating tumour cells. Nature 2016; 529(7586): 298-306.[http://dx.doi.org/10.1038/nature17038] [PMID: 26791720]

[13]   Zeeshan R, Mutahir Z. Cancer metastasis - tricks of the trade. Bosn J Basic Med Sci 2017; 17(3): 172-82.[PMID: 28278128]

[14]   Seyfried TN, Huysentruyt LC. On the origin of cancer metastasis. Crit Rev Oncog 2013; 18(1-2): 43-73.[http://dx.doi.org/10.1615/CritRevOncog.v18.i1-2.40] [PMID: 23237552]

[15]   Steeg PS. Targeting metastasis. Nat Rev Cancer 2016; 16(4): 201-18.[http://dx.doi.org/10.1038/nrc.2016.25] [PMID: 27009393]

[16]   Liu Q, Zhang H, Jiang X, Qian C, Liu Z, Luo D. Factors involved in cancer metastasis: a better understanding to "seed and soil" hypothesis. Mol Cancer 2017; 16(1): 176.[http://dx.doi.org/10.1186/s12943-017-0742-4] [PMID: 29197379]

[17]   Siegel RL, Miller KD, Jemal A. Cancer statistics, 2019. CA Cancer J Clin 2019; 69(1): 7-34.[http://dx.doi.org/10.3322/caac.21551] [PMID: 30620402]

[18]   Kotecha R, Takami A, Espinoza JL. Dietary phytochemicals and cancer chemoprevention: a review of the clinical evidence. Oncotarget 2016; 7(32): 52517-29.[http://dx.doi.org/10.18632/oncotarget.9593] [PMID: 27232756]

[19]   I.N.D.C. INCA2020.

[20]   Salari K, Kuppermann D, Preston MA, *et al.* Active surveillance of prostate cancer is a viable option for men younger than 60 years. J Urol 2019; 201(4): 721-7.[http://dx.doi.org/10.1097/JU.0000000000000031] [PMID: 30664083]

[21]   Steffen RE, Trajman A, Santos M, Caetano R. Rastreamento populacional para o câncer de próstata: mais riscos que benefícios. Physis 2018; 28e280209[http://dx.doi.org/10.1590/s0103-73312018280209]

[22]   Mimeault M, Batra SK. Frequent gene products and molecular pathways altered in prostate cancer- and metastasis-initiating cells and their progenies and novel promising multitargeted therapies. Mol Med 2011; 17(9-10): 949-64.[http://dx.doi.org/10.2119/molmed.2011.00115] [PMID: 21607288]

[23]   Vilamaior PS, Taboga SR, Carvalho HF. Postnatal growth of the ventral prostate in Wistar rats: a stereological and morphometrical study, The Anatomical Record Part A: Discoveries in Molecular, Cellular,

and Evolutionary Biology. An Official Publication of the American Association of Anatomists 2006; 288: 885-92.

[24] Taboga SR, Vilamaior PSL, Góes RM. Modulação androgênica e estrogênica na próstata: uma abordagem em modelos experimentais de roedores com enfoque na biologia cstrutural. Arq Bras Endocrinol Metabol 2009; 53(8): 946-55.[http://dx.doi.org/10.1590/S0004-27302009000800007] [PMID: 20126846]

[25] Yacoub JH, Oto A. MR imaging of prostate zonal anatomy. Radiol Clin North Am 2018; 56(2): 197-209.[http://dx.doi.org/10.1016/j.rcl.2017.10.003] [PMID: 29420976]

[26] Bianchi-Frias D, Damodarasamy M, Hernandez SA, *et al.* The aged microenvironment influences the tumorigenic potential of malignant prostate epithelial cells. Mol Cancer Res 2019; 17(1): 321-31.[http://dx.doi.org/10.1158/1541-7786.MCR-18-0522] [PMID: 30224545]

[27] Walz J, Epstein JI, Ganzer R, *et al.* A critical analysis of the current knowledge of surgical anatomy of the prostate related to optimisation of cancer control and preservation of continence and erection in candidates for radical prostatectomy: an update. Eur Urol 2016; 70(2): 301-11.[http://dx.doi.org/10.1016/j.eururo.2016.01.026] [PMID: 26850969]

[28] Rassweiler J, Laguna P, Chlosta P, *et al.* ESUT expert group on laparoscopy proposes uniform terminology during radical prostatectomy: we need to speak the same language. Eur Urol 2013; 64(1): 97-100.[http://dx.doi.org/10.1016/j.eururo.2013.01.014] [PMID: 23357350]

[29] Henry GH, Malewska A, Joseph DB, *et al.* A cellular anatomy of the normal adult human prostate and prostatic urethra Cell reports 2018; 252018: 3530-42.e3535

[30] Padgett KR, Swallen A, Pirozzi S, *et al.* Towards a universal MRI atlas of the prostate and prostate zones : Comparison of MRI vendor and image acquisition parameters. Strahlenther Onkol 2019; 195(2): 121-30.[http://dx.doi.org/10.1007/s00066-018-1348-5] [PMID: 30140944]

[31] Packer JR, Maitland NJ. The molecular and cellular origin of human prostate cancer. Biochim Biophys Acta 2016; 1863(6 Pt A): 1238-60.[http://dx.doi.org/10.1016/j.bbamcr.2016.02.016] [PMID: 26921821]

[32] Charas T, Vargas A, Zelefsky MJ. Imaging and Anatomic Considerations for Prostate and Pelvic Organs Contouring.Stereotactic Radiosurgery for Prostate Cancer 201955-73.[http://dx.doi.org/10.1007/978-3-319-92453-3_4]

[33] Alanazi AB, Alshalan AM, Alanazi OA, *et al.* Epidemiology of senile prostatic enlargement among elderly men in Arar, Kingdom of Saudi Arabia. Electron Physician 2017; 9(9): 5349-53.[http://dx.doi.org/10.19082/5349] [PMID: 29038720]

[34] Lu ZH, Ji LB, Zhao WL, *et al.* Differentiating Transition Zone Cancers From Benign Prostatic Hyperplasia by Histogram Analysis of Apparent Diffusion Coefficient Maps With Standard and Ultrahigh b-value Diffusion-weighted MR Imaging. J Comput Assist Tomogr 2019; 43(2): 235-41.[http://dx.doi.org/10.1097/RCT.0000000000000829] [PMID: 30475249]

[35] Lepor H. Focal Ablation of Prostate Cancer. Rev Urol 2018; 20(2): 107-11.[PMID: 30288150]

[36] Novara G, Galfano A, Berto RB, Ficarra V, Navarrete RV, Artibani W. Inflammation, apoptosis, and BPH: what is the evidence?, european urology supplements, 2006; 5(2006): 401-9.

[37] Shoji S, Hashimoto A, Nakamura T, *et al.* Novel application of three-dimensional shear wave elastography in the detection of clinically significant prostate cancer. Biomed Rep 2018; 8(4): 373-7.[http://dx.doi.org/10.3892/br.2018.1059] [PMID: 29541458]

[38] Chistiakov DA, Myasoedova VA, Grechko AV, Melnichenko AA, Orekhov AN. New biomarkers for diagnosis and prognosis of localized prostate cancer.Seminars in cancer biology 20189-16.[http://dx.doi.org/10.1016/j.semcancer.2018.01.012]

[39] Arora K, Barbieri CE. Molecular subtypes of prostate cancer. Curr Oncol Rep 2018; 20(8): 58.[http://dx.doi.org/10.1007/s11912-018-0707-9] [PMID: 29858674]

[40] Houlahan KE, Salmasi A, Sadun TY, *et al.* Molecular hallmarks of multiparametric magnetic resonance imaging visibility in prostate cancer. Eur Urol 2019; 76(1): 18-23.[http://dx.doi.org/10.1016/j.eururo.2018.12.036] [PMID: 30685078]

[41] Salumbides BC, Meyering SS. Changes in the Epigenetic Landscape of Prostate Cancer.Epigenetic Mechanisms in Cancer 201859-85.[http://dx.doi.org/10.1016/B978-0-12-809552-2.00003-6]

[42] Ozen M, Creighton CJ, Ozdemir M, Ittmann M. Widespread deregulation of microRNA expression in human prostate cancer. Oncogene 2008; 27(12): 1788-93.[http://dx.doi.org/10.1038/sj.onc.1210809] [PMID: 17891175]

[43] Stamey TA, McNeal JE, Yemoto CM, Sigal BM, Johnstone IM. Biological determinants of cancer progression in men with prostate cancer. JAMA 1999; 281(15): 1395-400.[http://dx.doi.org/10.1001/jama.281.15.1395] [PMID: 10217055]

[44] Damber JE, Aus G. Prostate cancer. Lancet 2008; 371(9625): 1710-21.[http://dx.doi.org/10.1016/S0140-6736(08)60729-1] [PMID: 18486743]

[45] Hoang DT, Iczkowski KA, Kilari D, See W, Nevalainen MT. Androgen receptor-dependent and -independent mechanisms driving prostate cancer progression: Opportunities for therapeutic targeting from multiple angles. Oncotarget 2017; 8(2): 3724-45.[http://dx.doi.org/10.18632/oncotarget.12554] [PMID: 27741508]

[46] Wang G, Zhao D, Spring DJ, DePinho RA. Genetics and biology of prostate cancer. Genes Dev 2018; 32(17-18): 1105-40.[http://dx.doi.org/10.1101/gad.315739.118] [PMID: 30181359]

[47] Zadra G, Photopoulos C, Loda M. The fat side of prostate cancer. Biochim Biophys Acta 2013; 1831(10): 1518-32.[http://dx.doi.org/10.1016/j.bbalip.2013.03.010] [PMID: 23562839]

[48] Aaron L, Franco OE, Hayward SW. Review of prostate anatomy and embryology and the etiology of benign prostatic hyperplasia. Urol Clin North Am 2016; 43(3): 279-88.[http://dx.doi.org/10.1016/j.ucl.2016.04.012] [PMID: 27476121]

[49] Bashir MN. Epidemiology of Prostate Cancer, Asian Pacific journal of cancer prevention. Asian Pac J Cancer Prev 2015; 16(13): 5137-41.[http://dx.doi.org/10.7314/APJCP.2015.16.13.5137] [PMID: 26225642]

[50] Rebbeck TR. Prostate cancer genetics: variation by race, ethnicity, and geography.Seminars in radiation oncology 20173-10.[http://dx.doi.org/10.1016/j.semradonc.2016.08.002]

[51] Robinson BD, Mosquera JM, Ro JY, Divatia M. Precision molecular pathology of prostate cancer 2018.[http://dx.doi.org/10.1007/978-3-319-64096-9]

[52] Ilic D, Djulbegovic M, Jung JH, et al. Prostate cancer screening with prostate-specific antigen (PSA) test: a systematic review and meta-analysis bmj 2018; 362(2018) k3519

[53] Epstein JI, Zelefsky MJ, Sjoberg DD, et al. A contemporary prostate cancer grading system: a validated alternative to the Gleason score. Eur Urol 2016; 69(3): 428-35.[http://dx.doi.org/10.1016/j.eururo.2015.06.046] [PMID: 26166626]

[54] Grönberg H, Isaacs SD, Smith JR, et al. Characteristics of prostate cancer in families potentially linked to the hereditary prostate cancer 1 (HPC1) locus. JAMA 1997; 278(15): 1251-5.[http://dx.doi.org/10.1001/jama.1997.03550150055035] [PMID: 9333266]

[55] Goulart AE. Impactos do silenciamento do RNA não codificante PCA3 em células de câncer de próstata 2014.

[56] Manguoğlu E, Güran S, Yamaç D, et al. Germline mutations of BRCA1 and BRCA2 genes in Turkish breast, ovarian, and prostate cancer patients. Cancer Genet Cytogenet 2010; 203(2): 230-7.[http://dx.doi.org/10.1016/j.cancergencyto.2010.07.125] [PMID: 21156238]

[57] Rivas C, Matheson L, Nayoan J, et al. Ethnicity and the prostate cancer experience: a qualitative metasynthesis. Psychooncology 2016; 25(10): 1147-56.[http://dx.doi.org/10.1002/pon.4222] [PMID: 27416079]

[58] Lima LR, da Silva ILC, Alves DC. Revista interdisciplinar ciências e saúde-rics. 2018; 4(2018).

[59] Perdana NR, Mochtar CA, Umbas R, Hamid AR. The risk factors of prostate cancer and its prevention: a literature review. Acta Med Indones 2016; 48(3): 228-38.[PMID: 27840359]

[60] Kinlock BL, Parker LJ, Bowie JV, Howard DL, LaVeist TA, Thorpe RJ, Jr. High levels of medical mistrust are associated with low quality of life among black and white men with prostate cancer. SAGE Publications Sage 2017.

[61] Wang Y, Cui R, Xiao Y, Fang J, Xu Q. Correction: effect of carotene and lycopene on the risk of prostate cancer: a systematic review and dose-response meta-analysis of observational studies. PLoS One 2015; 10(10)e0140415[http://dx.doi.org/10.1371/journal.pone.0140415] [PMID: 26448461]

[62] Robertson CN. Prostate cancer treatment options for men with significant urinary symptoms and enlarged prostates. Prostate Cancer 201875-80.[http://dx.doi.org/10.1007/978-3-319-78646-9_6]

[63] Galvão DA, Taaffe DR, Spry N, et al. Exercise preserves physical function in prostate cancer patients with bone metastases. Med Sci Sports Exerc 2018; 50(3): 393-9.[http://dx.doi.org/10.1249/MSS.0000000000001454] [PMID: 29036016]

[64] Liau J, Goldberg D, Arif-Tiwari H. Prostate Cancer Detection and Diagnosis: Role of Ultrasound with MRI Correlates. Curr Radiol Rep 2019; 7: 7.[http://dx.doi.org/10.1007/s40134-019-0318-8]

[65] Kirby R. The role of PSA in detection and management of prostate cancer. Practitioner 2016; 260(1792): 17-21, 3.[PMID: 27337755]

[66] Tonon TCA, Schoffen JPF. < b> Câncer de Próstata: Uma Revisão da Literatura. Saúde Pesqui 20092.

[67] Gomes R, Rebello LEFS, de Araújo FC, do Nascimento EF. A prevenção do câncer de próstata: uma revisão da literatura. Cien Saude Colet 2008; 13(1): 235-46.[http://dx.doi.org/10.1590/S1413-81232008000100027]

[PMID: 18813537]

[68]   Yacoub JH, Oto A. MR Imaging of Prostate Zonal Anatomy. Radiol Clin North Am 2018; 56(2): 197-209.[http://dx.doi.org/10.1016/j.rcl.2017.10.003] [PMID: 29420976]

[69]   Brierley JD, Gospodarowicz MK, Wittekind C. TNM classification of malignant tumours 2017.

[70]   Leidinger P, Hart M, Backes C, *et al.* Differential blood-based diagnosis between benign prostatic hyperplasia and prostate cancer: miRNA as source for biomarkers independent of PSA level, Gleason score, or TNM status. Tumour Biol 2016; 37(8): 10177-85.[http://dx.doi.org/10.1007/s13277-016-4883-7] [PMID: 26831660]

[71]   Stark JR, Perner S, Stampfer MJ, *et al.* Gleason score and lethal prostate cancer: does 3 + 4 = 4 + 3? J Clin Oncol 2009; 27(21): 3459-64.[http://dx.doi.org/10.1200/JCO.2008.20.4669] [PMID: 19433685]

[72]   Epstein JI, Allsbrook WC, Jr, Amin MB, Egevad LL, Committee IG. The 2005 International Society of Urological Pathology (ISUP) consensus conference on Gleason grading of prostatic carcinoma. Am J Surg Pathol 2005; 29(9): 1228-42.[http://dx.doi.org/10.1097/01.pas.0000173646.99337.b1] [PMID: 16096414]

[73]   Gleason DF. Classification of prostatic carcinomas. Cancer Chemother Rep 1966; 50(3): 125-8.[PMID: 5948714]

[74]   Gleason D. Histological grading and clinical staging of prostatic carcinoma, Urologic pathology. Prostate 1977171.

[75]   Gleason DF. Histologic grading of prostate cancer: a perspective. Hum Pathol 1992; 23(3): 273-9.[http://dx.doi.org/10.1016/0046-8177(92)90108-F] [PMID: 1555838]

[76]   Marshall CH, Fu W, Wang H, Baras AS, Lotan TL, Antonarakis ES. Prevalence of DNA repair gene mutations in localized prostate cancer according to clinical and pathologic features: association of Gleason score and tumor stage. Prostate Cancer Prostatic Dis 2019; 22(1): 59-65.[http://dx.doi.org/10.1038/s41391-018-0086-1] [PMID: 30171229]

[77]   Johnston WL, Catton CN, Swallow CJ. Unbiased data mining identifies cell cycle transcripts that predict non-indolent Gleason score 7 prostate cancer. BMC Urol 2019; 19(1): 4.[http://dx.doi.org/10.1186/s12894-018-0433-5] [PMID: 30616540]

[78]   Hassan O, Han M, Zhou A, *et al.* Incidence of extraprostatic extension at radical prostatectomy with pure Gleason score 3+ 3= 6 (grade group 1) cancer: implications for whether Gleason score 6 prostate cancer should be renamed" not cancer" and for selection criteria for active surveillance. J Urol 2018; 199(6): 1482-7.[http://dx.doi.org/10.1016/j.juro.2017.11.067] [PMID: 29154905]

[79]   Egevad L, Delahunt B, Srigley JR, Samaratunga H. International Society of Urological Pathology (ISUP) grading of prostate cancer - An ISUP consensus on contemporary grading. APMIS 2016; 124(6): 433-5.[http://dx.doi.org/10.1111/apm.12533] [PMID: 27150257]

[80]   Bloom JB, Hale GR, Gold SA, *et al.* Predicting Gleason group progression for men on prostate cancer active surveillance: Role of a negative confirmatory magnetic resonance imaging-ultrasound fusion biopsy. J Urol 2019; 201: 84-90.[http://dx.doi.org/10.1016/j.juro.2018.07.051]

[81]   Klocker H, Steiner E, Horninger W, *et al.* Thrombospondin 1 and cathepsin D improve the detection of high-grade prostate cancer and reduce the number of unnecessary prostate biopsies. Eur Urol Suppl 2018; 17e544[http://dx.doi.org/10.1016/S1569-9056(18)31224-7]

[82]   Elkhoury FF, Simopoulos DN, Marks LS. Targeted prostate biopsy in the era of active surveillance. Urology 2018; 112: 12-9.[http://dx.doi.org/10.1016/j.urology.2017.09.007] [PMID: 28962878]

[83]   Ito Y, Udo K, Vertosick EA, *et al.* Clinical usefulness of prostate and tumor volume related parameters following radical prostatectomy for localized prostate cancer. J Urol 2019; 201(3): 535-40.[http://dx.doi.org/10.1016/j.juro.2018.09.060] [PMID: 30300632]

[84]   Dickey SL, Grayson CJ. The quality of life among men receiving active surveillance for prostate cancer: an integrative review.Healthcare 201914.

[85]   Choy B, Pearce SM, Anderson BB, *et al.* Prognostic significance of percentage and architectural types of contemporary Gleason pattern 4 prostate cancer in radical prostatectomy. Am J Surg Pathol 2016; 40(10): 1400-6.[http://dx.doi.org/10.1097/PAS.0000000000000691] [PMID: 27379821]

[86]   Shipley WU, Seiferheld W, Lukka HR, *et al.* Radiation with or without antiandrogen therapy in recurrent prostate cancer. N Engl J Med 2017; 376(5): 417-28.[http://dx.doi.org/10.1056/NEJMoa1607529] [PMID: 28146658]

[87]   Dellis A, Zagouri F, Liontos M, Mitropoulos D, Bamias A, Papatsoris AG. Management of advanced prostate cancer: A systematic review of existing guidelines and recommendations. Cancer Treat Rev 2019; 73: 54-61.[http://dx.doi.org/10.1016/j.ctrv.2018.11.005] [PMID: 30623865]

[88] Cotter KA, Rubin MA. Sequence of events in prostate cancer. Nature 2018; 560(7720): 557-9.[http://dx.doi.org/10.1038/d41586-018-06029-5] [PMID: 30143757]

[89] Saad F, Hotte SJ. Guidelines for the management of castrate-resistant prostate cancer. Can Urol Assoc J 2010; 4(6): 380-4.[http://dx.doi.org/10.5489/cuaj.10167] [PMID: 21191494]

[90] Nader R, El Amm J, Aragon-Ching JB. Role of chemotherapy in prostate cancer. Asian J Androl 2018; 20(3): 221-9.[http://dx.doi.org/10.4103/aja.aja_40_17] [PMID: 29063869]

[91] Ceci F, Fanti S. PSMA-PET/CT imaging in prostate cancer: why and when. Clin Transl Imaging 2019; 7: 377-9.[http://dx.doi.org/10.1007/s40336-019-00348-x]

[92] Ceci F, Bianchi L, Borghesi M, *et al.* Prediction nomogram for ^{68}Ga-PSMA-11 PET/CT in different clinical settings of PSA failure after radical treatment for prostate cancer. Eur J Nucl Med Mol Imaging 2020; 47(1): 136-46.[http://dx.doi.org/10.1007/s00259-019-04505-2] [PMID: 31492993]

[93] Kato M, Kimura K, Hirakawa A, *et al.* Prognostic parameter for high risk prostate cancer patients at initial presentation. Prostate 2018; 78(1): 11-6.[http://dx.doi.org/10.1002/pros.23438] [PMID: 29094384]

[94] Mohler JL, Armstrong AJ, Bahnson RR, *et al.* Prostate cancer, version 1.2016. J Natl Compr Canc Netw 2016; 14(1): 19-30.[http://dx.doi.org/10.6004/jnccn.2016.0004] [PMID: 26733552]

[95] Kung C-P, Maggi LB, Jr, Weber JD. The role of RNA editing in cancer development and metabolic disorders. Front Endocrinol (Lausanne) 2018; 9: 762.[http://dx.doi.org/10.3389/fendo.2018.00762] [PMID: 30619092]

[96] Gerashchenko G, Kashuba V. Molecular profiling of prostate tumors. Biological Markers in Fundamental and Clinical Medicine 2018; 2: 25-5. [scientific journal].

[97] Leapman MS, Carroll PR. New genetic markers for prostate Cancer. Urol Clin North Am 2016; 43(1): 7-15.[http://dx.doi.org/10.1016/j.ucl.2015.08.002] [PMID: 26614025]

[98] Sfanos KS, Yegnasubramanian S, Nelson WG, De Marzo AM. The inflammatory microenvironment and microbiome in prostate cancer development. Nat Rev Urol 2018; 15(1): 11-24.[http://dx.doi.org/10.1038/nrurol.2017.167] [PMID: 29089606]

[99] Arora H, Panara K, Kuchakulla M, *et al.* Alterations of tumor microenvironment by nitric oxide impedes castration-resistant prostate cancer growth. Proc Natl Acad Sci USA 2018; 115(44): 11298-303.[http://dx.doi.org/10.1073/pnas.1812704115] [PMID: 30322928]

[100] Burnstein KL. Regulation of androgen receptor levels: implications for prostate cancer progression and therapy. J Cell Biochem 2005; 95(4): 657-69.[http://dx.doi.org/10.1002/jcb.20460] [PMID: 15861399]

[101] Kim J, Coetzee GA. Prostate specific antigen gene regulation by androgen receptor. J Cell Biochem 2004; 93(2): 233-41.[http://dx.doi.org/10.1002/jcb.20228] [PMID: 15368351]

[102] Srivastava A, Creek DJ. Discovery and validation of clinical biomarkers of cancer: a review combining metabolomics and proteomics. Proteomics 2019; 19(10)e1700448[http://dx.doi.org/10.1002/pmic.201700448] [PMID: 30353665]

[103] Havel JJ, Chowell D, Chan TA. The evolving landscape of biomarkers for checkpoint inhibitor immunotherapy. Nat Rev Cancer 2019; 19(3): 133-50.[http://dx.doi.org/10.1038/s41568-019-0116-x] [PMID: 30755690]

[104] Carneiro G, Radcenco AL, Evaristo J, Monnerat G. Novel strategies for clinical investigation and biomarker discovery: a guide to applied metabolomics. Horm Mol Biol Clin Investig 2019; 38(3): 38.[http://dx.doi.org/10.1515/hmbci-2018-0045] [PMID: 30653466]

[105] Liu TT, Thomas S, Mclean DT, *et al.* Prostate enlargement and altered urinary function are part of the aging process. Aging (Albany NY) 2019; 11(9): 2653-69.[http://dx.doi.org/10.18632/aging.101938] [PMID: 31085797]

[106] Ferreira LB, Palumbo A, de Mello KD, *et al.* PCA3 noncoding RNA is involved in the control of prostate-cancer cell survival and modulates androgen receptor signaling. BMC Cancer 2012; 12: 507.[http://dx.doi.org/10.1186/1471-2407-12-507] [PMID: 23130941]

[107] Neves AF, Dias-Oliveira JDD, Araújo TG, Marangoni K, Goulart LR. Prostate cancer antigen 3 (PCA3) RNA detection in blood and tissue samples for prostate cancer diagnosis. Clin Chem Lab Med 2013; 51(4): 881-7.[http://dx.doi.org/10.1515/cclm-2012-0392] [PMID: 23241599]

[108] Nakamura Y. Biomarkers for immune checkpoint inhibitor-mediated tumor response and adverse events. Front Med (Lausanne) 2019; 6: 119.[http://dx.doi.org/10.3389/fmed.2019.00119] [PMID: 31192215]

[109] Saini S. PSA and beyond: alternative prostate cancer biomarkers. Cell Oncol (Dordr) 2016; 39(2): 97-106.[http://dx.doi.org/10.1007/s13402-016-0268-6] [PMID: 26790878]

[110] Gugnoni M, Ciarrocchi A. Long noncoding RNA and epithelial mesenchymal transition in cancer. Int J Mol

]   Sci 2019; 20(8): 1924.[http://dx.doi.org/10.3390/ijms20081924] [PMID: 31003545]

[111   Koo KM, Mainwaring PN, Tomlins SA, Trau M. Merging new-age biomarkers and nanodiagnostics for
]   precision prostate cancer management. Nat Rev Urol 2019; 16(5): 302-17.[http://dx.doi.org/10.1038/s41585-019-0178-2] [PMID: 30962568]

[112   Lau D, Bobe AM, Khan AA. RNA sequencing of the tumor microenvironment in precision cancer
]   immunotherapy. Trends Cancer 2019; 5(3): 149-56.[http://dx.doi.org/10.1016/j.trecan.2019.02.006] [PMID: 30898262]

[113   Sumiyoshi T, Mizuno K, Yamasaki T, et al. Clinical utility of androgen receptor gene aberrations in
]   circulating cell-free DNA as a biomarker for treatment of castration-resistant prostate cancer. Sci Rep 2019;
       9(1): 4030.[http://dx.doi.org/10.1038/s41598-019-40719-y] [PMID: 30858508]

[114   Xiong T, Li J, Chen F, Zhang F. PCAT-1: A novel oncogenic long non-coding rna in human cancers. Int J
]   Biol Sci 2019; 15(4): 847-56.[http://dx.doi.org/10.7150/ijbs.30970] [PMID: 30906215]

[115   Zhao W, Ma X, Liu L, et al. SNHG20: A vital lncRNA in multiple human cancers. J Cell Physiol 2019; 234:
]   14519-25.[http://dx.doi.org/10.1002/jcp.28143] [PMID: 30644099]

[116   Moradi A, Srinivasan S, Clements J, Batra J. Beyond the biomarker role: prostate-specific antigen (PSA) in
]   the   prostate   cancer   microenvironment.   Cancer   Metastasis   Rev   2019;   38(3):   333-
       46.[http://dx.doi.org/10.1007/s10555-019-09815-3] [PMID: 31659564]

[117   Avgeris M, Mavridis K, Scorilas A. Kallikrein-related peptidase genes as promising biomarkers for prognosis
]   and   monitoring   of   human   malignancies.   Biol   Chem   2010;   391(5):   505-
       11.[http://dx.doi.org/10.1515/bc.2010.056] [PMID: 20302518]

[118   Mamoulakis C, Mavridis C, Georgiadis G, et al. Prostate Cancer Biomarkers. Biomarkers in Toxicology
]   2019869-81.[http://dx.doi.org/10.1016/B978-0-12-814655-2.00048-7]

[119   KLK3 kallikrein related peptidase 3 Homo sapiens (human) 2019.
]

[120   Otero JR, Gomez BG, Juanatey FC, Touijer KA. Prostate cancer biomarkers: an update.Urologic Oncology:
]   Seminars and Original Investigations 2014252-60.

[121   Lilja H. A kallikrein-like serine protease in prostatic fluid cleaves the predominant seminal vesicle protein. J
]   Clin Invest 1985; 76(5): 1899-903.[http://dx.doi.org/10.1172/JCI112185] [PMID: 3902893]

[122   Balk SP, Ko Y-J, Bubley GJ. Biology of prostate-specific antigen. J Clin Oncol 2003; 21(2): 383-
]   91.[http://dx.doi.org/10.1200/JCO.2003.02.083] [PMID: 12525533]

[123   dos Reis RB, Cassini MF. Antígeno Prostático Específico (PSA).
]

[124   Dijkstra S, Hendriks R, Leyten G, Mulders P, Schalken J. Biomarkers for prostate cancer. Management of
]   Prostate Cancer 201777-96.[http://dx.doi.org/10.1007/978-3-319-42769-0_5]

[125   Stravodimos KG, Petrolekas A, Kapetanakis T, et al. TRUS versus transabdominal ultrasound as a predictor
]   of enucleated adenoma weight in patients with BPH: a tool for standard preoperative work-up? Int Urol
       Nephrol 2009; 41(4): 767-71.[http://dx.doi.org/10.1007/s11255-009-9554-9] [PMID: 19350408]

[126   Lilja H, Ulmert D, Vickers AJ. Prostate-specific antigen and prostate cancer: prediction, detection and
]   monitoring. Nat Rev Cancer 2008; 8(4): 268-78.[http://dx.doi.org/10.1038/nrc2351] [PMID: 18337732]

[127   Kuriyama M, Wang MC, Papsidero LD, et al. Quantitation of prostate-specific antigen in serum by a
]   sensitive enzyme immunoassay. Cancer Res 1980; 40(12): 4658-62.[PMID: 6159971]

[128   Tokudome S, Ando R, Koda Y. Discoveries and application of prostate-specific antigen, and some proposals
]   to   optimize   prostate   cancer   screening.   Cancer   Manag   Res   2016;   8:   45-
       7.[http://dx.doi.org/10.2147/CMAR.S98326] [PMID: 27274309]

[129   Kim JW. In search of a new prostate-specific antigen. Int Neurourol J 2019; 23(1): 3-
]   4.[http://dx.doi.org/10.5213/inj.1920edi.004] [PMID: 30943688]

[130   N.C.I. NCIProstate-Specific Antigen (PSA). Test 2017.
]

[131   Hong   SK.   Kallikreins   as   biomarkers   for   prostate   cancer.   BioMed   Res   Int   2014;
]   2014526341[http://dx.doi.org/10.1155/2014/526341] [PMID: 24809052]

[132   Anceschi U, Tuderti G, Lugnani F, et al. Novel diagnostic biomarkers of prostate cancer: An update. Curr
]   Med   Chem   2019;   26(6):   1045-58.[http://dx.doi.org/10.2174/0929867325666180914115416]   [PMID:
       30215331]

[133   Mikolajczyk SD, Marks LS, Partin AW, Rittenhouse HG. Free prostate-specific antigen in serum is becoming
]   more complex. Urology 2002; 59(6): 797-802.[http://dx.doi.org/10.1016/S0090-4295(01)01605-3] [PMID:

12031356]

[134] Morgan T, Palapattu G, Wei J. Screening for prostate cancer—beyond total PSA, utilization of novel biomarkers. Curr Urol Rep 2015; 16(9): 63.[http://dx.doi.org/10.1007/s11934-015-0537-3] [PMID: 26169584]

[135] Khalifa AH, Cornfield JZ. PSA screening for prostate cancer in men under the age of 65: a review of current practice, open. J Urol 20188.

[136] Sartori DA, Chan DW. Biomarkers in prostate cancer: what's new? Curr Opin Oncol 2014; 26(3): 259-64.[http://dx.doi.org/10.1097/CCO.0000000000000065] [PMID: 24626128]

[137] McGrath S, Christidis D, Perera M, et al. Prostate cancer biomarkers: Are we hitting the mark? Prostate Int 2016; 4(4): 130-5.[http://dx.doi.org/10.1016/j.prnil.2016.07.002] [PMID: 27995111]

[138] Fossati N, Buffi NM, Haese A, et al. Preoperative prostate-specific antigen isoform p2PSA and its derivatives,% p2PSA and Prostate Health Index, predict pathologic outcomes in patients undergoing radical prostatectomy for prostate cancer: results from a multicentric European prospective study. Eur Urol 2015; 68(1): 132-8.[http://dx.doi.org/10.1016/j.eururo.2014.07.034] [PMID: 25139197]

[139] Canto EI, Singh H, Shariat SF, et al. Serum BPSA outperforms both total PSA and free PSA as a predictor of prostatic enlargement in men without prostate cancer. Urology 2004; 63(5): 905-10.[http://dx.doi.org/10.1016/j.urology.2003.12.037] [PMID: 15134977]

[140] Sriplakich S, Lojanapiwat B, Chongruksut W, et al. Prospective performance of the Prostate Health Index in prostate cancer detection in the first prostate biopsy of men with a total prostatic specific antigen of 4-10 ng/mL and negative digital rectal examination. Prostate Int 2018; 6(4): 136-9.[http://dx.doi.org/10.1016/j.prnil.2018.02.002] [PMID: 30505815]

[141] Bosch JL, Tilling K, Bohnen AM, Bangma CH, Donovan JL. Establishing normal reference ranges for prostate volume change with age in the population-based Krimpen-study: prediction of future prostate volume in individual men. Prostate 2007; 67(16): 1816-24.[http://dx.doi.org/10.1002/pros.20663] [PMID: 17935157]

[142] Anyango R, Ojwando J, Mwita C, Mugalo E. Diagnostic accuracy of the [-2]Pro-PSA and Prostate Health Index versus the Gleason score for determining the aggressiveness of prostate cancer: a systematic review protocol. JBI Database Syst Rev Implement Reports 2018; 16(11): 2066-71.[http://dx.doi.org/10.11124/JBISRIR-2017-003385] [PMID: 30024433]

[143] Mikolajczyk SD, Millar LS, Wang TJ, et al. "BPSA," a specific molecular form of free prostate-specific antigen, is found predominantly in the transition zone of patients with nodular benign prostatic hyperplasia. Urology 2000; 55(1): 41-5.[http://dx.doi.org/10.1016/S0090-4295(99)00372-6] [PMID: 10654892]

[144] Rhodes T, Jacobson DJ, McGree ME, et al. Longitudinal changes of benign prostate-specific antigen and [-2]proprostate-specific antigen in seven years in a community-based sample of men. Urology 2012; 79(3): 655-61.[http://dx.doi.org/10.1016/j.urology.2011.09.056] [PMID: 22386420]

[145] Rhodes T, Jacobson DJ, McGree ME, et al. Benign prostate specific antigen distribution and associations with urological outcomes in community dwelling black and white men. J Urol 2012; 187(1): 87-91.[http://dx.doi.org/10.1016/j.juro.2011.09.061] [PMID: 22093190]

[146] Wang Y, Liu XJ, Yao XD. Function of PCA3 in prostate tissue and clinical research progress on developing a PCA3 score. Chin J Cancer Res 2014; 26(4): 493-500.[PMID: 25232225]

[147] Volkin D. 2017 Summaries. Rev Urol 2017; 19(4): 252-60.[PMID: 29472829]

[148] Arriaga-Canon C, De La Rosa-Velázquez IA, González-Barrios R, et al. The use of long non-coding RNAs as prognostic biomarkers and therapeutic targets in prostate cancer. Oncotarget 2018; 9(29): 20872-90.[http://dx.doi.org/10.18632/oncotarget.25038] [PMID: 29755696]

[149] Salameh A, Lee AK, Cardó-Vila M, et al. PRUNE2 is a human prostate cancer suppressor regulated by the intronic long noncoding RNA PCA3. Proc Natl Acad Sci USA 2015; 112(27): 8403-8.[http://dx.doi.org/10.1073/pnas.1507882112] [PMID: 26080435]

[150] Lemos AEG, Ferreira LB, Batoreu NM, de Freitas PP, Bonamino MH, Gimba ERP. PCA3 long noncoding RNA modulates the expression of key cancer-related genes in LNCaP prostate cancer cells. Tumour Biol 2016; 37(8): 11339-48.[http://dx.doi.org/10.1007/s13277-016-5012-3] [PMID: 26960690]

[151] Wang T, Qu X, Jiang J, et al. Diagnostic significance of urinary long non-coding PCA3 RNA in prostate cancer. Oncotarget 2017; 8(35): 58577-86.[http://dx.doi.org/10.18632/oncotarget.17272] [PMID: 28938580]

[152] Mao Z, Ji A, Yang K, et al. Diagnostic performance of PCA3 and hK2 in combination with serum PSA for prostate cancer. Medicine (Baltimore) 2018; 97(42)e12806[http://dx.doi.org/10.1097/MD.0000000000012806] [PMID: 30334974]

[153] Jiang Z, Zhao Y, Tian Y. Comparison of diagnostic efficacy by two urine PCA3 scores in prostate cancer patients undergoing repeat biopsies Minerva urologica e nefrologica= The Italian journal of urology and nephrology 2019; 71(2019): 373-80.

[154] Rodríguez SVM, García-Perdomo HA. Diagnostic accuracy of prostate cancer antigen 3 (PCA3) prior to first prostate biopsy: A systematic review and meta-analysis. Can Urol Assoc J 2020; 14(5): E214-9.[PMID: 31793864]

[155] Abdellaoui Maane I, El Hadi H, Qmichou Z, et al. Evaluation of combined quantification of PCA3 and AMACR gene expression for molecular diagnosis of prostate cancer in Moroccan patients by RT-qPCR, Asian Pacific journal of cancer prevention. Asian Pac J Cancer Prev 2016; 17(12): 5229-35.[PMID: 28125866]

[156] Jiang N, Pan J, Fang S, et al. Liquid biopsy: Circulating exosomal long noncoding RNAs in cancer. Clin Chim Acta 2019; 495: 331-7.[http://dx.doi.org/10.1016/j.cca.2019.04.082] [PMID: 31054913]

[157] van der Toom EE, Axelrod HD, de la Rosette JJ, de Reijke TM, Pienta KJ, Valkenburg KC. Prostate-specific markers to identify rare prostate cancer cells in liquid biopsies. Nat Rev Urol 2019; 16(1): 7-22.[http://dx.doi.org/10.1038/s41585-018-0119-5] [PMID: 30479377]

[158] Becerra MF, Bhat A, Mouzannar A, Atluri VS, Punnen S. Serum and urinary biomarkers for detection and active surveillance of prostate cancer. Curr Opin Urol 2019; 29(6): 593-7.[http://dx.doi.org/10.1097/MOU.0000000000000670] [PMID: 31436568]

[159] Boerrigter E, Groen LN, Van Erp NP, Verhaegh GW, Schalken JA. Clinical utility of emerging biomarkers in prostate cancer liquid biopsies. Expert Rev Mol Diagn 20191-12.[PMID: 31577907]

[160] Eskra JN, Rabizadeh D, Pavlovich CP, Catalona WJ, Luo J. Approaches to urinary detection of prostate cancer. Prostate Cancer Prostatic Dis 2019; 22(3): 362-81.[http://dx.doi.org/10.1038/s41391-019-0127-4] [PMID: 30655600]

[161] Newcomb LF, Zheng Y, Faino AV, et al. Performance of PCA3 and TMPRSS2:ERG urinary biomarkers in prediction of biopsy outcome in the Canary Prostate Active Surveillance Study (PASS). Prostate Cancer Prostatic Dis 2019; 22(3): 438-45.[http://dx.doi.org/10.1038/s41391-018-0124-z] [PMID: 30664734]

[162] Kohaar I, Petrovics G, Srivastava S. A rich array of prostate cancer molecular biomarkers: opportunities and challenges. Int J Mol Sci 2019; 20(8): 1813.[http://dx.doi.org/10.3390/ijms20081813] [PMID: 31013716]

[163] Ankerst DP, Goros M, Tomlins SA, et al. Incorporation of urinary prostate cancer antigen 3 and tmprss2: Erg into prostate cancer prevention trial risk calculator. Eur Urol Focus 2019; 5(1): 54-61.[http://dx.doi.org/10.1016/j.euf.2018.01.010] [PMID: 29422418]

[164] Qin Z, Yao J, Xu L, et al. Diagnosis accuracy of PCA3 level in patients with prostate cancer: a systematic review with meta-analysis International braz j urol: official journal of the Brazilian Society of Urology 2019; 45(2019)

[165] Martínez-Piñeiro L, Schalken JA, Cabri P, Maisonobe P, de la Taille A, Group TS. Evaluation of urinary prostate cancer antigen-3 (PCA3) and TMPRSS2-ERG score changes when starting androgen-deprivation therapy with triptorelin 6-month formulation in patients with locally advanced and metastatic prostate cancer. BJU Int 2014; 114(4): 608-16.[http://dx.doi.org/10.1111/bju.12542] [PMID: 24806330]

[166] Gezer U, Tiryakioglu D, Bilgin E, Dalay N, Holdenrieder S. Androgen stimulation of PCA3 and miR-141 and their release from prostate cancer cells. Cell J 2015; 16(4): 488-93.[PMID: 25685739]

[167] Zheng K, Dou Y, He L, et al. Improved sensitivity and specificity for prostate cancer diagnosis based on the urine PCA3/PSA ratio acquired by sequence-specific RNA capture. Oncol Rep 2015; 34(5): 2439-44.[http://dx.doi.org/10.3892/or.2015.4266] [PMID: 26351770]

[168] Li Y, Hou CZ, Dong YL, Zhu L, Xu H. Long noncoding RNA LINP1 promoted proliferation and invasion of ovarian cancer via inhibiting KLF6. Eur Rev Med Pharmacol Sci 2020; 24(1): 36-42.[PMID: 31957816]

[169] Shaimardanova AA, Solovyeva VV, Chulpanova DS, James V, Kitaeva KV, Rizvanov AA. Extracellular vesicles in the diagnosis and treatment of central nervous system diseases. Neural Regen Res 2020; 15(4): 586-96.[http://dx.doi.org/10.4103/1673-5374.266908] [PMID: 31638080]

[170] Sharrocks AD. The ETS-domain transcription factor family. Nat Rev Mol Cell Biol 2001; 2(11): 827-37.[http://dx.doi.org/10.1038/35099076] [PMID: 11715049]

[171] Kron KJ, Murison A, Zhou S, et al. TMPRSS2-ERG fusion co-opts master transcription factors and activates NOTCH signaling in primary prostate cancer. Nat Genet 2017; 49(9): 1336-45.[http://dx.doi.org/10.1038/ng.3930] [PMID: 28783165]

[172] Tomlins SA, Rhodes DR, Perner S, et al. Recurrent fusion of TMPRSS2 and ETS transcription factor genes in prostate cancer science 2005; 3102005: 644-8.

[173] Perner S, Mosquera J-M, Demichelis F, et al. TMPRSS2-ERG fusion prostate cancer: an early molecular

] event associated with invasion. Am J Surg Pathol 2007; 31(6): 882-8.[http://dx.doi.org/10.1097/01.pas.0000213424.38503.aa] [PMID: 17527075]

[174 Perner S, Demichelis F, Beroukhim R, *et al.* TMPRSS2:ERG fusion-associated deletions provide insight into
] the heterogeneity of prostate cancer. Cancer Res 2006; 66(17): 8337-41.[http://dx.doi.org/10.1158/0008-5472.CAN-06-1482] [PMID: 16951139]

[175 Lin B, Ferguson C, White JT, *et al.* Prostate-localized and androgen-regulated expression of the membrane-
] bound serine protease TMPRSS2. Cancer Res 1999; 59(17): 4180-4.[PMID: 10485450]

[176 Chen Y-W, Lee M-S, Lucht A, *et al.* TMPRSS2, a serine protease expressed in the prostate on the apical
] surface of luminal epithelial cells and released into semen in prostasomes, is misregulated in prostate cancer
cells. Am J Pathol 2010; 176(6): 2986-96.[http://dx.doi.org/10.2353/ajpath.2010.090665] [PMID: 20382709]

[177 Yu J, Yu J, Mani R-S, *et al.* An integrated network of androgen receptor, polycomb, and TMPRSS2-ERG
] gene fusions in prostate cancer progression. Cancer Cell 2010; 17(5): 443-54.[http://dx.doi.org/10.1016/j.ccr.2010.03.018] [PMID: 20478527]

[178 Carver BS, Tran J, Gopalan A, *et al.* Aberrant ERG expression cooperates with loss of PTEN to promote
] cancer progression in the prostate. Nat Genet 2009; 41(5): 619-24.[http://dx.doi.org/10.1038/ng.370] [PMID: 19396168]

[179 King JC, Xu J, Wongvipat J, *et al.* Cooperativity of TMPRSS2-ERG with PI3-kinase pathway activation in
] prostate oncogenesis. Nat Genet 2009; 41(5): 524-6.[http://dx.doi.org/10.1038/ng.371] [PMID: 19396167]

[180 Hägglöf C, Hammarsten P, Strömvall K, *et al.* TMPRSS2-ERG expression predicts prostate cancer survival
] and associates with stromal biomarkers. PLoS One 2014; 9(2)e86824[http://dx.doi.org/10.1371/journal.pone.0086824] [PMID: 24505269]

[181 Tomlins SA, Laxman B, Varambally S, *et al.* Role of the TMPRSS2-ERG gene fusion in prostate cancer.
] Neoplasia 2008; 10(2): 177-88.[http://dx.doi.org/10.1593/neo.07822] [PMID: 18283340]

[182 Leyten GH, Hessels D, Smit FP, *et al.* Identification of a candidate gene panel for the early diagnosis of
] prostate cancer. Clin Cancer Res 2015; 21(13): 3061-70.[http://dx.doi.org/10.1158/1078-0432.CCR-14-3334]
[PMID: 25788493]

[183 Kimura S, D'Andrea D, Iwata T, *et al.* Expression of urokinase-type plasminogen activator system in non-
] metastatic prostate cancer. World J Urol 2019.[http://dx.doi.org/10.1007/s00345-019-03038-5] [PMID: 31797075]

[184 Han KY, Chen PN, Hong MC, *et al.* Naringenin Attenuated Prostate Cancer Invasion *via* Reversal of
] Epithelial-to-Mesenchymal Transition and Inhibited uPA Activity. Anticancer Res 2018; 38(12): 6753-8.[http://dx.doi.org/10.21873/anticanres.13045] [PMID: 30504386]

[185 Lippert S, Berg KD, Høyer-Hansen G, *et al.* Copenhagen uPAR prostate cancer (CuPCa) database: protocol
] and early results. Biomarkers Med 2016; 10(2): 209-16.[http://dx.doi.org/10.2217/bmm.15.114] [PMID: 26764285]

[186 Bakht MK, Lovnicki JM, Tubman J, *et al.* Differential expression of glucose transporters and hexokinases in
] prostate cancer with a neuroendocrine gene signature: a mechanistic perspective for FDG imaging of PSMA-
suppressed tumors. J Nucl Med 2019.[PMID: 31806771]

[187 Rasul S, Hacker M, Kretschmer-Chott E, *et al.* Clinical outcome of standardized (177)Lu-PSMA-617 therapy
] in metastatic prostate cancer patients receiving 7400 MBq every 4 weeks. Eur J Nucl Med Mol Imaging
2019.[PMID: 31781834]

[188 Umbricht CA, Köster U, Bernhardt P, *et al.* Alpha-PET for Prostate Cancer: Preclinical investigation using
] ^{149}Tb-PSMA-617. Sci Rep 2019; 9(1): 17800.[http://dx.doi.org/10.1038/s41598-019-54150-w] [PMID: 31780798]

[189 Yadav MP, Ballal S, Bal C, *et al.* Efficacy and Safety of 177Lu-PSMA-617 Radioligand Therapy in
] Metastatic Castration-Resistant Prostate Cancer Patients. Clin Nucl Med 2020; 45(1): 19-31.[http://dx.doi.org/10.1097/RLU.0000000000002833] [PMID: 31789908]

[190 Roberts A, Tripathi PP, Gandhi S. Graphene nanosheets as an electric mediator for ultrafast sensing of
] urokinase plasminogen activator receptor-A biomarker of cancer. Biosens Bioelectron 2019;
141111398[http://dx.doi.org/10.1016/j.bios.2019.111398] [PMID: 31176112]

[191 Lee SH, Hu W, Matulay JT, *et al.* Tumor evolution and drug response in patient-derived organoid models of
] bladder cancer. Cell 2018; 173: 515-528 e517.

[192 Witkowska-Patena E, Gizewska A, Dziuk M, Misko J, Budzynska A, Walecka-Mazur A. Diagnostic
] performance of 18F-PSMA-1007 PET/CT in biochemically relapsed patients with prostate cancer with PSA
levels </= 2.0 ng/ml. Prostate Cancer Prostatic Dis 2019.[http://dx.doi.org/10.1038/s41391-019-0194-6]

[PMID: 31780781]

[193 Priftakis D, Afaq A, Bomanji J. Imaging of prostate cancer recurrence in the vas deferens with 68Ga-PSMA
] PET/CT. Clin Nucl Med 2020; 45(1): 49-51.[http://dx.doi.org/10.1097/RLU.0000000000002837] [PMID: 31789910]

[194 Siva S, Udovicich C, Tran B, Zargar H, Murphy DG, Hofman MS. Expanding the role of small-molecule
] PSMA ligands beyond PET staging of prostate cancer. Nat Rev Urol 2020; 17(2): 107-18.[http://dx.doi.org/10.1038/s41585-019-0272-5] [PMID: 31937920]

[195 Zippel C, Ronski SC, Bohnet-Joschko S, Giesel FL, Kopka K. Current status of PSMA-radiotracers for
] prostate cancer: data analysis of prospective trials listed on clinicaltrials.gov. Pharmaceuticals (Basel) 2020;
13(1): 13.[http://dx.doi.org/10.3390/ph13010012] [PMID: 31940969]

[196 Farolfi A, Ilhan H, Gafita A, et al. Mapping prostate cancer lesions pre/post unsuccessful salvage lymph node
] dissection using repeat PSMA-PET. J Nucl Med 2019.[http://dx.doi.org/10.2967/jnumed.119.235374]

[197 Chang CS, Kokontis J, Liao ST. Molecular cloning of human and rat complementary DNA encoding
] androgen receptors. Science 1988; 240(4850): 324-6.[http://dx.doi.org/10.1126/science.3353726] [PMID: 3353726]

[198 McEwan IJ. Molecular mechanisms of androgen receptor-mediated gene regulation: structure-function
] analysis of the AF-1 domain. Endocr Relat Cancer 2004; 11(2): 281-93.[http://dx.doi.org/10.1677/erc.0.0110281] [PMID: 15163303]

[199 Anestis A, Zoi I, Papavassiliou AG, Karamouzis MV. Androgen Receptor in Breast Cancer-Clinical and
] Preclinical Research Insights Molecules 2020; 25

[200 Gelmann EP. Molecular biology of the androgen receptor. J Clin Oncol 2002; 20(13): 3001-15.[http://dx.doi.org/10.1200/JCO.2002.10.018] [PMID: 12089231]

[201 Lin HK, Wang L, Hu YC, Altuwaijri S, Chang C. Phosphorylation-dependent ubiquitylation and degradation
] of androgen receptor by Akt require Mdm2 E3 ligase. EMBO J 2002; 21(15): 4037-48.[http://dx.doi.org/10.1093/emboj/cdf406] [PMID: 12145204]

[202 Takayama K, Inoue S. Transcriptional network of androgen receptor in prostate cancer progression. Int J Urol
] 2013; 20(8): 756-68.[http://dx.doi.org/10.1111/iju.12146] [PMID: 23600948]

[203 Nickols NG, Dervan PB. Suppression of androgen receptor-mediated gene expression by a sequence-specific
] DNA-binding polyamide. Proc Natl Acad Sci USA 2007; 104(25): 10418-23.[http://dx.doi.org/10.1073/pnas.0704217104] [PMID: 17566103]

[204 Shafi AA, Yen AE, Weigel NL. Androgen receptors in hormone-dependent and castration-resistant prostate
] cancer. Pharmacol Ther 2013; 140(3): 223-38.[http://dx.doi.org/10.1016/j.pharmthera.2013.07.003] [PMID: 23859952]

[205 Denis LJ, Griffiths K. Endocrine treatment in prostate cancer. Semin Surg Oncol 2000; 18(1): 52-74.[http://dx.doi.org/10.1002/(SICI)1098-2388(200001/02)18:1<52::AID-SSU8>3.0.CO;2-6]   [PMID: 10617897]

[206 Pienta KJ, Bradley D. Mechanisms underlying the development of androgen-independent prostate cancer.
] Clin Cancer Res 2006; 12(6): 1665-71.[http://dx.doi.org/10.1158/1078-0432.CCR-06-0067] [PMID: 16551847]

[207 Teo MY, Rathkopf DE, Kantoff P. Treatment of Advanced Prostate Cancer. Annu Rev Med 2019; 70: 479-99.[http://dx.doi.org/10.1146/annurev-med-051517-011947] [PMID: 30691365]

[208 Penning TM. Mechanisms of drug resistance that target the androgen axis in castration resistant prostate
] cancer (CRPC). J Steroid Biochem Mol Biol 2015; 153: 105-13.[http://dx.doi.org/10.1016/j.jsbmb.2015.05.010] [PMID: 26032458]

[209 Cornford P, Bellmunt J, Bolla M, et al. EAU-ESTRO-SIOG Guidelines on Prostate Cancer. Part II:
] Treatment of Relapsing, Metastatic, and Castration-Resistant Prostate Cancer. Eur Urol 2017; 71(4): 630-42.[http://dx.doi.org/10.1016/j.eururo.2016.08.002] [PMID: 27591931]

[210 Feng Q, He B. Androgen Receptor Signaling in the Development of Castration-Resistant Prostate Cancer.
] Front Oncol 2019; 9: 858.[http://dx.doi.org/10.3389/fonc.2019.00858] [PMID: 31552182]

[211 Fujita K, Nonomura N. Role of Androgen Receptor in Prostate Cancer: A Review. World J Mens Health
] 2019; 37(3): 288-95.[http://dx.doi.org/10.5534/wjmh.180040] [PMID: 30209899]

[212 Yezi Zhu JL. Regulation of androgen receptor variants in prostate cancer. Asian J Urol 2020.
]

[213 Gaddipati JP, McLeod DG, Heidenberg HB, et al. Frequent detection of codon 877 mutation in the androgen
] receptor gene in advanced prostate cancers. Cancer Res 1994; 54(11): 2861-4.[PMID: 8187068]

[214] Gottlieb B, Beitel LK, Nadarajah A, Paliouras M, Trifiro M. The androgen receptor gene mutations database:
] 2012 update. Hum Mutat 2012; 33(5): 887-94.[http://dx.doi.org/10.1002/humu.22046] [PMID: 22334387]

[215] Heemers HV, Schmidt LJ, Kidd E, Raclaw KA, Regan KM, Tindall DJ. Differential regulation of steroid
] nuclear receptor coregulator expression between normal and neoplastic prostate epithelial cells. Prostate
2010; 70(9): 959-70.[http://dx.doi.org/10.1002/pros.21130] [PMID: 20166126]

[216 Edlind MP, Hsieh AC. PI3K-AKT-mTOR signaling in prostate cancer progression and androgen deprivation
] therapy resistance. Asian J Androl 2014; 16(3): 378-86.[http://dx.doi.org/10.4103/1008-682X.122876]
[PMID: 24759575]

[217 Hu R, Dunn TA, Wei S, *et al.* Ligand-independent androgen receptor variants derived from splicing of
] cryptic exons signify hormone-refractory prostate cancer. Cancer Res 2009; 69(1): 16-
22.[http://dx.doi.org/10.1158/0008-5472.CAN-08-2764] [PMID: 19117982]

[218 Li Y, Chan SC, Brand LJ, Hwang TH, Silverstein KA, Dehm SM. Androgen receptor splice variants mediate
] enzalutamide resistance in castration-resistant prostate cancer cell lines. Cancer Res 2013; 73(2): 483-
9.[http://dx.doi.org/10.1158/0008-5472.CAN-12-3630] [PMID: 23117885]

[219 Lu C, Luo J. Decoding the androgen receptor splice variants. Transl Androl Urol 2013; 2(3): 178-86.[PMID:
] 25356377]

[220 Cao B, Qi Y, Zhang G, *et al.* Androgen receptor splice variants activating the full-length receptor in
] mediating resistance to androgen-directed therapy. Oncotarget 2014; 5(6): 1646-
56.[http://dx.doi.org/10.18632/oncotarget.1802] [PMID: 24722067]

[221 Hu R, Lu C, Mostaghel EA, *et al.* Distinct transcriptional programs mediated by the ligand-dependent full-
] length androgen receptor and its splice variants in castration-resistant prostate cancer. Cancer Res 2012;
72(14): 3457-62.[http://dx.doi.org/10.1158/0008-5472.CAN-11-3892] [PMID: 22710436]

[222 Guo Z, Yang X, Sun F, *et al.* A novel androgen receptor splice variant is up-regulated during prostate cancer
] progression and promotes androgen depletion-resistant growth. Cancer Res 2009; 69(6): 2305-
13.[http://dx.doi.org/10.1158/0008-5472.CAN-08-3795] [PMID: 19244107]

[223 Jones D, Noble M, Wedge SR, Robson CN, Gaughan L. Aurora A regulates expression of AR-V7 in models
] of castrate resistant prostate cancer. Sci Rep 2017; 7: 40957.[http://dx.doi.org/10.1038/srep40957] [PMID:
28205582]

[224 Shao C, Yu B, Liu Y. Androgen receptor splicing variant 7: Beyond being a constitutively active variant. Life
] Sci 2019; 234116768[http://dx.doi.org/10.1016/j.lfs.2019.116768] [PMID: 31445027]

[225 Cato L, de Tribolet-Hardy J, Lee I, *et al.* Inactivation of androgen receptor coregulator ARA55 inhibits
] androgen receptor activity and agonist effect of antiandrogens in prostate cancer cells Proc Natl Acad Sci U S
A 2019; 100(2003): 5124-9.

[226 Zhang T, Karsh LI, Nissenblatt MJ, Canfield SE. Androgen Receptor Splice Variant, AR-V7, as a Biomarker
] of Resistance to Androgen Axis-Targeted Therapies in Advanced Prostate Cancer. Clin Genitourin Cancer
2020; 18(1): 1-10.[http://dx.doi.org/10.1016/j.clgc.2019.09.015] [PMID: 31653572]

[227 Rahman MM, Miyamoto H, Lardy H, Chang C. Inactivation of androgen receptor coregulator ARA55
] inhibits androgen receptor activity and agonist effect of antiandrogens in prostate cancer cells. Proc Natl
Acad Sci USA 2003; 100(9): 5124-9.[http://dx.doi.org/10.1073/pnas.0530097100] [PMID: 12700349]

[228 Benjamin Sunkel QW. Looking beyond Androgen Receptor Signaling in the Treatment of Advanced Prostate
] Cancer. Advances in Andrology 2014; 2014: 9.

[229 Robinson JL, Hickey TE, Warren AY, *et al.* Elevated levels of FOXA1 facilitate androgen receptor
] chromatin binding resulting in a CRPC-like phenotype. Oncogene 2014; 33(50): 5666-
74.[http://dx.doi.org/10.1038/onc.2013.508] [PMID: 24292680]

[230 Vidal SJ, Rodriguez-Bravo V, Quinn SA, *et al.* A targetable GATA2-IGF2 axis confers aggressiveness in
] lethal prostate cancer. Cancer Cell 2015; 27(2): 223-39.[http://dx.doi.org/10.1016/j.ccell.2014.11.013]
[PMID: 25670080]

[231 Chiang YT, Wang K, Fazli L, *et al.* GATA2 as a potential metastasis-driving gene in prostate cancer.
] Oncotarget 2014; 5(2): 451-61.[http://dx.doi.org/10.18632/oncotarget.1296] [PMID: 24448395]

[232 Böhm M, Locke WJ, Sutherland RL, Kench JG, Henshall SM. A role for GATA-2 in transition to an
] aggressive phenotype in prostate cancer through modulation of key androgen-regulated genes. Oncogene
2009; 28(43): 3847-56.[http://dx.doi.org/10.1038/onc.2009.243] [PMID: 19684615]

[233 Chaytor L, Simcock M, Nakjang S, *et al.* The Pioneering Role of GATA2 in Androgen Receptor Variant
] Regulation Is Controlled by Bromodomain and Extraterminal Proteins in Castrate-Resistant Prostate Cancer
Mol Cancer Res 2019; 17

[234 Leo C, Chen JD. The SRC family of nuclear receptor coactivators. Gene 2000; 245(1): 1-

]   11.[http://dx.doi.org/10.1016/S0378-1119(00)00024-X] [PMID: 10713439]

[235 Agoulnik IU, Vaid A, Bingman WE, III, *et al.* Role of SRC-1 in the promotion of prostate cancer cell growth
]   and tumor progression. Cancer Res 2005; 65(17): 7959-67.[http://dx.doi.org/10.1158/0008-5472.CAN-04-3541] [PMID: 16140968]

[236 Agoulnik IU, Weigel NL. Androgen receptor action in hormone-dependent and recurrent prostate cancer. J
]   Cell Biochem 2006; 99(2): 362-72.[http://dx.doi.org/10.1002/jcb.20811] [PMID: 16619264]

[237 Kim SM, Park JH, Kim KD, *et al.* Brassinin induces apoptosis in PC-3 human prostate cancer cells through
]   the suppression of PI3K/Akt/mTOR/S6K1 signaling cascades. Phytother Res 2014; 28(3): 423-
       31.[http://dx.doi.org/10.1002/ptr.5010] [PMID: 23686889]

[238 Hopkins BD, Hodakoski C, Barrows D, Mense SM, Parsons RE. PTEN function: the long and the short of it.
]   Trends Biochem Sci 2014; 39(4): 183-90.[http://dx.doi.org/10.1016/j.tibs.2014.02.006] [PMID: 24656806]

[239 Naderali E, Khaki AA, Rad JS, Ali-Hemmati A, Rahmati M, Charoudeh HN. Regulation and modulation of
]   PTEN activity. Mol Biol Rep 2018; 45(6): 2869-81.[http://dx.doi.org/10.1007/s11033-018-4321-6] [PMID:
       30145641]

[240 Vogelstein B, Lane D, Levine AJ. Surfing the p53 network. Nature 2000; 408(6810): 307-
]   10.[http://dx.doi.org/10.1038/35042675] [PMID: 11099028]

[241 Grasso CS, Wu YM, Robinson DR, *et al.* The mutational landscape of lethal castration-resistant prostate
]   cancer. Nature 2012; 487(7406): 239-43.[http://dx.doi.org/10.1038/nature11125] [PMID: 22722839]

[242 Denicourt C, Dowdy SF. Cip/Kip proteins: more than just CDKs inhibitors. Genes Dev 2004; 18(8): 851-
]   5.[http://dx.doi.org/10.1101/gad.1205304] [PMID: 15107401]

[243 Low CG, Luk IS, Lin D, *et al.* BIRC6 protein, an inhibitor of apoptosis: role in survival of human prostate
]   cancer cells. PLoS One 2013; 8(2)e55837[http://dx.doi.org/10.1371/journal.pone.0055837] [PMID:
       23409057]

[244 Dong X, Lin D, Low C, *et al.* Elevated expression of BIRC6 protein in non-small-cell lung cancers is
]   associated with cancer recurrence and chemoresistance Journal of thoracic oncology : official publication of
       the International Association for the Study of Lung Cancer 2013; 8(2013): 161-70.

[245 Pilling AB, Hwang C. Targeting prosurvival BCL2 signaling through Akt blockade sensitizes castration-
]   resistant   prostate   cancer   cells   to   enzalutamide.   Prostate   2019;   79(11):   1347-
       59.[http://dx.doi.org/10.1002/pros.23843] [PMID: 31228231]

[246 Thiery JP, Acloque H, Huang RY, Nieto MA. Epithelial-mesenchymal transitions in development and
]   disease. Cell 2009; 139(5): 871-90.[http://dx.doi.org/10.1016/j.cell.2009.11.007] [PMID: 19945376]

[247 Kalluri R, Weinberg RA. The basics of epithelial-mesenchymal transition. J Clin Invest 2009; 119(6): 1420-
]   8.[http://dx.doi.org/10.1172/JCI39104] [PMID: 19487818]

[248 Odero-Marah V, Hawsawi O, Henderson V, Sweeney J. Epithelial-Mesenchymal Transition (EMT) and
]   Prostate Cancer. Adv Exp Med Biol 2018; 1095: 101-10.[http://dx.doi.org/10.1007/978-3-319-95693-0_6]
       [PMID: 30229551]

[249 Garg M. Epithelial-mesenchymal transition - activating transcription factors - multifunctional regulators in
]   cancer. World J Stem Cells 2013; 5(4): 188-95.[http://dx.doi.org/10.4252/wjsc.v5.i4.188] [PMID: 24179606]

[250 Kong D, Sethi S, Li Y, *et al.* Androgen receptor splice variants contribute to prostate cancer aggressiveness
]   through induction of EMT and expression of stem cell marker genes. Prostate 2015; 75(2): 161-
       74.[http://dx.doi.org/10.1002/pros.22901] [PMID: 25307492]

[251 Wang Q, Li W, Zhang Y, *et al.* Androgen receptor regulates a distinct transcription program in androgen-
]   independent prostate cancer. Cell 2009; 138(2): 245-56.[http://dx.doi.org/10.1016/j.cell.2009.04.056] [PMID:
       19632176]

[252 Mellado B, Codony J, Ribal MJ, Visa L, Gascon P. Molecular biology of androgen-independent prostate
]   cancer: the role of the androgen receptor pathway Clinical & translational oncology : official publication of
       the Federation of Spanish Oncology Societies and of the National Cancer Institute of Mexico 2009; 11(2009):
       5-10.

[253 Ku SY, Gleave ME, Beltran H. Towards precision oncology in advanced prostate cancer. Nat Rev Urol 2019;
]   16(11): 645-54.[http://dx.doi.org/10.1038/s41585-019-0237-8] [PMID: 31591549]

[254 Massagué J. TGFβ signalling in context. Nat Rev Mol Cell Biol 2012; 13(10): 616-
]   30.[http://dx.doi.org/10.1038/nrm3434] [PMID: 22992590]

[255 Yang G, Yang X. Smad4-mediated TGF-beta signaling in tumorigenesis. Int J Biol Sci 2010; 6(1): 1-
]   8.[http://dx.doi.org/10.7150/ijbs.6.1] [PMID: 20087440]

[256 Cao Z, Kyprianou N. Mechanisms navigating the TGF-β pathway in prostate cancer. Asian J Urol 2015; 2(1):

]   11-8.[http://dx.doi.org/10.1016/j.ajur.2015.04.011] [PMID: 29051866]

[257   Jones E, Pu H, Kyprianou N. Targeting TGF-beta in prostate cancer: therapeutic possibilities during tumor
]   progression. Expert Opin Ther Targets 2009; 13(2): 227-34.[http://dx.doi.org/10.1517/14728220802705696]
        [PMID: 19236240]

[258   Zhang YE. Non-Smad Signaling Pathways of the TGF-β Family. Cold Spring Harb Perspect Biol 2017; 9(2):
]   9.[http://dx.doi.org/10.1101/cshperspect.a022129] [PMID: 27864313]

[259   Padua D, Massagué J. Roles of TGFbeta in metastasis. Cell Res 2009; 19(1): 89-
]   102.[http://dx.doi.org/10.1038/cr.2008.316] [PMID: 19050696]

[260   Kim ES, Sohn YW, Moon A. TGF-beta-induced transcriptional activation of MMP-2 is mediated by
]   activating transcription factor (ATF)2 in human breast epithelial cells. Cancer Lett 2007; 252(1): 147-
        56.[http://dx.doi.org/10.1016/j.canlet.2006.12.016] [PMID: 17258390]

[261   Xia W, Lo CM, Poon RYC, *et al.* Smad inhibitor induces CSC differentiation for effective
]   chemosensitization in cyclin D1- and TGF-β/Smad-regulated liver cancer stem cell-like cells. Oncotarget
        2017; 8(24): 38811-24.[http://dx.doi.org/10.18632/oncotarget.16402] [PMID: 28415588]

[262   Cardillo MR, Petrangeli E, Perracchio L, Salvatori L, Ravenna L, Di Silverio F. Transforming growth factor-
]   beta expression in prostate neoplasia. Anal Quant Cytol Histol 2000; 22(1): 1-10.[PMID: 10696454]

[263   Kang HY, Lin HK, Hu YC, Yeh S, Huang KE, Chang C. From transforming growth factor-beta signaling to
]   androgen action: identification of Smad3 as an androgen receptor coregulator in prostate cancer cells. Proc
        Natl Acad Sci USA 2001; 98(6): 3018-23.[http://dx.doi.org/10.1073/pnas.061305498] [PMID: 11248024]

[264   Inui S, Itami S. Molecular basis of androgenetic alopecia: From androgen to paracrine mediators through
]   dermal papilla. J Dermatol Sci 2011; 61(1): 1-6.[http://dx.doi.org/10.1016/j.jdermsci.2010.10.015] [PMID:
        21167691]

[265   Wang H, Song K, Sponseller TL, Danielpour D. Novel function of androgen receptor-associated protein
]   55/Hic-5 as a negative regulator of Smad3 signaling. J Biol Chem 2005; 280(7): 5154-
        62.[http://dx.doi.org/10.1074/jbc.M411575200] [PMID: 15561701]

[266   Lamouille S, Xu J, Derynck R. Molecular mechanisms of epithelial-mesenchymal transition. Nat Rev Mol
]   Cell Biol 2014; 15(3): 178-96.[http://dx.doi.org/10.1038/nrm3758] [PMID: 24556840]

[267   Zhu ML, Kyprianou N. Role of androgens and the androgen receptor in epithelial-mesenchymal transition
]   and invasion of prostate cancer cells. FASEB J 2010; 24(3): 769-77.[http://dx.doi.org/10.1096/fj.09-136994]
        [PMID: 19901020]

[268   Liu YN, Liu Y, Lee HJ, Hsu YH, Chen JH. Activated androgen receptor downregulates E-cadherin gene
]   expression and promotes tumor metastasis. Mol Cell Biol 2008; 28(23): 7096-
        108.[http://dx.doi.org/10.1128/MCB.00449-08] [PMID: 18794357]

[269   Butti R, Das S, Gunasekaran VP, Yadav AS, Kumar D, Kundu GC. Receptor tyrosine kinases (RTKs) in
]   breast cancer: signaling, therapeutic implications and challenges. Mol Cancer 2018; 17(1):
        34.[http://dx.doi.org/10.1186/s12943-018-0797-x] [PMID: 29455658]

[270   Di Lorenzo G, Tortora G, D'Armiento FP, *et al.* Expression of epidermal growth factor receptor correlates
]   with disease relapse and progression to androgen-independence in human prostate cancer. Clin Cancer Res
        2002; 8(11): 3438-44.[PMID: 12429632]

[271   Traish AM, Morgentaler A. Epidermal growth factor receptor expression escapes androgen regulation in
]   prostate cancer: a potential molecular switch for tumour growth. Br J Cancer 2009; 101(12): 1949-
        56.[http://dx.doi.org/10.1038/sj.bjc.6605376] [PMID: 19888222]

[272   Shah RB, Ghosh D, Elder JT. Epidermal growth factor receptor (ErbB1) expression in prostate cancer
]   progression: correlation with androgen independence. Prostate 2006; 66(13): 1437-
        44.[http://dx.doi.org/10.1002/pros.20460] [PMID: 16741920]

[273   Pignon JC, Koopmansch B, Nolens G, Delacroix L, Waltregny D, Winkler R. Androgen receptor controls
]   EGFR and ERBB2 gene expression at different levels in prostate cancer cell lines. Cancer Res 2009; 69(7):
        2941-9.[http://dx.doi.org/10.1158/0008-5472.CAN-08-3760] [PMID: 19318561]

[274   Bonaccorsi L, Nosi D, Muratori M, Formigli L, Forti G, Baldi E. Altered endocytosis of epidermal growth
]   factor receptor in androgen receptor positive prostate cancer cell lines. J Mol Endocrinol 2007; 38(1-2): 51-
        66.[http://dx.doi.org/10.1677/jme.1.02155] [PMID: 17242169]

[275   Migliaccio A, Castoria G, Di Domenico M, *et al.* Crosstalk between EGFR and extranuclear steroid
]   receptors. Ann N Y Acad Sci 2006; 1089: 194-200.[http://dx.doi.org/10.1196/annals.1386.006] [PMID:
        17261767]

[276   Nordstrand A, Bergström SH, Thysell E, *et al.* Inhibition of the insulin-like growth factor-1 receptor
]   potentiates acute effects of castration in a rat model for prostate cancer growth in bone. Clin Exp Metastasis

2017; 34(3-4): 261-71.[http://dx.doi.org/10.1007/s10585-017-9848-8] [PMID: 28447314]

[277] Denduluri SK, Idowu O, Wang Z, *et al.* Insulin-like growth factor (IGF) signaling in tumorigenesis and the development of cancer drug resistance. Genes Dis 2015; 2(1): 13-25.[http://dx.doi.org/10.1016/j.gendis.2014.10.004] [PMID: 25984556]

[278] Gennigens C, Menetrier-Caux C, Droz JP. Insulin-Like Growth Factor (IGF) family and prostate cancer. Crit Rev Oncol Hematol 2006; 58(2): 124-45.[http://dx.doi.org/10.1016/j.critrevonc.2005.10.003] [PMID: 16387509]

[279] Sánchez-Tilló E, Lázaro A, Torrent R, *et al.* ZEB1 represses E-cadherin and induces an EMT by recruiting the SWI/SNF chromatin-remodeling protein BRG1. Oncogene 2010; 29(24): 3490-500.[http://dx.doi.org/10.1038/onc.2010.102] [PMID: 20418909]

[280] Mooney SM, Parsana P, Hernandez JR, *et al.* The presence of androgen receptor elements regulates ZEB1 expression in the absence of androgen receptor. J Cell Biochem 2015; 116(1): 115-23.[http://dx.doi.org/10.1002/jcb.24948] [PMID: 25160502]

[281] Wu JD, Haugk K, Woodke L, Nelson P, Coleman I, Plymate SR. Interaction of IGF signaling and the androgen receptor in prostate cancer progression. J Cell Biochem 2006; 99(2): 392-401.[http://dx.doi.org/10.1002/jcb.20929] [PMID: 16639715]

[282] Veikkola T, Karkkainen M, Claesson-Welsh L, Alitalo K. Regulation of angiogenesis *via* vascular endothelial growth factor receptors. Cancer Res 2000; 60(2): 203-12.[PMID: 10667560]

[283] George DJ, Halabi S, Shepard TF, *et al.* Prognostic significance of plasma vascular endothelial growth factor levels in patients with hormone-refractory prostate cancer treated on Cancer and Leukemia Group B 9480. Clin Cancer Res 2001; 7(7): 1932-6.[PMID: 11448906]

[284] Stewart RJ, Panigrahy D, Flynn E, Folkman J. Vascular endothelial growth factor expression and tumor angiogenesis are regulated by androgens in hormone responsive human prostate carcinoma: evidence for androgen dependent destabilization of vascular endothelial growth factor transcripts. J Urol 2001; 165(2): 688-93.[http://dx.doi.org/10.1097/00005392-200102000-00095] [PMID: 11176459]

[285] Eisermann K, Broderick CJ, Bazarov A, Moazam MM, Fraizer GC. Androgen up-regulates vascular endothelial growth factor expression in prostate cancer cells *via* an Sp1 binding site. Mol Cancer 2013; 12: 7.[http://dx.doi.org/10.1186/1476-4598-12-7] [PMID: 23369005]

[286] Christensen JG, Burrows J, Salgia R. c-Met as a target for human cancer and characterization of inhibitors for therapeutic intervention. Cancer Lett 2005; 225(1): 1-26.[http://dx.doi.org/10.1016/j.canlet.2004.09.044] [PMID: 15922853]

[287] Knudsen BS, Edlund M. Prostate cancer and the met hepatocyte growth factor receptor. Adv Cancer Res 2004; 91: 31-67.[http://dx.doi.org/10.1016/S0065-230X(04)91002-0] [PMID: 15327888]

[288] McKay MM, Morrison DK. Integrating signals from RTKs to ERK/MAPK. Oncogene 2007; 26(22): 3113-21.[http://dx.doi.org/10.1038/sj.onc.1210394] [PMID: 17496910]

[289] Oka H, Chatani Y, Kohno M, Kawakita M, Ogawa O. Constitutive activation of the 41- and 43-kDa mitogen-activated protein (MAP) kinases in the progression of prostate cancer to an androgen-independent state. Int J Urol 2005; 12(10): 899-905.[http://dx.doi.org/10.1111/j.1442-2042.2005.01164.x] [PMID: 16323984]

[290] Chmelar R, Buchanan G, Need EF, Tilley W, Greenberg NM. Androgen receptor coregulators and their involvement in the development and progression of prostate cancer. Int J Cancer 2007; 120(4): 719-33.[http://dx.doi.org/10.1002/ijc.22365] [PMID: 17163421]

[291] Lee HJ, Bao J, Miller A, *et al.* Structure-based Discovery of Novel Small Molecule Wnt Signaling Inhibitors by Targeting the Cysteine-rich Domain of Frizzled. J Biol Chem 2015; 290(51): 30596-606.[http://dx.doi.org/10.1074/jbc.M115.673202] [PMID: 26504084]

[292] Lin HK, Yeh S, Kang HY, Chang C. Akt suppresses androgen-induced apoptosis by phosphorylating and inhibiting androgen receptor. Proc Natl Acad Sci USA 2001; 98(13): 7200-5.[http://dx.doi.org/10.1073/pnas.121173298] [PMID: 11404460]

[293] Xu K, Liu P, Wei W. mTOR signaling in tumorigenesis. Biochim Biophys Acta 2014; 1846(2): 638-54.[PMID: 25450580]

[294] Hay N, Sonenberg N. Upstream and downstream of mTOR. Genes Dev 2004; 18(16): 1926-45.[http://dx.doi.org/10.1101/gad.1212704] [PMID: 15314020]

[295] Massie CE, Lynch A, Ramos-Montoya A, *et al.* The androgen receptor fuels prostate cancer by regulating central metabolism and biosynthesis. EMBO J 2011; 30(13): 2719-33.[http://dx.doi.org/10.1038/emboj.2011.158] [PMID: 21602788]

[296] Audet-Walsh É, Dufour CR, Yee T, *et al.* Nuclear mTOR acts as a transcriptional integrator of the androgen signaling pathway in prostate cancer. Genes Dev 2017; 31(12): 1228-

42.[http://dx.doi.org/10.1101/gad.299958.117] [PMID: 28724614]

[297] Haura EB. Journal of thoracic oncology : official publication of the International Association for the Study of Lung Cancer 12006; (2006): 403-5.

[298] Tatarov O, Mitchell TJ, Seywright M, Leung HY, Brunton VG, Edwards J. SRC family kinase activity is up-regulated in hormone-refractory prostate cancer. Clin Cancer Res 2009; 15(10): 3540-9.[http://dx.doi.org/10.1158/1078-0432.CCR-08-1857] [PMID: 19447874]

[299] Cai H, Babic I, Wei X, Huang J, Witte ON. Invasive prostate carcinoma driven by c-Src and androgen receptor synergy. Cancer Res 2011; 71(3): 862-72.[http://dx.doi.org/10.1158/0008-5472.CAN-10-1605] [PMID: 21135112]

[300] Aaronson DS, Horvath CM. A road map for those who don't know JAK-STAT. Science 2002; 296(5573): 1653-5.[http://dx.doi.org/10.1126/science.1071545] [PMID: 12040185]

[301] Siegsmund MJ, Yamazaki H, Pastan I. Interleukin 6 receptor mRNA in prostate carcinomas and benign prostate hyperplasia. J Urol 1994; 151(5): 1396-9.[http://dx.doi.org/10.1016/S0022-5347(17)35267-9] [PMID: 7512667]

[302] Okamoto M, Lee C, Oyasu R. Interleukin-6 as a paracrine and autocrine growth factor in human prostatic carcinoma cells *in vitro*. Cancer Res 1997; 57(1): 141-6.[PMID: 8988055]

[303] Chen T, Wang LH, Farrar WL. Interleukin 6 activates androgen receptor-mediated gene expression through a signal transducer and activator of transcription 3-dependent pathway in LNCaP prostate cancer cells. Cancer Res 2000; 60(8): 2132-5.[PMID: 10786674]

[304] Ueda T, Mawji NR, Bruchovsky N, Sadar MD. Ligand-independent activation of the androgen receptor by interleukin-6 and the role of steroid receptor coactivator-1 in prostate cancer cells. J Biol Chem 2002; 277(41): 38087-94.[http://dx.doi.org/10.1074/jbc.M203313200] [PMID: 12163482]

[305] Lin DL, Whitney MC, Yao Z, Keller ET. Interleukin-6 induces androgen responsiveness in prostate cancer cells through up-regulation of androgen receptor expression. Clin Cancer Res 2001; 7(6): 1773-81.[PMID: 11410519]

[306] Matsuda T, Junicho A, Yamamoto T, *et al.* Cross-talk between signal transducer and activator of transcription 3 and androgen receptor signaling in prostate carcinoma cells. Biochem Biophys Res Commun 2001; 283(1): 179-87.[http://dx.doi.org/10.1006/bbrc.2001.4758] [PMID: 11322786]

[307] Yamamoto T, Sato N, Sekine Y, *et al.* Molecular interactions between STAT3 and protein inhibitor of activated STAT3, and androgen receptor. Biochem Biophys Res Commun 2003; 306(2): 610-5.[http://dx.doi.org/10.1016/S0006-291X(03)01026-X] [PMID: 12804609]

[308] Ara T, Declerck YA. Interleukin-6 in bone metastasis and cancer progression. Eur J Cancer 2010; 46(7): 1223-31.[http://dx.doi.org/10.1016/j.ejca.2010.02.026] [PMID: 20335016]

[309] Rojas A, Liu G, Coleman I, *et al.* IL-6 promotes prostate tumorigenesis and progression through autocrine cross-activation of IGF-IR. Oncogene 2011; 30(20): 2345-55.[http://dx.doi.org/10.1038/onc.2010.605] [PMID: 21258401]

[310] Hu F, Zhao Y, Yu Y, *et al.* Docetaxel-mediated autophagy promotes chemoresistance in castration-resistant prostate cancer cells by inhibiting STAT3. Cancer Lett 2018; 416: 24-30.[http://dx.doi.org/10.1016/j.canlet.2017.12.013] [PMID: 29246644]

[311] Moon RT, Bowerman B, Boutros M, Perrimon N. The promise and perils of Wnt signaling through beta-catenin. Science 2002; 296(5573): 1644-6.[http://dx.doi.org/10.1126/science.1071549] [PMID: 12040179]

[312] Eastman Q, Grosschedl R. Regulation of LEF-1/TCF transcription factors by Wnt and other signals. Curr Opin Cell Biol 1999; 11(2): 233-40.[http://dx.doi.org/10.1016/S0955-0674(99)80031-3] [PMID: 10209158]

[313] Rao TP, Kühl M. An updated overview on Wnt signaling pathways: a prelude for more. Circ Res 2010; 106(12): 1798-806.[http://dx.doi.org/10.1161/CIRCRESAHA.110.219840] [PMID: 20576942]

[314] Wang G, Wang J, Sadar MD. Crosstalk between the androgen receptor and beta-catenin in castrate-resistant prostate cancer. Cancer Res 2008; 68(23): 9918-27.[http://dx.doi.org/10.1158/0008-5472.CAN-08-1718] [PMID: 19047173]

[315] Sun Y, Campisi J, Higano C, *et al.* Treatment-induced damage to the tumor microenvironment promotes prostate cancer therapy resistance through WNT16B. Nat Med 2012; 18(9): 1359-68.[http://dx.doi.org/10.1038/nm.2890] [PMID: 22863786]

[316] Hu W, Wang Z, Zhang S, *et al.* IQGAP1 promotes pancreatic cancer progression and epithelial-mesenchymal transition (EMT) through Wnt/β-catenin signaling. Sci Rep 2019; 9(1): 7539.[http://dx.doi.org/10.1038/s41598-019-44048-y] [PMID: 31101875]

[317] Hayden MS, Ghosh S. Signaling to NF-kappaB. Genes Dev 2004; 18(18): 2195-

]   224.[http://dx.doi.org/10.1101/gad.1228704] [PMID: 15371334]

[318   Sizemore N, Lerner N, Dombrowski N, Sakurai H, Stark GR. Distinct roles of the Ikappa B kinase alpha and
]   beta subunits in liberating nuclear factor kappa B (NF-kappa B) from Ikappa B and in phosphorylating the
         p65 subunit of NF-kappa B. J Biol Chem 2002; 277(6): 3863-9.[http://dx.doi.org/10.1074/jbc.M110572200]
         [PMID: 11733537]

[319   Li Y, Ahmed F, Ali S, Philip PA, Kucuk O, Sarkar FH. Inactivation of nuclear factor kappaB by soy
]   isoflavone genistein contributes to increased apoptosis induced by chemotherapeutic agents in human cancer
         cells. Cancer Res 2005; 65(15): 6934-42.[http://dx.doi.org/10.1158/0008-5472.CAN-04-4604] [PMID:
         16061678]

[320   McCall P, Bennett L, Ahmad I, et al. NFκB signalling is upregulated in a subset of castrate-resistant prostate
]   cancer patients and correlates with disease progression. Br J Cancer 2012; 107(9): 1554-
         63.[http://dx.doi.org/10.1038/bjc.2012.372] [PMID: 23093296]

[321   Ishiguro H, Akimoto K, Nagashima Y, et al. aPKClambda/iota promotes growth of prostate cancer cells in an
]   autocrine manner through transcriptional activation of interleukin-6. Proc Natl Acad Sci USA 2009; 106(38):
         16369-74.[http://dx.doi.org/10.1073/pnas.0907044106] [PMID: 19805306]

[322   Péant B, Diallo JS, Lessard L, et al. Regulation of IkappaB kinase epsilon expression by the androgen
]   receptor and the nuclear factor-kappaB transcription factor in prostate cancer. Mol Cancer Res 2007; 5(1):
         87-94.[http://dx.doi.org/10.1158/1541-7786.MCR-06-0144] [PMID: 17259348]

[323   Péant B, Gilbert S, Le Page C, et al. IκB-Kinase-epsilon (IKKε) over-expression promotes the growth of
]   prostate cancer through the C/EBP-β dependent activation of IL-6 gene expression. Oncotarget 2017; 8(9):
         14487-501.[http://dx.doi.org/10.18632/oncotarget.11629] [PMID: 27577074]

[324   Hutti JE, Shen RR, Abbott DW, et al. Phosphorylation of the tumor suppressor CYLD by the breast cancer
]   oncogene IKKepsilon promotes cell transformation. Mol Cell 2009; 34(4): 461-
         72.[http://dx.doi.org/10.1016/j.molcel.2009.04.031] [PMID: 19481526]

[325   Jin R, Yamashita H, Yu X, et al. Inhibition of NF-kappa B signaling restores responsiveness of castrate-
]   resistant prostate cancer cells to anti-androgen treatment by decreasing androgen receptor-variant expression.
         Oncogene 2015; 34(28): 3700-10.[http://dx.doi.org/10.1038/onc.2014.302] [PMID: 25220414]

[326   J Clin Oncol 2016; 34: 1402-18.[http://dx.doi.org/10.1200/JCO.2015.64.2702] [PMID: 26903579]
]

[327   Hong JH, Kim IY. Nonmetastatic castration-resistant prostate cancer. Korean J Urol 2014; 55(3): 153-
]   60.[http://dx.doi.org/10.4111/kju.2014.55.3.153] [PMID: 24648868]

[328   El-Amm J, Aragon-Ching JB. The Current Landscape of Treatment in Non-Metastatic Castration-Resistant
]   Prostate Cancer. Clin Med Insights Oncol 2019;
         131179554919833927[http://dx.doi.org/10.1177/1179554919833927] [PMID: 30872920]

[329   Chandrasekar T, Yang JC, Gao AC, Evans CP. Mechanisms of resistance in castration-resistant prostate
]   cancer (CRPC). Transl Androl Urol 2015; 4(3): 365-80.[PMID: 26814148]

[330   Sridhar SS, Freedland SJ, Gleave ME, et al. Castration-resistant prostate cancer: from new pathophysiology
]   to new treatment. Eur Urol 2014; 65(2): 289-99.[http://dx.doi.org/10.1016/j.eururo.2013.08.008] [PMID:
         23957948]

[331   Chen Y, Clegg NJ, Scher HI. Anti-androgens and androgen-depleting therapies in prostate cancer: new
]   agents for an established target. Lancet Oncol 2009; 10(10): 981-91.[http://dx.doi.org/10.1016/S1470-
         2045(09)70229-3] [PMID: 19796750]

[332   Teply BA, Hauke RJ. Chemotherapy options in castration-resistant prostate cancer Indian journal of urology :
]   IJU : journal of the Urological Society of India 2016; 32(2016): 262-70.

[333   Rice MA, Malhotra SV, Stoyanova T. Second-Generation Antiandrogens: From Discovery to Standard of
]   Care in Castration Resistant Prostate Cancer. Front Oncol 2019; 9:
         801.[http://dx.doi.org/10.3389/fonc.2019.00801] [PMID: 31555580]

[334   Galsky MD, Dritselis A, Kirkpatrick P, Oh WK. Cabazitaxel. Nat Rev Drug Discov 2010; 9(9): 677-
]   8.[http://dx.doi.org/10.1038/nrd3254] [PMID: 20811375]

[335   de Bono JS, Oudard S, Ozguroglu M, et al. Prednisone plus cabazitaxel or mitoxantrone for metastatic
]   castration-resistant prostate cancer progressing after docetaxel treatment: a randomised open-label trial.
         Lancet 2010; 376(9747): 1147-54.[http://dx.doi.org/10.1016/S0140-6736(10)61389-X] [PMID: 20888992]

[336   Attard G, Reid AH, A'Hern R, et al. Selective inhibition of CYP17 with abiraterone acetate is highly active
]   in the treatment of castration-resistant prostate cancer. J Clin Oncol 2009; 27(23): 3742-
         8.[http://dx.doi.org/10.1200/JCO.2008.20.0642] [PMID: 19470933]

[337   Bedoya DJ, Mitsiades N. Abiraterone acetate, a first-in-class CYP17 inhibitor, establishes a new treatment

[
]	paradigm in castration-resistant prostate cancer. Expert Rev Anticancer Ther 2012; 12(1): 1-3.[http://dx.doi.org/10.1586/era.11.196] [PMID: 22149426]

[338
]	Pal SK, Patel J, He M, *et al.* Identification of mechanisms of resistance to treatment with abiraterone acetate or enzalutamide in patients with castration-resistant prostate cancer (CRPC). Cancer 2018; 124(6): 1216-24.[http://dx.doi.org/10.1002/cncr.31161] [PMID: 29266182]

[339
]	Vasaitis TS, Bruno RD, Njar VC. CYP17 inhibitors for prostate cancer therapy. J Steroid Biochem Mol Biol 2011; 125(1-2): 23-31.[http://dx.doi.org/10.1016/j.jsbmb.2010.11.005] [PMID: 21092758]

[340
]	Luo J, Beer TM, Graff JN. Treatment of Nonmetastatic Castration-Resistant Prostate Cancer, Oncology, 302016.

[341
]	Gul A, Garcia JA, Barata PC. Treatment of non-metastatic castration-resistant prostate cancer: focus on apalutamide. Cancer Manag Res 2019; 11: 7253-62.[http://dx.doi.org/10.2147/CMAR.S165706] [PMID: 31534371]

[342
]	Parker C, Nilsson S, Heinrich D, *et al.* Alpha emitter radium-223 and survival in metastatic prostate cancer. N Engl J Med 2013; 369(3): 213-23.[http://dx.doi.org/10.1056/NEJMoa1213755] [PMID: 23863050]

[343
]	Deshayes E, Roumiguie M, Thibault C, *et al.* Radium 223 dichloride for prostate cancer treatment. Drug Des Devel Ther 2017; 11: 2643-51.[http://dx.doi.org/10.2147/DDDT.S122417] [PMID: 28919714]

[344
]	Parker C, Heidenreich A, Nilsson S, Shore N. Current approaches to incorporation of radium-223 in clinical practice. Prostate Cancer Prostatic Dis 2018; 21(1): 37-47.[http://dx.doi.org/10.1038/s41391-017-0020-y] [PMID: 29298991]

[345
]	Emmett L, Willowson K, Violet J, Shin J, Blanksby A, Lee J. Lutetium [177] PSMA radionuclide therapy for men with prostate cancer: a review of the current literature and discussion of practical aspects of therapy. J Med Radiat Sci 2017; 64(1): 52-60.[http://dx.doi.org/10.1002/jmrs.227] [PMID: 28303694]

[346
]	Kantoff PW, Higano CS, Shore ND, *et al.* Sipuleucel-T immunotherapy for castration-resistant prostate cancer. N Engl J Med 2010; 363(5): 411-22.[http://dx.doi.org/10.1056/NEJMoa1001294] [PMID: 20818862]

[347
]	George DJ, Nabhan C, DeVries T, Whitmore JB, Gomella LG. Survival Outcomes of Sipuleucel-T Phase III Studies: Impact of Control-Arm Cross-Over to Salvage Immunotherapy. Cancer Immunol Res 2015; 3(9): 1063-9.[http://dx.doi.org/10.1158/2326-6066.CIR-15-0006] [PMID: 25943532]

[348
]	Gaya JM, Ahallal Y, Sanchez-Salas R, *et al.* Current, new and novel therapy for castration-resistant prostate cancer. Expert Rev Anticancer Ther 2013; 13(7): 819-27.[http://dx.doi.org/10.1586/14737140.2013.811154] [PMID: 23875660]

[349
]	Knudsen KE, Kelly WK. Outsmarting androgen receptor: creative approaches for targeting aberrant androgen signaling in advanced prostate cancer. Expert Rev Endocrinol Metab 2011; 6(3): 483-93.[http://dx.doi.org/10.1586/eem.11.33] [PMID: 22389648]

[350
]	Oh SJ, Erb HH, Hobisch A, Santer FR, Culig Z. Sorafenib decreases proliferation and induces apoptosis of prostate cancer cells by inhibition of the androgen receptor and Akt signaling pathways. Endocr Relat Cancer 2012; 19(3): 305-19.[http://dx.doi.org/10.1530/ERC-11-0298] [PMID: 22383427]

[351
]	Yamashita S, Lai KP, Chuang KL, *et al.* ASC-J9 suppresses castration-resistant prostate cancer growth through degradation of full-length and splice variant androgen receptors. Neoplasia 2012; 14(1): 74-83.[http://dx.doi.org/10.1593/neo.111436] [PMID: 22355276]

[352
]	Zengerling F, Streicher W, Schrader AJ, *et al.* Effects of sorafenib on C-terminally truncated androgen receptor variants in human prostate cancer cells. Int J Mol Sci 2012; 13(9): 11530-42.[http://dx.doi.org/10.3390/ijms130911530] [PMID: 23109869]

[353
]	Newman DJ, Cragg GM. Natural products as sources of new drugs over the 30 years from 1981 to 2010. J Nat Prod 2012; 75(3): 311-35.[http://dx.doi.org/10.1021/np200906s] [PMID: 22316239]

[354
]	Cragg GM, Newman DJ. Natural products: a continuing source of novel drug leads. Biochim Biophys Acta 2013; 1830(6): 3670-95.[http://dx.doi.org/10.1016/j.bbagen.2013.02.008] [PMID: 23428572]

[355
]	Cheuka PM, Mayoka G, Mutai P, Chibale K. The Role of Natural Products in Drug Discovery and Development against Neglected Tropical Diseases. Molecules 2016; 22(1): 22.[http://dx.doi.org/10.3390/molecules22010058] [PMID: 28042865]

[356
]	Thomford NE, Senthebane DA, Rowe A, *et al.* Natural Products for Drug Discovery in the 21st Century: Innovations for Novel Drug Discovery. Int J Mol Sci 2018; 19(6): 19.[http://dx.doi.org/10.3390/ijms19061578] [PMID: 29799486]

[357
]	Zaynab M, Fatima M, Abbas S, *et al.* Role of secondary metabolites in plant defense against pathogens. Microb Pathog 2018; 124: 198-202.[http://dx.doi.org/10.1016/j.micpath.2018.08.034] [PMID: 30145251]

[358
]	Krishnamurti C, Rao SC. The isolation of morphine by Serturner. Indian J Anaesth 2016; 60(11): 861-

] 2.[http://dx.doi.org/10.4103/0019-5049.193696] [PMID: 27942064]

[359 Sharma P, McClees SF, Afaq F. Pomegranate for Prevention and Treatment of Cancer: An Update.
] Molecules 2017; 22(1): 22.[http://dx.doi.org/10.3390/molecules22010177] [PMID: 28125044]

[360 Periasamy G, Teketelew G, Gebrelibanos M, *et al*. Betulinic acid and its derivatives as anti-cancer agent: a
] review. Arch Appl Sci Res 2014; 6: 47-58.

[361 Hordyjewska A, Ostapiuk A, Horecka A. Betulin and betulinic acid in cancer research. Journal of Pre-
] Clinical and Clinical Research 2018; 12: 72-5.[http://dx.doi.org/10.26444/jpccr/92743]

[362 Shankar E, Zhang A, Franco D, Gupta S. Betulinic acid-mediated apoptosis in human prostate cancer cells
] involves p53 and nuclear factor-kappa B (NF-κB) pathways. Molecules 2017; 22(2):
264.[http://dx.doi.org/10.3390/molecules22020264] [PMID: 28208611]

[363 Zhang X, Hu J, Chen Y. Betulinic acid and the pharmacological effects of tumor suppression (Review). Mol
] Med Rep 2016; 14(5): 4489-95.[http://dx.doi.org/10.3892/mmr.2016.5792] [PMID: 27748864]

[364 Sharma G, Kar S, Palit S, Das PK. 18β-glycyrrhetinic acid induces apoptosis through modulation of
] Akt/FOXO3a/Bim pathway in human breast cancer MCF-7 cells. J Cell Physiol 2012; 227(5): 1923-
31.[http://dx.doi.org/10.1002/jcp.22920] [PMID: 21732363]

[365 Hawthorne S, Gallagher S. Effects of glycyrrhetinic acid and liquorice extract on cell proliferation and
] prostate-specific antigen secretion in LNCaP prostate cancer cells. J Pharm Pharmacol 2008; 60(5): 661-
6.[http://dx.doi.org/10.1211/jpp.60.5.0013] [PMID: 18416944]

[366 Shetty AV, Thirugnanam S, Dakshinamoorthy G, *et al*. 18α-glycyrrhetinic acid targets prostate cancer cells
] by down-regulating inflammation-related genes. Int J Oncol 2011; 39(3): 635-40.[PMID: 21637916]

[367 Hussain H, Green IR, Ali I, *et al*. Ursolic acid derivatives for pharmaceutical use: a patent review (2012-
] 2016). Expert Opin Ther Pat 2017; 27(9): 1061-72.[http://dx.doi.org/10.1080/13543776.2017.1344219]
[PMID: 28637397]

[368 Yang C, Li W, Li C, Zhou Z, Xiao Y, Yan X. Metabolism of ganoderic acids by a Ganoderma lucidum
] cytochrome P450 and the 3-keto sterol reductase ERG27 from yeast. Phytochemistry 2018; 155: 83-
92.[http://dx.doi.org/10.1016/j.phytochem.2018.07.009] [PMID: 30077898]

[369 Gill BS, Navgeet , Mehra R, Kumar V, Kumar S. Ganoderic acid, lanostanoid triterpene: a key player in
] apoptosis. Invest New Drugs 2018; 36(1): 136-43.[http://dx.doi.org/10.1007/s10637-017-0526-0] [PMID:
29081024]

[370 Gill BS, Kumar S, Navgeet . Evaluating anti-oxidant potential of ganoderic acid A in STAT 3 pathway in
] prostate cancer. Mol Biol Rep 2016; 43(12): 1411-22.[http://dx.doi.org/10.1007/s11033-016-4074-z] [PMID:
27640015]

[371 Siddique HR, Mishra SK, Karnes RJ, Saleem M. Lupeol, a novel androgen receptor inhibitor: implications in
] prostate cancer therapy. Clin Cancer Res 2011; 17(16): 5379-91.[http://dx.doi.org/10.1158/1078-0432.CCR-
11-0916] [PMID: 21712449]

[372 Tsai F-S, Lin L-W, Wu C-R. Lupeol and its role in chronic diseases.Drug Discovery from Mother Nature
] 2016145-75.[http://dx.doi.org/10.1007/978-3-319-41342-6_7]

[373 Vithana MD, Singh Z, Johnson SK. Regulation of the levels of health promoting compounds: lupeol,
] mangiferin and phenolic acids in the pulp and peel of mango fruit: a review. J Sci Food Agric 2019; 99(8):
3740-51.[http://dx.doi.org/10.1002/jsfa.9628] [PMID: 30723909]

[374 Huang S-P, Ho T-M, Yang C-W, *et al*. Chemopreventive potential of ethanolic extracts of luobuma leaves
] (Apocynum venetum L.) in androgen insensitive prostate cancer. Nutrients 2017; 9(9):
948.[http://dx.doi.org/10.3390/nu9090948] [PMID: 28846663]

[375 Oh HN, Seo JH, Lee MH, *et al*. Oridonin induces apoptosis in oral squamous cell carcinoma probably
] through the generation of reactive oxygen species and the p38/JNK MAPK pathway. Int J Oncol 2018; 52(5):
1749-59.[http://dx.doi.org/10.3892/ijo.2018.4319] [PMID: 29568920]

[376 Chen S, Gao J, Halicka HD, Traganos F, Darzynkiewicz Z. Down-regulation of androgen-receptor and PSA
] by phytochemicals. Int J Oncol 2008; 32(2): 405-11.[http://dx.doi.org/10.3892/ijo.32.2.405] [PMID:
18202763]

[377 Xia R, Chen SX, Qin Q, *et al*. Oridonin Suppresses Proliferation of Human Ovarian Cancer Cells *via*
] Blockage of mTOR Signaling. Asian Pac J Cancer Prev 2016; 17(2): 667-
71.[http://dx.doi.org/10.7314/APJCP.2016.17.2.667] [PMID: 26925661]

[378 Hu HZ, Yang YB, Xu XD, *et al*. Oridonin induces apoptosis *via* PI3K/Akt pathway in cervical carcinoma
] HeLa cell line. Acta Pharmacol Sin 2007; 28(11): 1819-26.[http://dx.doi.org/10.1111/j.1745-
7254.2007.00667.x] [PMID: 17959034]

[379 Konstat-Korzenny E, Ascencio-Aragón JA, Niezen-Lugo S, Vázquez-López R. Artemisinin and its synthetic
] derivatives as a possible therapy for cancer. Med Sci (Basel) 2018; 6(1): 19.[http://dx.doi.org/10.3390/medsci6010019] [PMID: 29495461]

[380 Steely AM, Willoughby JA, Sr, Sundar SN, Aivaliotis VI, Firestone GL. Artemisinin disrupts androgen
] responsiveness of human prostate cancer cells by stimulating the 26S proteasome-mediated degradation of the androgen receptor protein. Anticancer Drugs 2017; 28(9): 1018-31.[http://dx.doi.org/10.1097/CAD.0000000000000547] [PMID. 28708672]

[381 Camara M, de Cortes Sánchez-Mata M, Fernandez-Ruiz V, Cámara RM, Manzoor S, Caceres JO. Lycopene:
] A review of chemical and biological activity related to beneficial health effects.Studies in natural products chemistry 2013383-426.

[382 Rackley JD, Clark PE, Hall MC. Complementary and alternative medicine for advanced prostate cancer. Urol
] Clin North Am 2006; 33(2): 237-246, viii. [viii.].[http://dx.doi.org/10.1016/j.ucl.2005.12.007] [PMID: 16631462]

[383 Zu K, Mucci L, Rosner BA, et al. Dietary lycopene, angiogenesis, and prostate cancer: a prospective study in
] the prostate-specific antigen era. J Natl Cancer Inst 2014; 106(2)djt430[http://dx.doi.org/10.1093/jnci/djt430] [PMID: 24463248]

[384 Yang CM, Yen YT, Huang CS, Hu ML. Growth inhibitory efficacy of lycopene and β-carotene against
] androgen-independent prostate tumor cells xenografted in nude mice. Mol Nutr Food Res 2011; 55(4): 606-12.[http://dx.doi.org/10.1002/mnfr.201000308] [PMID: 21462328]

[385 Chen ML, Lin YH, Yang CM, Hu ML. Lycopene inhibits angiogenesis both *in vitro* and *in vivo* by inhibiting
] MMP-2/uPA system through VEGFR2-mediated PI3K-Akt and ERK/p38 signaling pathways. Mol Nutr Food Res 2012; 56(6): 889-99.[http://dx.doi.org/10.1002/mnfr.201100683] [PMID: 22707264]

[386 Wan L, Tan HL, Thomas-Ahner JM, et al. Dietary tomato and lycopene impact androgen signaling- and
] carcinogenesis-related gene expression during early TRAMP prostate carcinogenesis. Cancer Prev Res (Phila) 2014; 7(12): 1228-39.[http://dx.doi.org/10.1158/1940-6207.CAPR-14-0182] [PMID: 25315431]

[387 Barber NJ, Barber J. Lycopene and prostate cancer. Prostate Cancer Prostatic Dis 2002; 5(1): 6-
] 12.[http://dx.doi.org/10.1038/sj.pcan.4500560] [PMID: 15195123]

[388 Maldonado E, Torres FR, Martínez M, Pérez-Castorena AL. 18-Acetoxywithanolides from Physalis
] chenopodifolia1. Planta Med 2004; 70(1): 59-64.[http://dx.doi.org/10.1055/s-2004-815457] [PMID: 14765295]

[389 Chen L-X, He H, Qiu F. Natural withanolides: an overview. Nat Prod Rep 2011; 28(4): 705-
] 40.[http://dx.doi.org/10.1039/c0np00045k] [PMID: 21344104]

[390 Xu YM, Bunting DP, Liu MX, Bandaranayake HA, Gunatilaka AA. 17β-Hydroxy-18-acetoxywithanolides
] from aeroponically grown Physalis crassifolia and their potent and selective cytotoxicity for prostate cancer cells. J Nat Prod 2016; 79(4): 821-30.[http://dx.doi.org/10.1021/acs.jnatprod.5b00911] [PMID: 27071003]

[391 Xu Y-M, Liu MX, Grunow N, et al. Discovery of potent 17β-hydroxywithanolides for castration-resistant
] prostate cancer by high-throughput screening of a natural products library for androgen-induced gene expression inhibitors. J Med Chem 2015; 58(17): 6984-93.[http://dx.doi.org/10.1021/acs.jmedchem.5b00867] [PMID: 26305181]

[392 Imran M, Rauf A, Abu-Izneid T, et al. Luteolin, a flavonoid, as an anticancer agent: A review. Biomed
] Pharmacother 2019; 112108612[http://dx.doi.org/10.1016/j.biopha.2019.108612] [PMID: 30798142]

[393 Reipas KM, Law JH, Couto N, et al. Luteolin is a novel p90 ribosomal S6 kinase (RSK) inhibitor that
] suppresses Notch4 signaling by blocking the activation of Y-box binding protein-1 (YB-1). Oncotarget 2013; 4(2): 329-45.[http://dx.doi.org/10.18632/oncotarget.834] [PMID: 23593654]

[394 Zhang J, Kuang Y, Wang Y, Xu Q, Ren Q. Notch-4 silencing inhibits prostate cancer growth and EMT *via*
] the NF-κB pathway. Apoptosis 2017; 22(6): 877-84.[http://dx.doi.org/10.1007/s10495-017-1368-0] [PMID: 28374086]

[395 Han K, Meng W, Zhang JJ, et al. Luteolin inhibited proliferation and induced apoptosis of prostate cancer
] cells through miR-301. OncoTargets Ther 2016; 9: 3085-94.[http://dx.doi.org/10.2147/OTT.S102862] [PMID: 27307749]

[396 Han K, Lang T, Zhang Z, et al. Luteolin attenuates Wnt signaling *via* upregulation of FZD6 to suppress
] prostate cancer stemness revealed by comparative proteomics. Sci Rep 2018; 8(1): 8537.[http://dx.doi.org/10.1038/s41598-018-26761-2] [PMID: 29867083]

[397 Salehi B, Venditti A, Sharifi-Rad M, et al. The therapeutic potential of apigenin. Int J Mol Sci 2019; 20(6):
] 1305.[http://dx.doi.org/10.3390/ijms20061305] [PMID: 30875872]

[398 Shukla S, Kanwal R, Shankar E, et al. Apigenin blocks IKKα activation and suppresses prostate cancer

] progression. Oncotarget 2015; 6(31): 31216-32.[http://dx.doi.org/10.18632/oncotarget.5157] [PMID: 26435478]

[399 Shukla S, MacLennan GT, Flask CA, *et al.* Blockade of beta-catenin signaling by plant flavonoid apigenin
] suppresses prostate carcinogenesis in TRAMP mice. Cancer Res 2007; 67(14): 6925-35.[http://dx.doi.org/10.1158/0008-5472.CAN-07-0717] [PMID: 17638904]

[400 Kaur P, Shukla S, Gupta S. Plant flavonoid apigenin inactivates Akt to trigger apoptosis in human prostate
] cancer: an *in vitro* and *in vivo* study. Carcinogenesis 2008; 29(11): 2210-7.[http://dx.doi.org/10.1093/carcin/bgn201] [PMID: 18725386]

[401 Shukla S, Gupta S. Apigenin suppresses insulin-like growth factor I receptor signaling in human prostate
] cancer: an *in vitro* and *in vivo* study. Mol Carcinog 2009; 48(3): 243-52.[http://dx.doi.org/10.1002/mc.20475] [PMID: 18726972]

[402 Tsai CH, Lin FM, Yang YC, *et al.* Herbal extract of Wedelia chinensis attenuates androgen receptor activity
] and orthotopic growth of prostate cancer in nude mice. Clin Cancer Res 2009; 15(17): 5435-44.[http://dx.doi.org/10.1158/1078-0432.CCR-09-0298] [PMID: 19690196]

[403 Tsai CH, Tzeng SF, Hsieh SC, *et al.* A standardized herbal extract mitigates tumor inflammation and
] augments chemotherapy effect of docetaxel in prostate cancer. Sci Rep 2017; 7(1): 15624.[http://dx.doi.org/10.1038/s41598-017-15934-0] [PMID: 29142311]

[404 Cione E, La Torre C, Cannataro R, Caroleo MC, Plastina P, Gallelli L. Quercetin, Epigallocatechin Gallate,
] Curcumin, and Resveratrol: From Dietary Sources to Human MicroRNA Modulation. Molecules 2019; 25(1): 63.[http://dx.doi.org/10.3390/molecules25010063] [PMID: 31878082]

[405 Rauf A, Patel S, Imran M, *et al.* Honokiol: An anticancer lignan. Biomed Pharmacother 2018; 107: 555-
] 62.[http://dx.doi.org/10.1016/j.biopha.2018.08.054] [PMID: 30114639]

[406 Rauf A, Imran M, Khan IA, *et al.* Anticancer potential of quercetin: A comprehensive review. Phytother Res
] 2018; 32(11): 2109-30.[http://dx.doi.org/10.1002/ptr.6155] [PMID: 30039547]

[407 Hashemzaei M, Delarami Far A, Yari A, *et al.* Anticancer and apoptosis-inducing effects of quercetin *in vitro*
] and *in vivo*. Oncol Rep 2017; 38(2): 819-28.[http://dx.doi.org/10.3892/or.2017.5766] [PMID: 28677813]

[408 Aalinkeel R, Bindukumar B, Reynolds JL, *et al.* The dietary bioflavonoid, quercetin, selectively induces
] apoptosis of prostate cancer cells by down-regulating the expression of heat shock protein 90. Prostate 2008; 68(16): 1773-89.[http://dx.doi.org/10.1002/pros.20845] [PMID: 18726985]

[409 Saporita AJ, Ai J, Wang Z. The Hsp90 inhibitor, 17-AAG, prevents the ligand-independent nuclear
] localization of androgen receptor in refractory prostate cancer cells. Prostate 2007; 67(5): 509-20.[http://dx.doi.org/10.1002/pros.20541] [PMID: 17221841]

[410 Mahmoud AM, Zhu T, Parray A, *et al.* Differential effects of genistein on prostate cancer cells depend on
] mutational status of the androgen receptor. PLoS One 2013; 8(10)e78479[http://dx.doi.org/10.1371/journal.pone.0078479] [PMID: 24167630]

[411 Jagadeesh S, Kyo S, Banerjee PP. Genistein represses telomerase activity *via* both transcriptional and
] posttranslational mechanisms in human prostate cancer cells. Cancer Res 2006; 66(4): 2107-15.[http://dx.doi.org/10.1158/0008-5472.CAN-05-2494] [PMID: 16489011]

[412 Wang G, Zhang D, Yang S, Wang Y, Tang Z, Fu X. Co-administration of genistein with doxorubicin-loaded
] polypeptide nanoparticles weakens the metastasis of malignant prostate cancer by amplifying oxidative damage. Biomater Sci 2018; 6(4): 827-35.[http://dx.doi.org/10.1039/C7BM01201B] [PMID: 29480308]

[413 Hawula ZJ, Wallace DF, Subramaniam VN, Rishi G. Therapeutic Advances in Regulating the
] Hepcidin/Ferroportin Axis. Pharmaceuticals (Basel) 2019; 12(4): 170.[http://dx.doi.org/10.3390/ph12040170] [PMID: 31775259]

[414 Basak S, Pookot D, Noonan EJ, Dahiya R. Genistein down-regulates androgen receptor by modulating
] HDAC6-Hsp90 chaperone function. Mol Cancer Ther 2008; 7(10): 3195-202.[http://dx.doi.org/10.1158/1535-7163.MCT-08-0617] [PMID: 18852123]

[415 Zhang S, Wang Y, Chen Z, *et al.* Genistein enhances the efficacy of cabazitaxel chemotherapy in metastatic
] castration-resistant prostate cancer cells. Prostate 2013; 73(15): 1681-9.[http://dx.doi.org/10.1002/pros.22705] [PMID: 23999913]

[416 Li F, Zhu YF, Chen JY, Zhou J, He YQ, Yu XP. Geinsten inhibits the proliferation of VCaP castration-
] resistant prostate cancer cells Zhonghua nan ke xue = National journal of andrology 2016; 22(2016): 1065-70.

[417 Terzioglu-Usak S, Yildiz MT, Goncu B, Ozten-Kandas N. Achieving the balance: Biphasic effects of
] genistein on PC-3 cells. J Food Biochem 2019; 43(8)e12951[http://dx.doi.org/10.1111/jfbc.12951] [PMID: 31368541]

[418
]
Polachi N, Bai G, Li T, *et al.* Modulatory effects of silibinin in various cell signaling pathways against liver disorders and cancer - A comprehensive review. Eur J Med Chem 2016; 123: 577-95.[http://dx.doi.org/10.1016/j.ejmech.2016.07.070] [PMID: 27517806]

[419
]
Jahanafrooz Z, Motamed N, Rinner B, Mokhtarzadeh A, Baradaran B. Silibinin to improve cancer therapeutic, as an apoptotic inducer, autophagy modulator, cell cycle inhibitor, and microRNAs regulator. Life Sci 2018; 213: 236-47.[http://dx.doi.org/10.1016/j.lfs.2018.10.009] [PMID: 30308184]

[420
]
Deep G, Kumar R, Jain AK, Agarwal C, Agarwal R. Silibinin inhibits fibronectin induced motility, invasiveness and survival in human prostate carcinoma PC3 cells *via* targeting integrin signaling. Mutat Res 2014; 768: 35-46.[http://dx.doi.org/10.1016/j.mrfmmm.2014.05.002] [PMID: 25285031]

[421
]
Kavitha CV, Deep G, Gangar SC, Jain AK, Agarwal C, Agarwal R. Silibinin inhibits prostate cancer cells-and RANKL-induced osteoclastogenesis by targeting NFATc1, NF-κB, and AP-1 activation in RAW264.7 cells. Mol Carcinog 2014; 53(3): 169-80.[http://dx.doi.org/10.1002/mc.21959] [PMID: 23115104]

[422
]
Dinda B, Dinda S, DasSharma S, Banik R, Chakraborty A, Dinda M. Therapeutic potentials of baicalin and its aglycone, baicalein against inflammatory disorders. Eur J Med Chem 2017; 131: 68-80.[http://dx.doi.org/10.1016/j.ejmech.2017.03.004] [PMID: 28288320]

[423
]
Cheng C-S, Chen J, Tan H-Y, Wang N, Chen Z, Feng Y. Scutellaria baicalensis and cancer treatment: Recent progress and perspectives in biomedical and clinical studies. Am J Chin Med 2018; 46(1): 25-54.[http://dx.doi.org/10.1142/S0192415X18500027] [PMID: 29316796]

[424
]
Xu D, Chen Q, Liu Y, Wen X. Baicalein suppresses the androgen receptor (AR)-mediated prostate cancer progression *via* inhibiting the AR N-C dimerization and AR-coactivators interaction. Oncotarget 2017; 8(62): 105561-73.[http://dx.doi.org/10.18632/oncotarget.22319] [PMID: 29285272]

[425
]
Chen S, Ruan Q, Bedner E, *et al.* Effects of the flavonoid baicalin and its metabolite baicalein on androgen receptor expression, cell cycle progression and apoptosis of prostate cancer cell lines. Cell Prolif 2001; 34(5): 293-304.[http://dx.doi.org/10.1046/j.0960-7722.2001.00213.x] [PMID: 11591177]

[426
]
Guo Z, Hu X, Xing Z, *et al.* Baicalein inhibits prostate cancer cell growth and metastasis *via* the caveolin-1/AKT/mTOR pathway. Mol Cell Biochem 2015; 406(1-2): 111-9.[http://dx.doi.org/10.1007/s11010-015-2429-8] [PMID: 25957503]

[427
]
Fu C, Guan G, Wang H. The anticancer effect of sanguinarine: a review. Curr Pharm Des 2018; 24(24): 2760-4.[http://dx.doi.org/10.2174/1381612824666180829100601] [PMID: 30156147]

[428
]
Galadari S, Rahman A, Pallichankandy S, Thayyullathil F. Molecular targets and anticancer potential of sanguinarine-a benzophenanthridine alkaloid. Phytomedicine 2017; 34: 143-53.[http://dx.doi.org/10.1016/j.phymed.2017.08.006] [PMID: 28899497]

[429
]
Luo H, Vong CT, Chen H, *et al.* Naturally occurring anti-cancer compounds: shining from Chinese herbal medicine. Chin Med 2019; 14: 48.[http://dx.doi.org/10.1186/s13020-019-0270-9] [PMID: 31719837]

[430
]
Calvaruso M, Pucci G, Musso R, *et al.* Nutraceutical Compounds as Sensitizers for Cancer Treatment in Radiation Therapy. Int J Mol Sci 2019; 20(21): 5267.[http://dx.doi.org/10.3390/ijms20215267] [PMID: 31652849]

[431
]
Cha T-L, Qiu L, Chen C-T, Wen Y, Hung M-C. Emodin down-regulates androgen receptor and inhibits prostate cancer cell growth. Cancer Res 2005; 65(6): 2287-95.[http://dx.doi.org/10.1158/0008-5472.CAN-04-3250] [PMID: 15781642]

[432
]
Kallifatidis G, Hoy JJ, Lokeshwar BL. Bioactive natural products for chemoprevention and treatment of castration-resistant prostate cancer.Seminars in cancer biology 2016160-9.[http://dx.doi.org/10.1016/j.semcancer.2016.06.003]

[433
]
Ok S, Kim SM, Kim C, *et al.* Emodin inhibits invasion and migration of prostate and lung cancer cells by downregulating the expression of chemokine receptor CXCR4. Immunopharmacol Immunotoxicol 2012; 34(5): 768-78.[http://dx.doi.org/10.3109/08923973.2012.654494] [PMID: 22299827]

[434
]
Jasiński M, Jasińska L, Ogrodowczyk M. Resveratrol in prostate diseases - a short review. Cent European J Urol 2013; 66(2): 144-9.[PMID: 24579014]

[435
]
Rauf A, Imran M, Butt MS, Nadeem M, Peters DG, Mubarak MS. Resveratrol as an anti-cancer agent: A review. Crit Rev Food Sci Nutr 2018; 58(9): 1428-47.[http://dx.doi.org/10.1080/10408398.2016.1263597] [PMID: 28001084]

[436
]
Jang Y-G, Go R-E, Hwang K-A, Choi K-C. Resveratrol inhibits DHT-induced progression of prostate cancer cell line through interfering with the AR and CXCR4 pathway. J Steroid Biochem Mol Biol 2019; 192105406[http://dx.doi.org/10.1016/j.jsbmb.2019.105406] [PMID: 31185279]

[437
]
Al Aameri RFH, Sheth S, Alanisi EMA, *et al.* Tonic suppression of PCAT29 by the IL-6 signaling pathway in prostate cancer: Reversal by resveratrol. PLoS One 2017;

12(5)e0177198[http://dx.doi.org/10.1371/journal.pone.0177198] [PMID: 28467474]

[438] Benitez DA, Hermoso MA, Pozo-Guisado E, Fernández-Salguero PM, Castellón EA. Regulation of cell survival by resveratrol involves inhibition of NF κ B-regulated gene expression in prostate cancer cells. Prostate 2009; 69(10): 1045-54.[http://dx.doi.org/10.1002/pros.20953] [PMID: 19301309]

[439] López-Guarnido O, Urquiza-Salvat N, Saiz M, et al. Bioactive compounds of the Mediterranean diet and prostate cancer. Aging Male 2018; 21(4): 251-60.[http://dx.doi.org/10.1080/13685538.2018.1430129] [PMID: 29375002]

[440] Elshaer M, Chen Y, Wang XJ, Tang X. Resveratrol: An overview of its anti-cancer mechanisms. Life Sci 2018; 207: 340-9.[http://dx.doi.org/10.1016/j.lfs.2018.06.028] [PMID: 29959028]

[441] Harper CE, Patel BB, Wang J, Arabshahi A, Eltoum IA, Lamartiniere CA. Resveratrol suppresses prostate cancer progression in transgenic mice. Carcinogenesis 2007; 28(9): 1946-53.[http://dx.doi.org/10.1093/carcin/bgm144] [PMID: 17675339]

[442] Banik K, Ranaware AM, Deshpande V, et al. Honokiol for cancer therapeutics: A traditional medicine that can modulate multiple oncogenic targets. Pharmacol Res 2019; 144: 192-209.[http://dx.doi.org/10.1016/j.phrs.2019.04.004] [PMID: 31002949]

[443] Ong CP, Lee WL, Tang YQ, Yap WH. Honokiol: A Review of Its Anticancer Potential and Mechanisms. Cancers (Basel) 2019; 12(1): 48.[http://dx.doi.org/10.3390/cancers12010048] [PMID: 31877856]

[444] Shigemura K, Arbiser JL, Sun SY, et al. Honokiol, a natural plant product, inhibits the bone metastatic growth of human prostate cancer cells. Cancer 2007; 109(7): 1279-89.[http://dx.doi.org/10.1002/cncr.22551] [PMID: 17326044]

[445] Kong Z-L, Tzeng S-C, Liu Y-C. Cytotoxic neolignans: an SAR study. Bioorg Med Chem Lett 2005; 15(1): 163-6.[http://dx.doi.org/10.1016/j.bmcl.2004.10.011] [PMID: 15582432]

[446] Hahm ER, Karlsson AI, Bonner MY, Arbiser JL, Singh SV. Honokiol inhibits androgen receptor activity in prostate cancer cells. Prostate 2014; 74(4): 408-20.[http://dx.doi.org/10.1002/pros.22762] [PMID: 24338950]

[447] Halasi M, Hitchinson B, Shah BN, et al. Honokiol is a FOXM1 antagonist. Cell Death Dis 2018; 9(2): 84.[http://dx.doi.org/10.1038/s41419-017-0156-7] [PMID: 29367668]

[448] Mantzorou M, Pavlidou E, Vasios G, Tsagalioti E, Giaginis C. Effects of curcumin consumption on human chronic diseases: A narrative review of the most recent clinical data. Phytother Res 2018; 32(6): 957-75.[http://dx.doi.org/10.1002/ptr.6037] [PMID: 29468820]

[449] Schmidt KT, Figg WD. The potential role of curcumin in prostate cancer: the importance of optimizing pharmacokinetics in clinical studies. Transl Cancer Res 2016; 5 (Suppl. 6): S1107-10.[http://dx.doi.org/10.21037/tcr.2016.11.04] [PMID: 30613476]

[450] Choi HY, Lim JE, Hong JH. Curcumin interrupts the interaction between the androgen receptor and Wnt/β-catenin signaling pathway in LNCaP prostate cancer cells. Prostate Cancer Prostatic Dis 2010; 13(4): 343-9.[http://dx.doi.org/10.1038/pcan.2010.26] [PMID: 20680030]

[451] Tomeh MA, Hadianamrei R, Zhao X. A review of curcumin and its derivatives as anticancer agents. Int J Mol Sci 2019; 20(5): 1033.[http://dx.doi.org/10.3390/ijms20051033] [PMID: 30818786]

[452] Hour TC, Chen J, Huang CY, Guan JY, Lu SH, Pu YS. Curcumin enhances cytotoxicity of chemotherapeutic agents in prostate cancer cells by inducing p21(WAF1/CIP1) and C/EBPbeta expressions and suppressing NF-kappaB activation. Prostate 2002; 51(3): 211-8.[http://dx.doi.org/10.1002/pros.10089] [PMID: 11967955]

[453] Mori A, Lehmann S, O'Kelly J, et al. Capsaicin, a component of red peppers, inhibits the growth of androgen-independent, p53 mutant prostate cancer cells. Cancer Res 2006; 66(6): 3222-9.[http://dx.doi.org/10.1158/0008-5472.CAN-05-0087] [PMID: 16540674]

[454] Díaz-Laviada I. Effect of capsaicin on prostate cancer cells. Future Oncol 2010; 6(10): 1545-50.[http://dx.doi.org/10.2217/fon.10.117] [PMID: 21062154]

[455] Zhu M, Yu X, Zheng Z, Huang J, Yang X, Shi H. Capsaicin suppressed activity of prostate cancer stem cells by inhibition of Wnt/β-catenin pathway. Phytother Res 2019.[PMID: 31782192]

[456] Cho S-C, Lee H, Choi BY. An updated review on molecular mechanisms underlying the anticancer effects of capsaicin. Food Sci Biotechnol 2017; 26(1): 1-13.[http://dx.doi.org/10.1007/s10068-017-0001-x] [PMID: 30263503]

[457] Friedman JR, Nolan NA, Brown KC, et al. Anticancer activity of natural and synthetic capsaicin analogs. J Pharmacol Exp Ther 2018; 364(3): 462-73.[http://dx.doi.org/10.1124/jpet.117.243691] [PMID: 29246887]

[458] Guerra B, Issinger O-G. Natural compounds and derivatives as Ser/Thr protein kinase modulators and inhibitors. Pharmaceuticals (Basel) 2019; 12(1): 4.[http://dx.doi.org/10.3390/ph12010004] [PMID:

30609679]

[459] Sarveswaran S, Gautam SC, Ghosh J. Wedelolactone, a medicinal plant-derived coumestan, induces caspase-dependent apoptosis in prostate cancer cells *via* downregulation of PKCε without inhibiting Akt. Int J Oncol 2012; 41(6): 2191-9.[http://dx.doi.org/10.3892/ijo.2012.1664] [PMID: 23076676]

[460] Sarveswaran S, Gautam S, Ghosh J. Wedelolactone, a medicinal plant-derived coumestan, induces caspase-dependent apoptosis in prostate cancer cells *via* down-regulation of PKC-epsilon without inhibiting Akt. 2013.

[461] Lee PMY, Ng CF, Liu ZM, *et al.* Reduced prostate cancer risk with green tea and epigallocatechin 3-gallate intake among Hong Kong Chinese men. Prostate Cancer Prostatic Dis 2017; 20(3): 318-22.[http://dx.doi.org/10.1038/pcan.2017.18] [PMID: 28417981]

[462] Yeo C, Han DS, Lee HJ, Lee EO. Epigallocatechin-3-Gallate Suppresses Vasculogenic Mimicry through Inhibiting the Twist/VE-Cadherin/AKT Pathway in Human Prostate Cancer PC-3 Cells. Int J Mol Sci 2020; 21(2): 21.[http://dx.doi.org/10.3390/ijms21020439] [PMID: 31936664]

[463] Chen J, Zhang L, Li C, Chen R, Liu C, Chen M. Lipophilized Epigallocatechin Gallate Derivative Exerts Anti-Proliferation Efficacy through Induction of Cell Cycle Arrest and Apoptosis on DU145 Human Prostate Cancer Cells. Nutrients 2019; 12(1): 12.[http://dx.doi.org/10.3390/nu12010092] [PMID: 31905647]

[464] Khan N, Bharali DJ, Adhami VM, *et al.* Oral administration of naturally occurring chitosan-based nanoformulated green tea polyphenol EGCG effectively inhibits prostate cancer cell growth in a xenograft model. Carcinogenesis 2014; 35(2): 415-23.[http://dx.doi.org/10.1093/carcin/bgt321] [PMID: 24072771]

[465] Zeng Y, Ma J, Xu L, Wu D. Natural product gossypol and its derivatives in precision cancer medicine. Curr Med Chem 2019; 26(10): 1849-73.[http://dx.doi.org/10.2174/0929867324666170523123655] [PMID: 28545375]

[466] Xu J, Zhu G-Y, Cao D, Pan H, Li Y-W. Gossypol overcomes EGFR-TKIs resistance in non-small cell lung cancer cells by targeting YAP/TAZ and EGFR$^{L858R/T790M}$. Biomed Pharmacother 2019; 115108860[http://dx.doi.org/10.1016/j.biopha.2019.108860] [PMID: 31055235]

[467] Lu Y, Li J, Dong C-E, Huang J, Zhou H-B, Wang W. Recent advances in gossypol derivatives and analogs: a chemistry and biology view. Future Med Chem 2017; 9(11): 1243-75.[http://dx.doi.org/10.4155/fmc-2017-0046] [PMID: 28722469]

[468] Jin CL, Chen ML, Wang Y, Kang XC, Han GY, Xu SL. Preparation of novel (-)-gossypol nanoparticles and the effect on growth inhibition in human prostate cancer PC-3 cells *in vitro*. Exp Ther Med 2015; 9(3): 675-8.[http://dx.doi.org/10.3892/etm.2015.2172] [PMID: 25667612]

[469] Aggarwal M, Saxena R, Asif N, *et al.* p53 mutant-type in human prostate cancer cells determines the sensitivity to phenethyl isothiocyanate induced growth inhibition. J Exp Clin Cancer Res 2019; 38(1): 307.[http://dx.doi.org/10.1186/s13046-019-1267-z] [PMID: 31307507]

[470] Singh KB, Hahm ER, Rigatti LH, Normolle DP, Yuan JM, Singh SV. Inhibition of Glycolysis in Prostate Cancer Chemoprevention by Phenethyl Isothiocyanate. Cancer Prev Res (Phila) 2018; 11(6): 337-46.[http://dx.doi.org/10.1158/1940-6207.CAPR-17-0389] [PMID: 29545400]

[471] Ceci C, Lacal PM, Tentori L, De Martino MG, Miano R, Graziani G. Experimental evidence of the antitumor, antimetastatic and antiangiogenic activity of ellagic acid. Nutrients 2018; 10(11): 1756.[http://dx.doi.org/10.3390/nu10111756] [PMID: 30441769]

[472] Gupta P, Mohammad T, Khan P, *et al.* Evaluation of ellagic acid as an inhibitor of sphingosine kinase 1: A targeted approach towards anticancer therapy. Biomed Pharmacother 2019; 118109245[http://dx.doi.org/10.1016/j.biopha.2019.109245] [PMID: 31352240]

[473] Singh SK, Apata T, Gordetsky JB, Singh R. Docetaxel Combined with Thymoquinone Induces Apoptosis in Prostate Cancer Cells *via* Inhibition of the PI3K/AKT Signaling Pathway. Cancers (Basel) 2019; 11(9): 11.[http://dx.doi.org/10.3390/cancers11091390] [PMID: 31540423]

[474] Imran M, Rauf A, Khan IA, *et al.* Thymoquinone: A novel strategy to combat cancer: A review. Biomed Pharmacother 2018; 106: 390-402.[http://dx.doi.org/10.1016/j.biopha.2018.06.159] [PMID: 29966985]

[475] Roell D, Baniahmad A. The natural compounds atraric acid and N-butylbenzene-sulfonamide as antagonists of the human androgen receptor and inhibitors of prostate cancer cell growth. Mol Cell Endocrinol 2011; 332(1-2): 1-8.[http://dx.doi.org/10.1016/j.mce.2010.09.013] [PMID: 20965230]

[476] Komakech R, Kang Y, Lee J-H, Omujal F. A review of the potential of phytochemicals from Prunus africana (Hook f.) Kalkman stem bark for chemoprevention and chemotherapy of prostate cancer. Evid Based Complement Alternat Med 2017; 20173014019[http://dx.doi.org/10.1155/2017/3014019] [PMID: 28286531]

[477] Li Y, Sarkar FH. Role of BioResponse 3, 3′-diindolylmethane in the treatment of human prostate cancer:

[   ] clinical experience. Med Princ Pract 2016; 25 (Suppl. 2): 11-7.[http://dx.doi.org/10.1159/000439307] [PMID: 26501150]

[478] Sunkari S, Bonam SR, Rao AVS, *et al.* Synthesis and biological evaluation of new bisindole-imidazopyridine hybrids as apoptosis inducers. Bioorg Chem 2019; 87: 484-94.[http://dx.doi.org/10.1016/j.bioorg.2019.03.061] [PMID: 30927589]

[479] Draz H, Goldberg AA, Tomlinson Guns ES, Fazli L, Safe S, Sanderson JT. Autophagy inhibition improves the chemotherapeutic efficacy of cruciferous vegetable-derived diindolymethane in a murine prostate cancer xenograft model. Invest New Drugs 2018; 36(4): 718-25.[http://dx.doi.org/10.1007/s10637-018-0595-8] [PMID: 29607466]

[480] Singh D, Arora R, Bhatia A, Singh H, Singh B, Arora S. Molecular targets in cancer prevention by 4-(methylthio)butyl isothiocyanate - A comprehensive review. Life Sci 2020; 241117061[http://dx.doi.org/10.1016/j.lfs.2019.117061] [PMID: 31794774]

[481] Khurana N, Kim H, Chandra PK, *et al.* Multimodal actions of the phytochemical sulforaphane suppress both AR and AR-V7 in 22Rv1 cells: Advocating a potent pharmaceutical combination against castration-resistant prostate cancer. Oncol Rep 2017; 38(5): 2774-86.[http://dx.doi.org/10.3892/or.2017.5932] [PMID: 28901514]

Inhibition of Key Protein-Protein Interactions by Small Molecules for Cancer Drug Design

Aykut Özgür[1], Lütfi Tutar[2], Mehmet Gümüş[3], İrfan Koca[4], [*], Servet Tunoğlu[5], Ezgi Nurdan Yenilmez Tunoğlu[5], Yusuf Tutar[6], [7], [*]

[1] Tokat Gaziosmanpaşa University, Artova Vocational School, Department of Veterinary Medicine, Laboratory and Veterinary Health Program, Tokat, Turkey

[2] Ahi Evran University, Faculty of Science, Department of Molecular Biology and Genetics, Kırşehir, Turkey

[3] Yozgat Bozok University, Akdağmadeni Health College, Yozgat, Turkey

[4] Yozgat Bozok University, Faculty of Arts and Sciences, Department of Chemistry, Yozgat, Turkey

[5] Istanbul University, Aziz Sancar Institutes of Health, Division of Molecular Medicine, Istanbul, Turkey

[6] University of Health Sciences, Hamidiye Institute of Health Sciences, Division of Molecular Oncology, Istanbul, Turkey

[7] Hamidiye Faculty of Pharmacy, Department of Basic Pharmaceutical Sciences, Division of Biochemistry, Istanbul, Turkey

Abstract

Human genome sequencing has revealed the complex nature of the human proteome. Researchers have been focused on mapping the proteome to find the right target for drug design. Inhibition of target proteins may be complemented by redundant forms of the proteins in the pathogenesis of diseases. Therefore, it is important to determine key proteins and their coordinating and/or cooperating partner proteins in protein pathways to design innovative chemotherapeutics. Computational and experimental studies indicated that approximately 200.000 protein-protein interactions (PPIs) have been predicted, with only about 8% identified in humans. PPIs play key roles in many important cellular processes, and

104

especially their up-regulation is closely associated with each step of the tumurogenesis in cancer cells. Therefore, the identification of protein interactions helps researchers to design drugs for target specific cancer treatment. To understand the relations between tumorigenesis and p53-MDM2, c-MYC-MAX, Bcl-2/Bcl-xL, Hsp90-Hsp70, β-catenin-TCF4, and Menin-MLL interactions are an important approach to design specific chemotherapeutics for

the treatment of individuals with cancer. This work focuses on key protein interactions on protein signaling pathways and designed inhibitors at these specific junctions in the literature.

Keywords: Apoptosis, Cancer, Drug design, Oncology, Protein-protein interactions.

*** Corresponding authors Yusuf Tutar:** University of Health Sciences, Hamidiye Institute of Health Sciences, Department of Molecular Medicine, İstanbul, Turkey; Tel: +90 216 418 96 16, Fax: +90 216 418 96 20; E-mail: yusuf.tutar@sbu.edu.tr & **İrfan KOCA:** Yozgat Bozok University, Faculty of Arts and Sciences, Department of Chemistry, Yozgat, Turkey; Tel: +90 543 513 67 65, Fax: +90 543 513 67 65; E-mail: koca.irfan@gmail.com

INTRODUCTION

PPIs control essential cellular processes that are involved in several biochemical events such as receptor-ligand interactions, down-stream cell signaling cascade, and DNA transcription initiation [1, 2]. Interestingly, protein isoforms or their family members can display adverse effects from pro-apoptotic to anti-apoptotic response. This diverse function may be performed by coordinating with different partner proteins. Further, isoform or other members of the protein family may complement inhibited target protein function [3, 4]. These escape strategies provide an opportunity for cancer cells to bypass a metabolic barrier. Shortcuts and bypass mechanisms of metabolic diseases have yet to be elucidated, but key interactions must be targeted. However, current strategies focus on specific PPIs where the function is explicitly defined, and inhibition of the sites block desired metabolic event. Since several functions involve PPI complexes, inhibition of this process has gleaned interest in drug design of several human diseases. Genomics and proteomics studies revealed key PPIs targets for metabolic processes: c-Myc-

Max, p53-MDM2, Bcl-2/Bcl-xL, β-Catenin/TCF4, Hsp90-Hsp70, and MENIN-MLL. The interaction networks reorganize in different diseases, and further, mutations that inhibit protein function may impact PPI networks [5⁻10]. Pharmaceutical studies to decipher PPI networks have been extensively searched by the pharmaceutical industry and research groups.

During the past century, many PPIs inhibitors have been clinically successful in the treatment of autoimmune diseases (abatacept, belatacept, and belimumab) and cancer (ipilimumab, nivolumab, pembrolizumab, atezolizumab, durvalumab, and avelumab) [11]. Designing small molecules to inhibit PPIs is a difficult task since many limitations are present to design target specific PPIs inhibitors. PPIs are stabilized by large interfaces, and further, these interfaces have a variety of binding sites. Allosteric changes help PPI, and perturbation of allosteric changes by a small molecule leads to loss of interaction with a partner protein. However, many inhibitors have not been reported yet [12, 13]. Mutational analysis of protein interfaces indicated that some critical residues (hot spots) at the PPI interface play vital roles in the binding of small inhibitors. These residues show a tendency to localization at the center of the interface, to be hydrophobic, and to show conformational adaptivity. Most of the clinical-stage inhibitors are designed that target PPI where the hot spot residues are clustered in a small binding site. Therefore, experimental assays have been developed to analyze critical residues in PPIs-based drug design studies [14, 15]. Critical residues at the PPIs interface can be detected by the alanine scanning approach in which target residue is converted to functionally "inert" amino acid alanine. Alanine scanning technique monitors the effect of interfacial residue mutations, and alterations of key residues may have major destabilizing effects. These hot spots may also be detected by *in silico* analysis, and the sites are critical in drug design [16, 17].

In this study, we focus on the biological activities of the significant PPIs and therapeutic activities of small inhibitors of the PPIs in target specific cancer drug discovery.

p53-MDM2 INTERACTION

Transcription factor p53 controls a major cellular pathway and prevents cancer development as a tumor suppressor. p53 is activated upon oncogenic stress and plays vital roles in the regulation of apoptosis, DNA repair, and cell cycle-related genes. Activation of p53 leads to cell cycle arrest, and this function plays an essential role in cancer protection. The arrest provides enough time for the repair mechanism to complete its function, and then cells are pushed to mitosis and replication. p53 also participates in the DNA repair mechanism, and if DNA cannot be repaired then, p53 drives the cell to apoptosis. Thus, this prevents potentially carcinogenic damaged DNA expansion. Since p53 is a tumor suppressor, it is inactivated in most cancer types. Modulating p53 activation by interfering with its regulation by mouse double minute (MDM2) is a potentially neat strategy for drug design research [18‑20].

At the normal state of cells, MDM2 protein negatively regulates p53 protein. If p53 level increases, MDM2 binds to p53 and inhibits its transactivation domain activity. Further, MDM2 is an E3 ligase and targets p53-ubiquitin dependent degradation (Fig. 1). MDM2 regulates p53 stability and activity, and several human cancer cells overproduce MDM2. The MDM2-p53 feedback loop is deregulated in cancer cells overexpressing MDM2 that leads to inefficient growth arrest and/or apoptosis. Therefore, blocking p53-MDM2 interaction releases p53 and restores its cell cycle arrest and pro-apoptotic activity [21‑23]. Small molecule designs to perturb this interaction have drawn the attention of the pharmaceutical industry.

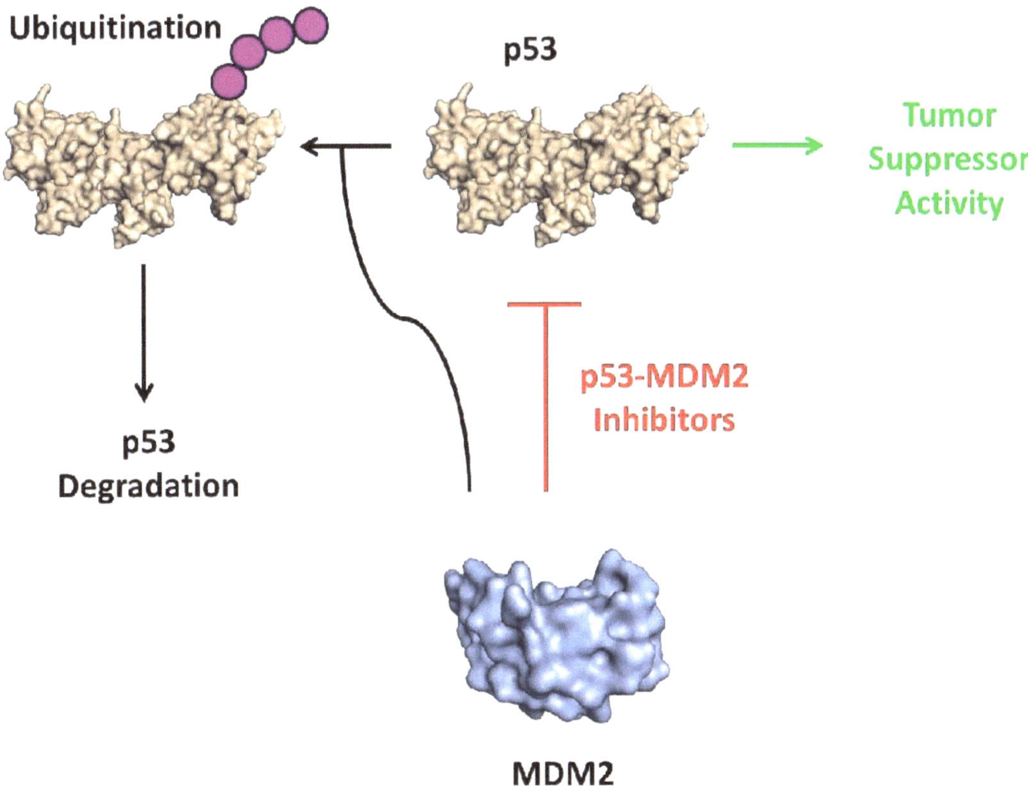

Fig. (1))

Interaction of p53-MDM2 and its inhibition with inhibitors.

Small-Molecule Inhibitors of the p53–MDM2 Interaction

p53 is a tumor suppressor nuclear transcription factor and induces apoptosis and regulates the cellular response to DNA damage in cancer cells. The MDM2 protein is a potent negative regulator of the p53, and aberrant expression of MDM2 plays significant roles in tumorigenesis and drug resistance. MDM2 binds to the p53 and MDM2-p53 complex masks the p53 transcription activation region and decreases p53 activity [18, 24]. Therefore, the development of MDM2-p53 inhibitors has been a significant therapeutic aspect in target specific cancer drug design. To date, numerous compounds have been evaluated as MDM2-p53 inhibitors in pre-clinical and clinical studies against a wide variety of cancer types [24-26].

Nutlins are a class of cis-imidazoline derivative small compounds, which are the first selective and potent small-molecule inhibitors of p53-MDM2 activity (Fig. 2). Nutlins inhibit the interaction between p53 and MDM2 and stabilize p53 activity in cancer cells. To date, anticancer activities of the nutlins (particularly Nutlin-3) have been evaluated against a wide variety of cancer types *in vitro* and *in vivo* studies. Subsequently, Hoffman–La Roche company has developed more effective and selective alternative compounds (RG7112 and RG-7388) to Nutlin in cancer treatment [27-29].

Structure of Nutlin.

RG7112 (formerly RO5045337) and RG7388 (formerly R05503781) (Fig. 3) are orally bioavailable p53-MDM2 inhibitors that selectively interact with the p53 pocket on the surface of MDM2 [29, 30]. Among p53-MDM2 inhibitors, RG7112 is the first clinical evaluated inhibitor in clinical cancer studies. According to clinical phase-I studies, RG7112 exhibited potent anticancer activity in patients with hematologic malignancies and advanced solid tumors [31]. In a pre-clinical study, Vu and co-workers reported the optimization working that led to the exploration of a new member of the Nutlin family of this MDM2 inhibitor. In this study combination of dimethyl substitution of the imidazoline scaffold and modification of the methoxy group by tertbutyl group led to the exploration of MDM2 inhibitor [32]. RG7388 is second-generation clinical inhibitor that inhibits p53-MDM2 interaction selectively [29]. In osteosarcoma xenografts in nude mice, RG7388 inhibits p53-MDM2 binding and activates p53 activity, leading to stimulation of cell cycle arrest and apoptosis [33]. RG7388 is undergoing clinical phase-I studies in patients with acute myeloid leukemia, multiple myeloma, neuroblastoma, non-small cell lung cancer, colorectal cancer, and glioblastoma [34].

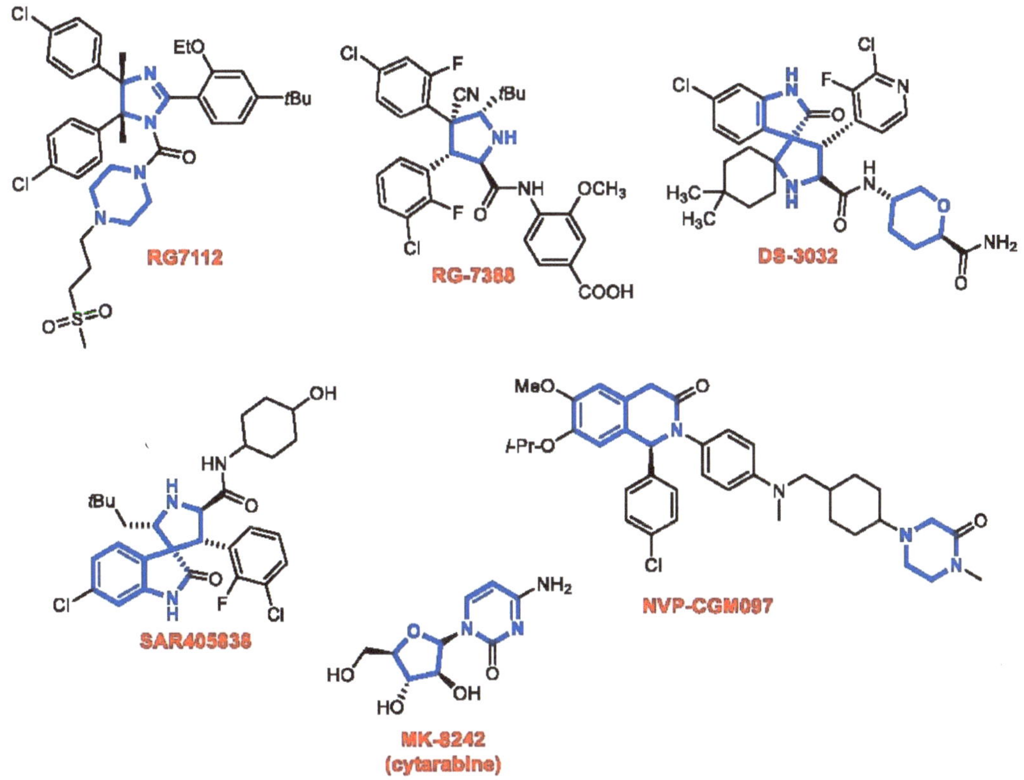

Fig. (3))
Structure of important p53-MDM2 inhibitors.

SAR405838 (Fig. 3) is an orally available spirooxindole derivative that selectively shows antagonist effect against p53-MDM2 activity [35]. Anticancer activities of the SAR405838 have been tested in pre-clinical and clinical studies as a p53-MDM2 inhibitor. To characterize the pharmacokinetic profile, SAR405838 was tested in clinical phase-I studies on patients with solid tumors alone and in combination with pimasertib [36]. To understand acquired resistance mechanisms of the SAR405838, several mutations of the p53 were observed in leukemia and osteosarcoma cells [37].

Holzer and collaborators developed a potent, selective, and new clinical candidate p53-MDM2 inhibitor (NVP-CGM097), which is a dihydroisoquinolinone derivative for treating cancer (Fig. 3). NVP-CGM097 was identified as an MDM2 inhibitor, and pharmacokinetic and pharmacodynamic properties of NVP-CGM097, mechanism of action, scientific rationale, binding mode, *in vivo* pharmacology/toxicology properties were reported in preclinical study. Furthermore, this p53-MDM2 inhibitor is recently undergoing phase 1 clinical trials in patients with advanced solid tumors [38].

MK-8242 (cytrabine) (Fig. 3) is an orally bioavailable HDM2 (human homolog of murine double minute 2) inhibitor including 3,4-dihydropyrimidine and tetrahydrofuran scaffolds. MK-8242 inhibits the binding of the HDM2 protein to the p53 and stimulates apoptosis in cancer cells. MK-8242 was evaluated in the clinical phase-I study for the treatment of acute myelogenous leukemia (AML) and advanced solid tumors by Merck Sharp & Dohme Corp. MK-8242 was administrated orally twice a day on days 1 to 7 in 21-day cycles in wild-type TP53 advanced solid tumors patients [39]. At the recommended phase II dose of 400 mg twice a day, MK-8242 induced the p53 pathway with acceptable safety. Available data and the observed clinical activity contributed to further study of HDM2 inhibitors in liposarcoma [40].

AM-8553 and AMG-232 are potent MDM2-p53 inhibitors bearing a piperidinone scaffold (Fig. 4). Upon oral administration, AM-8553 and AMG-232 bind to the MDM2 and prevent its binding to the transcriptional activation domain of the p53. Among piperidinone derivative compounds, AMG-232 has a high potential to inhibit MDM2–p53 interaction in pre-clinical and clinical studies [41]. *In vitro* and *in vivo* studies reported that AMG-232 interacts with the MDM2 with picomolar affinity (K_D: 450 pM) and inhibits cancer cell proliferation, and provides cell-cycle arrest with activation of p53 [41, 42]. Clinical phase-I studies of the AMG-232 was employed in patients with acute myeloid leukemia and multiple myeloma alone and in combinations with other FDA-approved drugs. In the recently completed clinical phase-II study, anticancer activity of the AMG-232 was evaluated in mctastatic melanoma alone and in combinations with trametinib and dabrafenib. Moreover, the clinical efficiency of the AMG-232 is being tested in patients with acute myeloid leukemia, brain cancer, multiple myeloma, and soft tissue sarcoma [43].

Fig. (4))
Structure of AM-8553 and AMG-232.

c-MYC-MAX INTERACTION

c-Myc, L-Myc, S-Myc, and N-Myc are important members of the Myc protein family and regulate cell cycle progression, apoptosis, and cellular transformation in cancer cells. c-Myc is defined as proto-oncogene, and overexpression of the c-Myc is associated with poor prognosis of cancer cells. To perform biological functions, c-Myc require heterodimerization with its activation partner Max. However, recent findings indicate that c-Myc is also involved in biological processes with RNA polymerase III-dependent transcription instead of Max. Therefore, inhibition of c-Myc dimerization and interaction between c-Myc/Max dimers and DNA are significant strategies to block tumorigenesis in cancer cells (Fig. 5) [5, 44¯47].

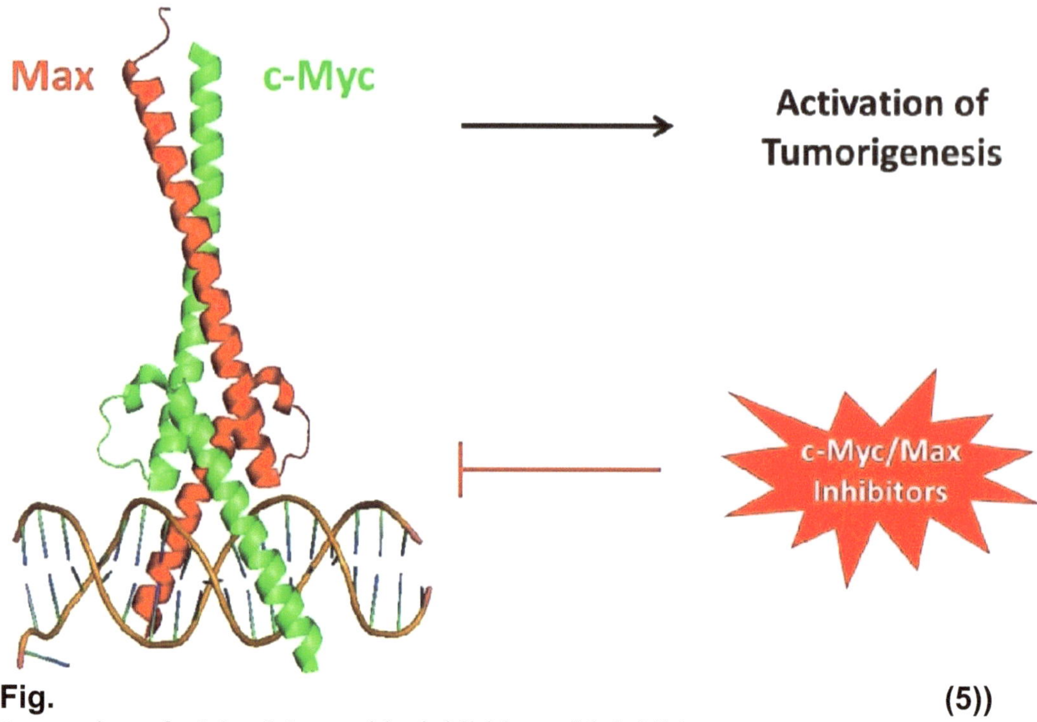

Fig. (5))
Interaction of c-Myc-Max and its inhibition with inhibitors.

Small-Molecule Inhibitors of the c-Myc-Max Interaction

IIA4B20, IIA6B17, IIA4B11, IA4B20, and IA4B6 are isoindoline-5,6-dicarboxamide derivative small compounds that exhibit inhibitory properties against c-Myc/Max dimerization *in vitro* and *in vivo* studies. In Myc-induced oncogenic transformation of chicken embryo fibroblast cells, especially IIA4B20 and IIA6B17 (Fig. **6**) reduced cell proliferation and inhibited Myc-Max dimerization at the highest concentrations [48]. Lu and co-workers reported that IIA6B17 selectively inhibits c-Myc-dependent transcriptional activity in NB11 cells expressing high levels of c-Myc and may also disrupt the interaction of c-Myc-Max [49].

Fig. (6))

Structure of IIA6B17 and IIA4B20.

Yin and co-workers investigated seven compounds (10058-F4, 10009-G9, 10050-C10, 10074-A4, 10074-G5, 10031-B8 and 10075-G5), each having different scaffolds to inhibit c-Myc/Max interaction (Fig. 7). All these compounds decreased the proliferation of fibroblast cells and c-Myc-dependent transcriptional activity. It was also found that four of these compounds (10058-F4, 10009-G9, 10050-C10, and 10074-A4) inhibited tumor growth in mice [50].

In a further study, different 10058-F4 analogs were designed with alteration of both six-member ethylbenzylidine and the five-member rhodanine rings (Fig. 7). 10058-F4 (IC_{50}: 49 µM) and its analogs, especially 12RH-NCN-1 (IC_{50}: 38 µM) and 28RH-NCN-1 (IC_{50}: 29 µM) decreased cell proliferation of human promyelocytic leukemia cells (HL-60). These compounds bind specifically to monomeric c-Myc and disrupt c-Myc-Max interaction and DNA binding of c-Myc [51].

Fig. (7))

Structure of important c-Myc-Max inhibitors.

In another study, novel 10058-F4 derivatives, which include peptide bond and nitrobenzofurazan moiety were synthesized (Fig. 8), and the correlation between c-Myc binding affinity and anti-proliferative profile of the compounds was determined in human promyelocytic leukemia and Burkitt's lymphoma cells. Results demonstrated that novel compounds effectively inhibited cell proliferation and DNA binding of c-Myc [52].

Fig. (8))

Structure of 10058-F4 derivative c-Myc-Max inhibitor.

Kiessling and co-workers designed two novel and potent compounds, Mycro1 and Mycro2, to inhibit interactions between the bHLHZip proteins c-Myc and Max. Mycro1 and Mcyro2 block c-Myc-Max dimerization in the low micromolar concentration range (Fig. **9**). To determine the structure-activity relationship against c-Myc-Max dimerization and to design Myc/Max dimerization inhibitor with improved properties, Kiessling and co-workers screened over one thousand compounds which have various functional group relating pyrazolo[1,5-a]- pyrimidine library based on the structures of Mycro1 and Mycro2. In this study, five compounds (2–6) were tested to inhibit DNA binding of c-Myc/Max. The obtained results indicated that compound 5 exhibited significant cellular specificity profiles as compared to the c-Myc inhibitors Mycro1 and Mycro2 [53].

Four α-acylamino amide derivative compounds have been reported by Xu *et al.* for inhibition of c-Myc–Max interaction and cellular functions of c-Myc (Fig. **10**). These compounds were selected from 285 compounds based on their properties such as planarity, aromatic scaffold, and four distinct molecules were selected. Initial screening of the compounds was carried out by fluorescence resonance energy transfer (FRET). The tested derivatives were examined by FRET assays to confirm the electrophoretic mobility shift assay (EMSA) results, and at 7.6 μM, the compounds inhibited dimerization at the range of 66% (NY2276) and 36% (NY2280) [54].

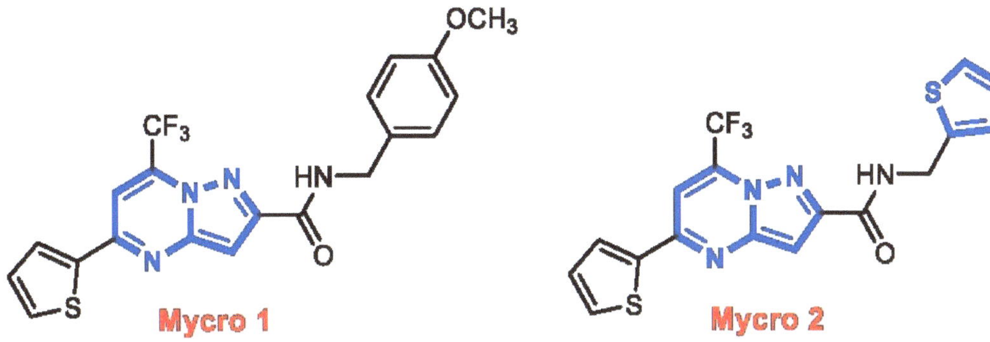

Fig.   **(9))**

Structure of Mycro1 and Mycro2.

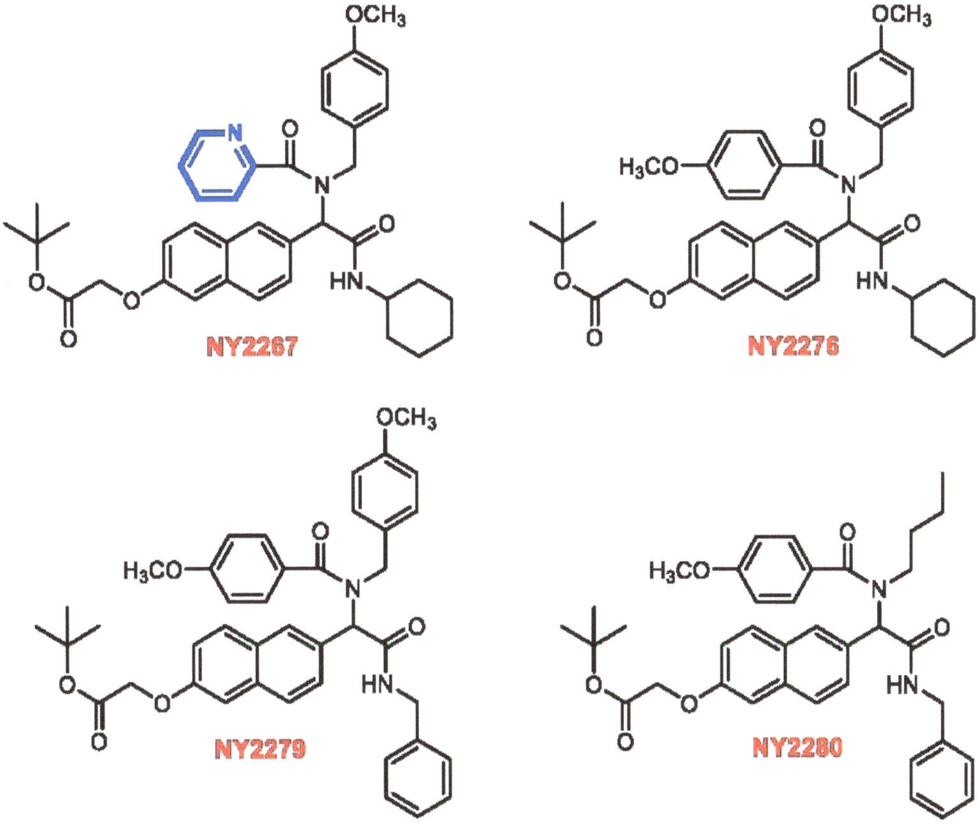

Fig.   **(10))**

Structure of NY2267, NY2276, NY2279 AND NY2280.

In a recent study by Han and co-workers, a compound library was generated with multiple filtrations, including PAINS (pan-assay interference compounds) filter and ZINC database to determine c-Myc/Max inhibitors. Among determined compounds, MCYi361 increased Myc phosphorylation and proteasome-mediated Myc degradation. Thus, MCYi361 inhibited *in-vivo* tumor growth in mice with favorable pharmacokinetic profiles. Also,

MCYi975 exhibited remarkable tolerability at higher concentrations compared to MCYi361 [55].

MYCMI-6 is a selective inhibitor of c-Myc/MAX interaction, and it was identified by a cell-based protein interaction screen. MYCMI-6 binds Myc with a K_D of 1.6 ± 0.5 µM and inhibits cell proliferation in a c-Myc-dependent manner with IC_{50} concentrations as low as 0.5 µM. In the c-Myc-driven xenograft tumor model, MYCMI-6 induces apoptosis, and blocks cancer cell growth in tumor tissues [56].

Bcl-2/Bcl-xL INTERACTION

Bcl-2 family of proteins plays significant roles in the regulation of the intrinsic apoptotic pathway. Aberrant expressions of Bcl-2 and Bcl-xL in cancer cells are essential in resistance to current therapeutic agents and inhibition of apoptosis [3, 57‒59]. Genetically instable cancer cells destroy normal cell homeostasis and give rise to defects in both cellular growth and programmed cell death. Defects in programmed cell death may not remove damaged and excess-unnecessary cells.

Cancer cells dysregulate apoptotic signaling pathways by suppressing proapoptotic proteins and overexpress antiapoptotic proteins. Bcl-2 family has both proapoptotic (Bax, Bak, Bad, Bik, Bid, Bim, Hrk, Bmf, Noxa, and Puma) and antiapoptotic (Bcl-2, BclxL, Bcl-w, Mcl-1, and Bcl2-A1) protein members [60]. Proapoptotic proteins induce permeabilization of mitochondrial membrane and release cyctocrome C and caspases to propagate death signals, resulting in a proteolytic cascade that degrades cytosolic-nuclear structures and promotes the formation of apoptotic bodies. Antiapoptotic proteins bind to proapoptotic proteins and help cell survival and suppress apoptotic signal (Fig. 11). Antiapoptotic Bcl-2 family members provide resistance to chemotherapy by this mechanism. Therefore, inhibition of antiapoptotic Bcl-2 family members are great interest to drug design [61‒63].

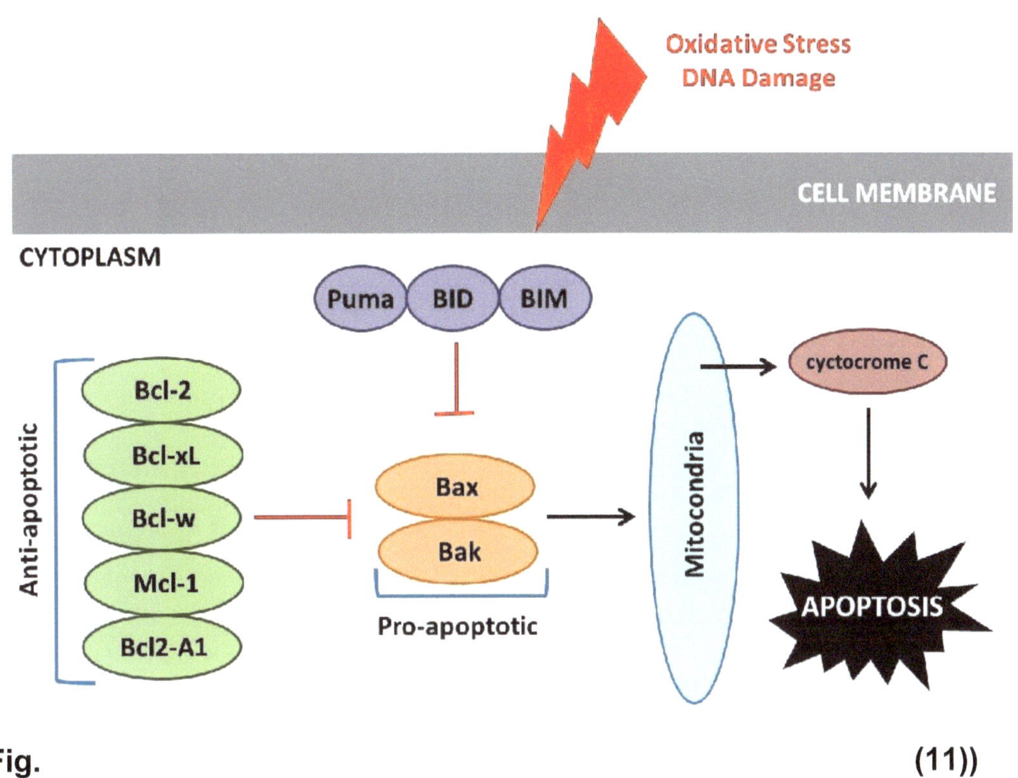

Fig. (11))

Interaction of Bcl-2/Bcl-xL and its role in apoptosis.

Small-Molecule Inhibitors of Bcl-2/Bcl-xL Interaction

Bcl-2 and Bcl-xL, which are key apoptosis regulators, have been an important biological target for cancer drug design. ABT-737, and its analogue ABT-263 (navitoclax) (Fig. 12) are potent Bcl-2/Bcl-xL inhibitors which are connected to Bcl-2 and Bcl-xL with high affinities and to Mcl-1 with weak affinity [64, 65]. ABT-737 is the first small inhibitor of Bcl-2/Bcl-xL interaction. ABT-737 binds selectively to Bcl2 and Bcl-xL, and blocks the sequestration of proapoptotic molecules, and stimulates apoptotic pathways in cancer cells. Unfortunately, ABT-737 has not been evaluated in clinical trials due to its low oral bioavailability and resistance to apoptosis [65, 66]. To outcome this limitation, orally bioavailable ABT-727 analog, ABT-263, was designed and synthesized to inhibit Bcl-2/Bcl-xL interaction. Anticancer activities of ABT-263 have been evaluated in clinical trials in many different types of cancer patients since 2009 [65, 67]. Further, a selective and orally bioavailable inhibitor of Bcl-2/Bcl-xL interaction, ABT-199 (Fig. 13), was designed for the treatment of BCL-2–dependent hematological cancers [68].

Fig. (12))

Structure of ABT-737 AND ABT-263.

Sleebs *et al.* designed and synthesized novel quinazoline-based heterocyclic compounds alternative to ABT-727 and ABT-263. These quinazoline analogs interact with high binding affinities to Bcl-2 and Bcl-xL and with weak affinity to Mcl-1 and exhibit significant anti-proliferative activities against small-cell lung carcinoma cell lines at concentration ranges [69].

WEHI-539 (Fig. 13) is benzothiazole-hydrazone derivative small molecule that binds very tightly to Bcl-xL (K_d: <1nM) and stimulates BAK-dependent apoptosis in murine embryonic fibroblasts (MEFs) cells [70].

Fig. (13))

Structure of ABT-199 and WEHI-539.

Zhou *et al.* suggested a series of compounds to inhibit Bcl-2 and Bcl-xL. Compounds are sulfonamide derivatives and containing different substituents such as piperidine, morpholine, pyrrole, and aryl groups. *In vitro* experiment results indicated that compound 21 binds to Bcl-xL and Bcl-2 (Ki < 1 nM) and inhibits cell proliferation of H146 and H1417 cell lines (small-cell lung cancer cells) with IC$_{50}$ values of 60–90 nM (H146 and H1417). Furthermore, compound 21 induces apoptotic pathways at 30–100 nM concentrations in the H146 cell line [71]. Also, Zhou *et al.* designed and optimized small molecule inhibitors of Bcl-2 and Bcl-xL containing a 4,5-diphenyl-1*H*-pyrrole-3-carboxylic acid core structure. The results revealed that compounds 14 and 15 interacted with Bcl-2 and Bcl-xL with subnanomolar K$_i$ values, and decreased cell proliferation with low nanomolar IC$_{50}$ values in multiple small-cell lung cancer cell lines by inducing apoptotic pathways. Also, compound 14 exhibited significant anticancer activity in H146 small-cell lung cancer xenograft model [71].

Wang and coworkers designed BM-1197 as an effective dual inhibitor of Bcl-2 and Bcl-xL (Fig. 14). In this study, the anticancer activity of BM-1197 was tested in human small cell lung cancer cell line panels. BM-1197 interacts with Bcl-2 and Bcl-xL proteins with Ki values less than 1 nM and shows >1,000-fold selectivity over Mcl-1. B1197 showed strong growth-inhibitory activity in small cell lung cancer cell lines *via* activation of the caspase cascade and apoptotic mechanisms. BM-1197 provides durable tumor regression in H146 small-cell lung cancer xenograft model in intense combined immunodeficiency (SCID) mice due to its favorable pharmacokinetic properties and solubility. Obtained results showed that BM-1197 was an encouraging dual Bcl-2/Bcl-xL inhibitor which guarantees further investigation as a new anticancer drug [72].

Fig. (14))
Structure of BM-1074 and BM-1197.

Bruncko and co-workers reported the discovery of a selective Bcl-xL antagonist which the biarylacyl-sulfonamide compounds that strengthens the antitumor activity of chemotherapy and radiation. These compounds were identified that used *N*-phenylpiperazine or 4-substituted *N*-phenylpiperidine templates as three distinct structural series. They investigated the use of structure-guided projection to detect a deep hydrophobic binding pocket on the surface of these proteins to improve the first dual, subnanomolar inhibitors of Bcl-xL and Bcl-2. The results revealed that compound **17** (Fig. 15), that is a biarylacylsulphonamide derivative, showed single agent efficacy against human follicular lymphoma cell lines that overexpress Bcl-2 [73].

Fig. (15))

Structure of biarylacylsulphonamide derivative Bcl-2/Bcl-xL inhibitor.

Hsp90/Hsp70 INTERACTION

Cancer cells metabolic rates are higher than that of healthy cells and faster growth rates cause accumulation of unfolded proteins. However, proteins must be in their native (properly folded) state in order to perform their functions. Otherwise, accumulation of unfolded proteins drive cell to apoptosis but cancer cell escapes from apoptosis mechanism by overexpressing anti apoptotic heat shock protein 70 (Hsp70) and 90 (Hsp90) [10, 74‑76]. Hsp70 and Hsp90 cooperate to fold substrate proteins (Fig. 16). Hsp70 process unfolded substrate proteins by seven residues each time and then send the substrate to Hsp90 for folding at the domain level. After Hsp90 processing, if the substrate protein folded properly, then it is ready to perform its biochemical function. However, if it is not processed to its proper three-dimensional forms then, it is sent to proteasomal degradation by Hsp cascade. Therefore, cancer cells overexpress Hsp proteins to compensate defects in protein folding at their higher metabolic rates [76‑78]. Several studies have been performed to inhibit Hsp90 protein. This protein is expressed abundantly in the cells and it expression increases at several different cancer types. Geldanamycine based small molecules are in clinical trials and common properties of these drugs are induced Hsp70 expression. Since Hsp70 complements Hsp90 function, it is convenient to inhibit both Hsps simultaneously or break up Hsp90-Hsp70 complex with a novel approach [76, 79]. Recent Hsp70 inhibitors or dual inhibitors are promising and suppress both Hsp90 and Hsp70 simultaneously [80]. Moreover, several researches suggested that inhibition of interaction between Hsps and their co-chaperones is an effective strategy in treatment of cancer [81].

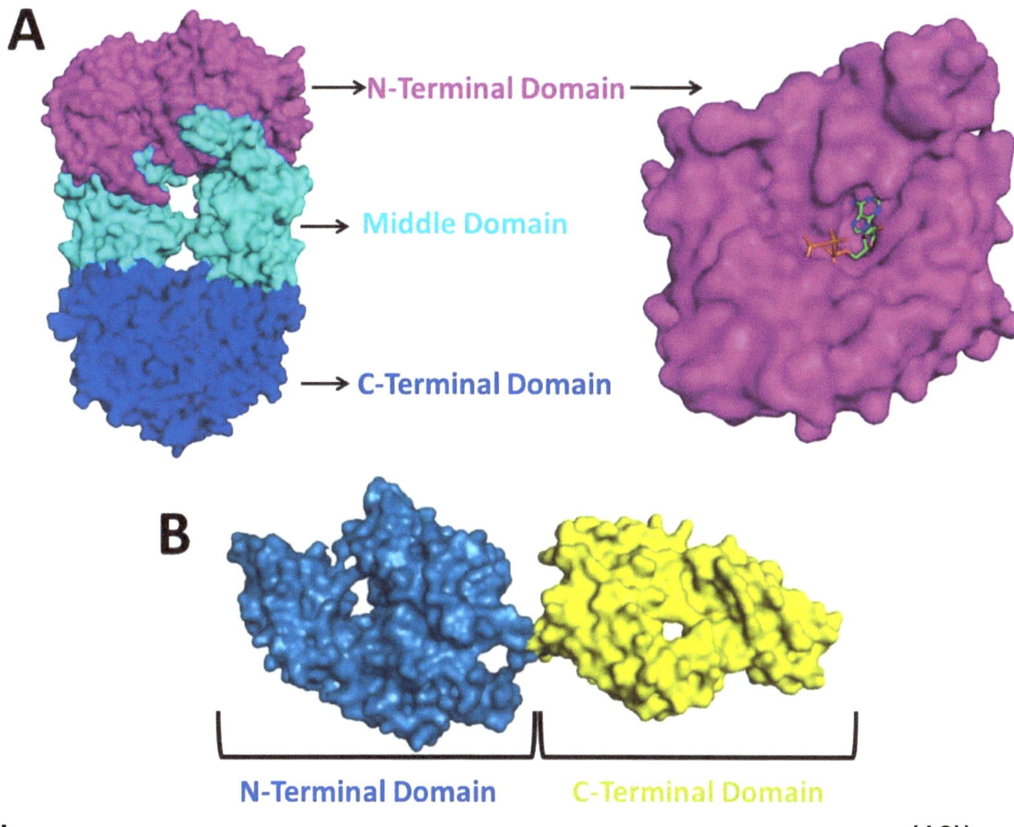

Fig. **(16))**
A) Structure of Hsp90 and Hsp90 N-terminal domain. **B)** Structure of Hsp70. Both proteins have ATPase (N Terminal) and substrate binding domain (C Terminal).

Small-Molecule Inhibitors of the Hsp70/Hsp90 Interaction

Recent work in our lab designed small molecule inhibitors to decrease Hsp90-Hsp70 complex not only by direct binding to active Hsp center but also by intercalating to interface surfaces. The inhibitors further binds to key co-chaperones and totally suppress Hsp90-Hsp70 function. Therefore, these molecules phase work will be started right after their completion of preclinical studies.

To inhibit Hsp90 chaperone activity, the new hybrid compounds (**18**) contains both thiazole and coumarine scaffolds were designed and synthesized by Koca and co-workers (Fig. 17). Dimerization of Hsp90 is an essential step in proper folding of oncogenic client proteins. These coumarine analogs displayed anticancer activities against human colon and liver cancer cell lines (DLD-1 and HepG2) at low concentrations. To understand the anti-proliferative effect of the compounds, structural and functional differences of the Hsp90 were determined with proteomic and *in silico* assays. The compounds interacted with dimerization region of the Hsp90 and disrupted proper conformation of C-terminal domain of Hsp90. These differences induced inhibition of Hsp90 interactions with Hop, Hsp40, and Hsp70 in cancer cells [82].

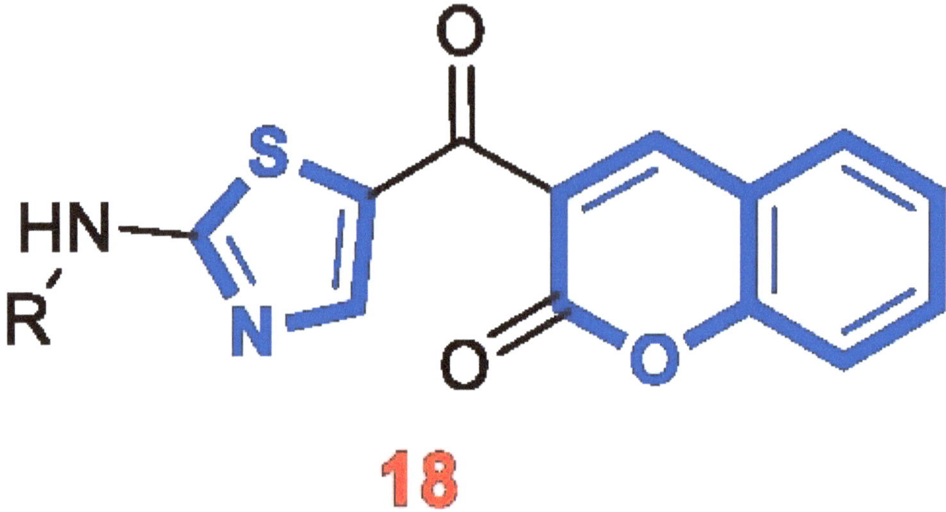

Fig.   **(17))**

Structure of thiazole and coumarine scaffolds-containing inhibitors of Hsp90-Hsp70.

In another study, thiazolyl diazepine compounds (**19**) were designed and synthetized as selective Hsp90 inhibitors (Fig. 18). Compounds exhibited significant anticancer activities against human breast (MCF-7) and human endothelial cells (HUVEC). Molecular docking assay demonstrated that diazepine derivatives selectively bind to the ATPase domain of the Hsp90 with binding energies ranging from -6.57 to -7.99 kcal/mol. Especially, compound D5 binds to Hsp90 with Kd value of 3,93 μM and with estimated free energy of binding -7.99 (kcal/mol). The compound D5 suppresses HSP90AA1 (Hsp90α), HSP90B1 (Grp94) and key genes (cell cycle receptors; PLK2 and TERT, kinases; PI3KC3 and PRKCE, and growth factors; IGF1, IGF2, KDR, and PDGFRA) on oncogenic pathways. Hsp90α (cytosol) and Grp94 (endoplasmic reticulum) are overexpressed in cancer cells and they are involved in all phases of tumorigenesis. The compound inhibits Hsp90 ATPase function and proper folding of Hsp90 client proteins and their interactions of

Hsp90. Inhibition of Hsp90 induces apoptotic pathways in cancer cells, and therefore benzodiazepine derivatives are potent drug templates to design target specific Hsp90 inhibitors [83].

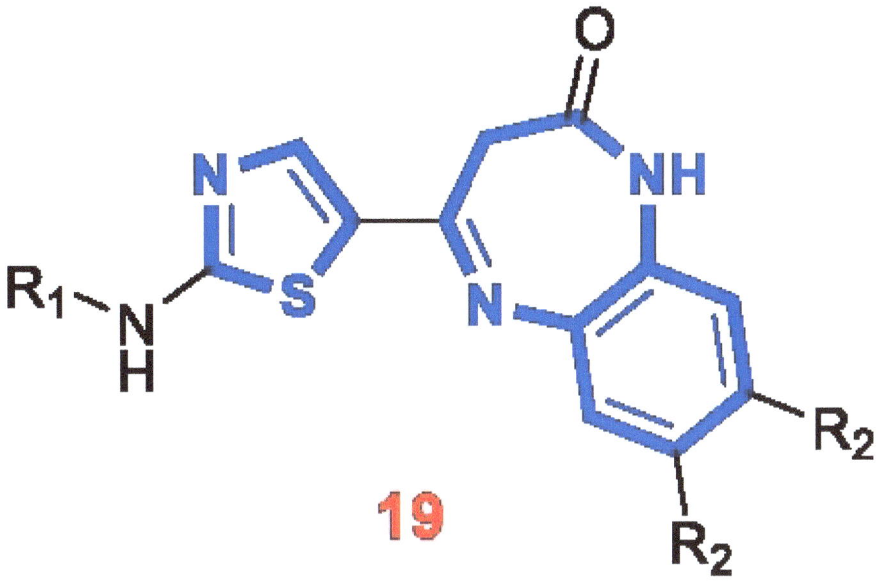

Fig. (18))
Structure of thiazolyl diazepine derivative Hsp90 inhibitors.

Koca and co-workers designed and synthesized pyrimidinyl acyl thiourea derivatives (**20**) as potent Hsp90 inhibitors in the treatment of breast cancer and its bone metastases (Fig. 19). The compounds inhibited proliferation of human breast (MCF-7) and bone (Saos-2) cells. *In silico* and experimental studies indicated that the compounds were localized in ATP binding site of Hsp90 and blocked ATPase activity of Hsp90. Additionally, these pyrimidinyl acyl thiourea derivatives down-regulated ER-α, KRT8, Notch-1, MMP2, CTNNB1, Bcl-2, MAPK3, Twist1, Rassf1, and Abcg2 in MCF-7 cells [84].

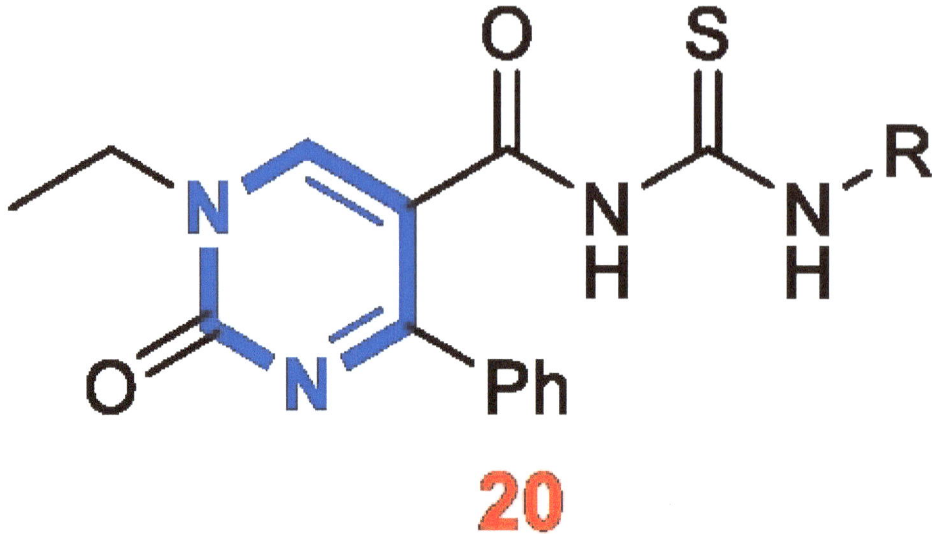

Fig. (19))

Structure of pyrimidinyl acyl thiourea derivative Hsp90 inhibitors.

Hsp70 is known to cooperate with many co-chaperones such as Bcl-2–associated athanogene 3 (Bag-3) in tumor formation. Bag-3 is over-expressed in wide variety of cancer types and it has been shown to collaborate with Hsp70 in up-regulation of oncogenic multiple signaling pathways. Therefore, inhibition of Hsp70-Bag-3 PPI has been significant approach to design target specific cancer drugs [85, 86]. In this context, YM-01, JG-98, and YM01-biotin were evaluated as potent Hsp70-Bag-3 inhibitors and their anticancer activities were examined in xenograft and *in vitro* models (Fig. 20). Overall, these compounds selectively interact with Hsp70-Bag-3 complex and block cancer cell proliferation and related signaling pathways [87].

Fig. (20))

Structure of important inhibitors of Hsp70-Bag3 interaction.

Similar to Hsp70-Bag-3 interaction, targeting Hsp90 and its co-chaperones interactions is remarkable strategy in cancer drug design. C-terminus of heat shock cognate protein 70 (HSC70)–interacting protein (Cdc37) is a ubiquitous co-chaperone of Hsp90 which participates in proper folding of oncogenic client proteins with Hsp90 [88, 89]. Wang *et al.* identified DDO-5936 as a potent small-molecule inhibitor of the Hsp90-Cdc37 interaction in colorectal cancer (Fig. 21). Both *in vitro* and *in vivo* experiments indicated that, DDO-5936 disrupted the Hsp90-Cdc37 interaction and blocked blocking proliferation of colorectal cancer cells. Additionally, DDO-5936 was down-regulated Hsp90 kinase clients in HCT116 cells [90].

β-catenin/TCF4 INTERACTION

Wnt signaling pathway and its aberrant regulation is a keystone in almost all steps of tumorigenesis. β-catenin is an important biological component of the Wnt pathway, and overexpression and activation of β-catenin are associated with tumor formation and survival (Fig. 22). The tumor suppressor adenomatous polyposis coli (APC), glycogen synthase kinase 3β (GSK3β), casein kinase 1α (CK1α) and the scaffold protein AXIN are upstream regulators which are regulated activation and expression of β-catenin. β-catenin binds to T-cell factor 4 (TCF4) after its translocation from cytosol to nucleus in cells. Therefore, inhibition of β-catenin/TCF4 interaction has been significant target in cancer drug design [91¯94].

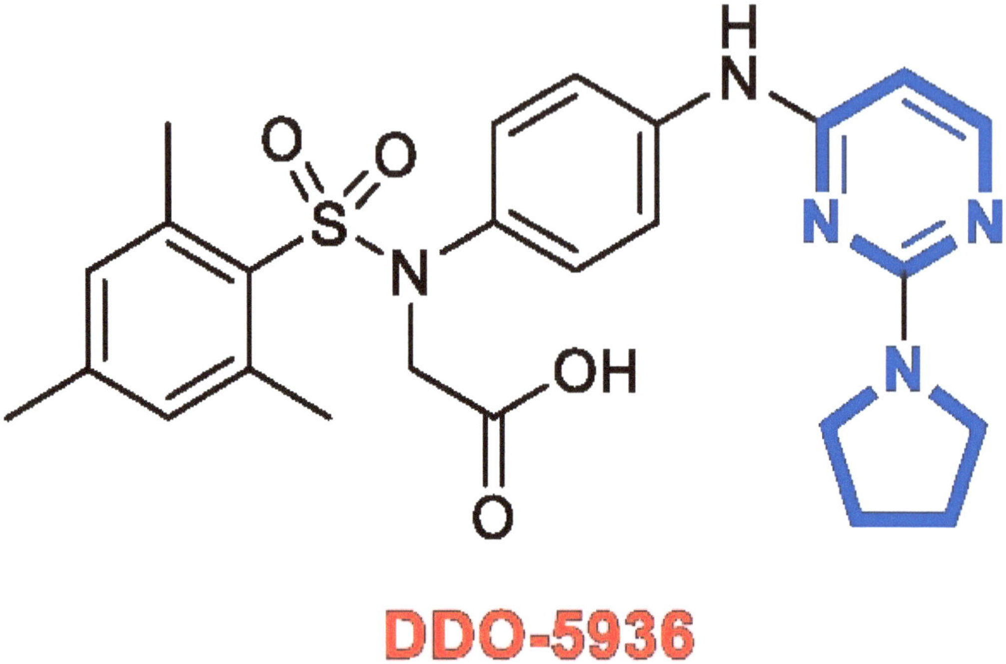

DDO-5936

Fig. (21))
Structure of DDO-5936.

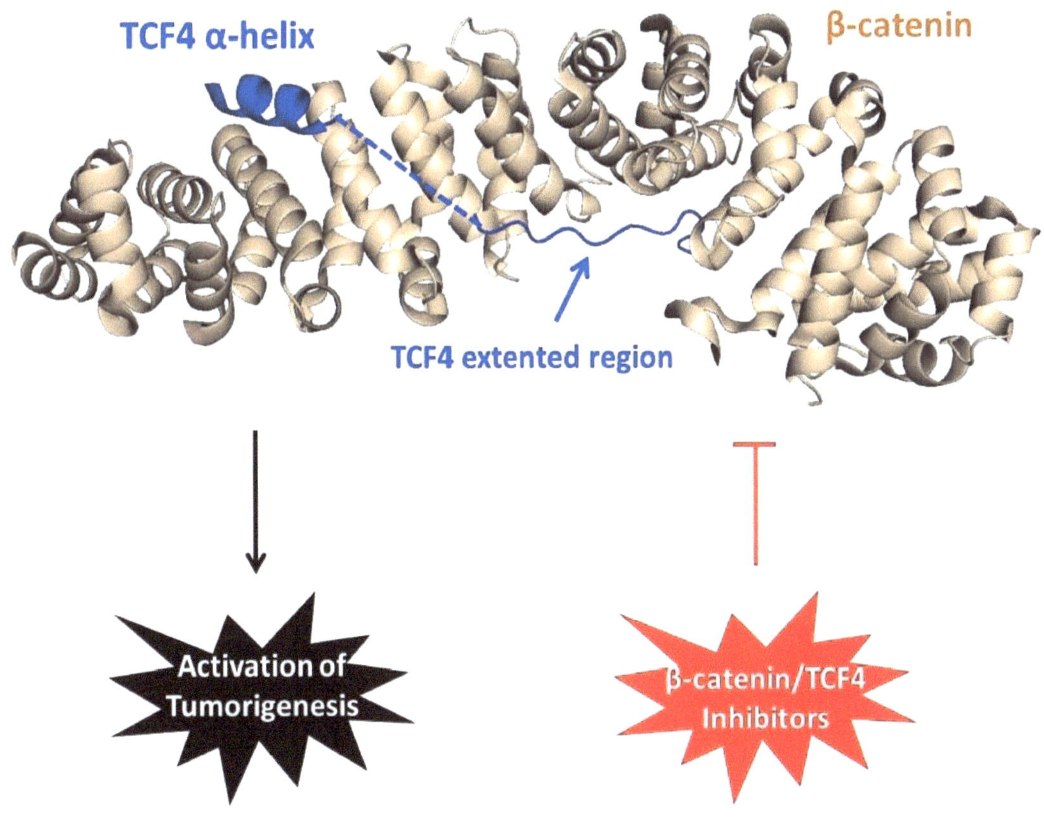

Fig. (22))

Interaction of β-catenin/TCF4 and its inhibition with small molecules.

Small-Molecule Inhibitors of the β-Catenin/TCF4 Interaction

β-catenin undertakes significant roles in Wnt signaling pathways with interacting with TCF4. Aberrant expression level of the β-catenin is determined in cancer cells and mediates anti-apoptotic pathways and cancer cell proliferations. For this reason, β-catenin/TCF4 signaling represents considerable a tempting target for cancer treatment [94, 95].

Lepourcelet *et al.* screened about 7000 natural compounds by ELISA technique in a high-throughput assay for detection of effective β-catenin/TCF4 inhibitors, and six potent compounds were identified with IC_{50} values less than 10 μM in human colorectal cancer cell lines (HCT-116, HT-29 and SW480), including PKF115-584, PKF222-815, CGP049090, PKF118-744, PKF118-310, and ZTM000990. These selected compounds mainly blocked β-catenin/TCF4 interaction and especially KF115-584, PKF222-815 and CGP049090 (Fig. 23) disrupted the interaction of β-catenin/APC. Also, KF115-584 and PKF222-815 inhibited the binding of TCF4 proteins to DNA [96].

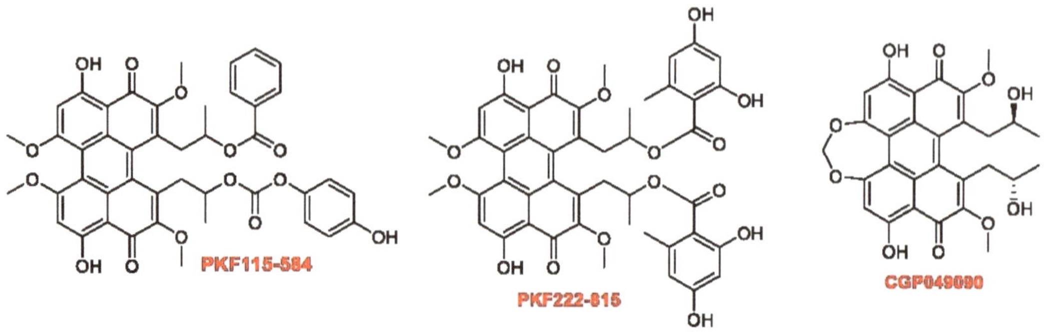

Fig. (23))

Structure of PKF115-584, PFK222-815 and CGP49090.

Gonsalves and co-workers reported potent three β-catenin/TCF4 inhibitors, iCRT3, iCRT5 and iCRT14 (Fig. 24), using RNAi-based modifier screening method. These compounds inhibited interaction of β-catenin with TCF4 at micromolar concentrations in various mammalian and cancer cell lines. Moreover, the compounds inhibited expression of downstream target genes of β-cat including WISP-1, Axin-2, CycD1 and c-Myc in cancer cells [97].

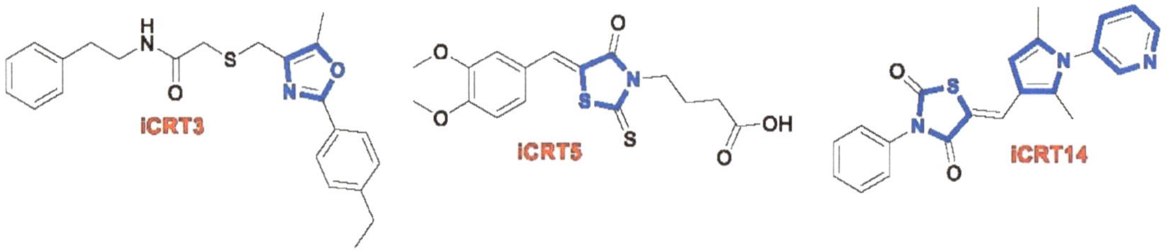

Fig. (24))

Structure of iCRT3, iCRT5 and iCRT14.

NC043 (Fig. 25), a potent inhibitor of β-catenin/TCF4 interaction, was discovered by screening a small molecule library of 4000 compounds. Anticancer activities of the NC043 were evaluated in SW480 and Caco-2 cell lines. NC043 decreased expression level of Wnt target genes (Axin2, Cyclin D1, surviving, Cdc25c and Cdc2) and arrested SW480 cells at the G2/M phase of the cell cycle and stimulated apoptosis in a dose-dependent manner. Also, NC043 did not affect the protein level of the soluble β-catenin, but blocked β-catenin/TCF4 interaction in SW480 cell line. In a xenograft model, treatment with NC043 (90 µg/kg for 17 days) significantly decreased tumor volume and tumor weight [98].

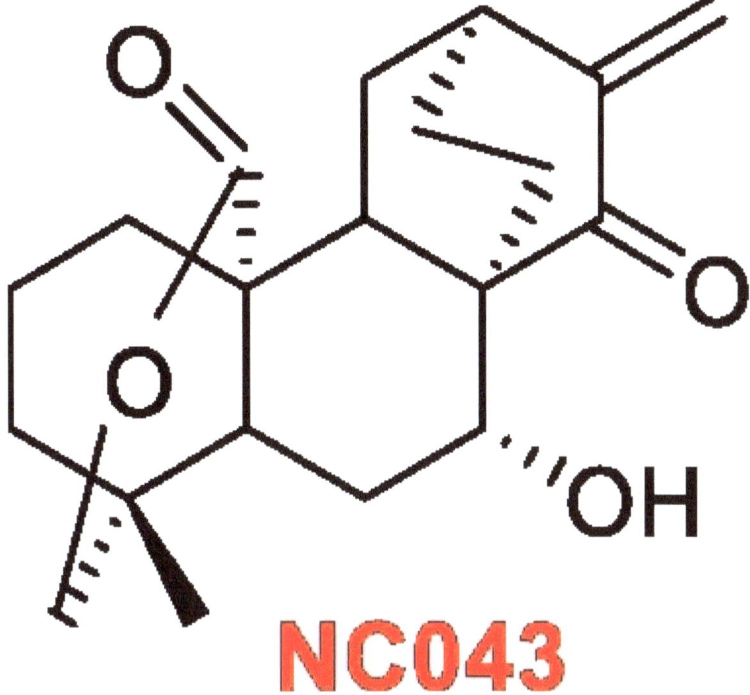

Fig. (25))

Structure of NC043.

CWP232228 (Fig. 26) was designed as an inhibitor of β-catenin/TCF4 interaction in the nucleus and down-regulated target genes of the Wnt/ β-catenin signaling pathways. *In vitro* and *in vivo* studies reported that CWP232228 exhibited anti-proliferative activities against liver and breast cancer cells. Insulin-like growth factor-I (IGF-I) signaling is associated with tumorigenesis in breast and the dysregulation of IGF-I lead to radio-resistance and tumor recurrence in primary breast cancers. In this context, CWP232228 may disrupt IGF-I signaling in breast cancer stem cells [99].

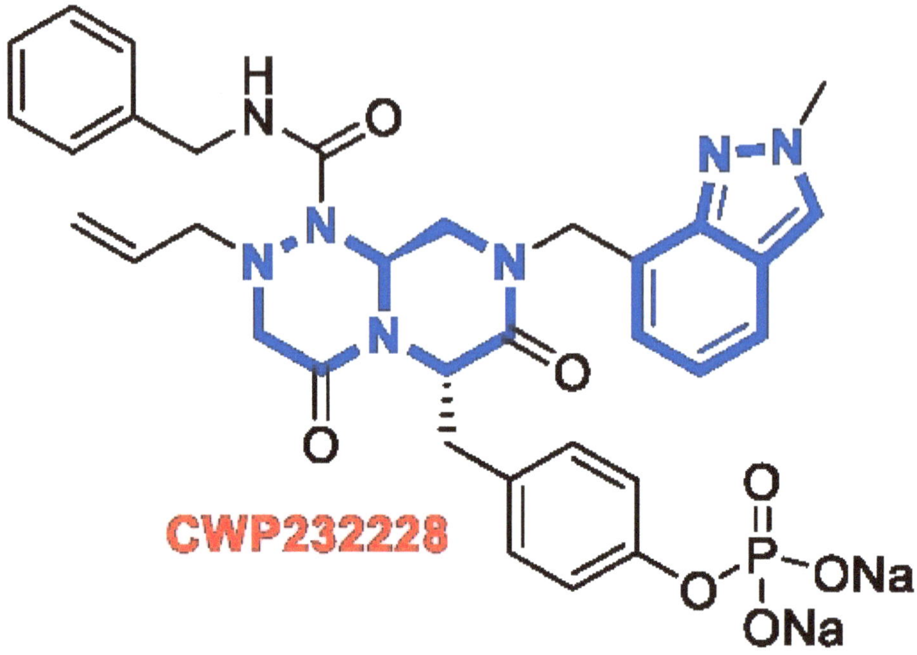

Fig. (26))
Structure of CWP232228.

Menin/MLL INTERACTION

Menin is a co-factor of MLL (mixed lineage leukemia) fusion proteins and targeting Menin/MLL interaction is significant to develop specific inhibitors for leukemia treatment. Menin is generally localized in nucleus and binds to N-terminal domain of the MLL.

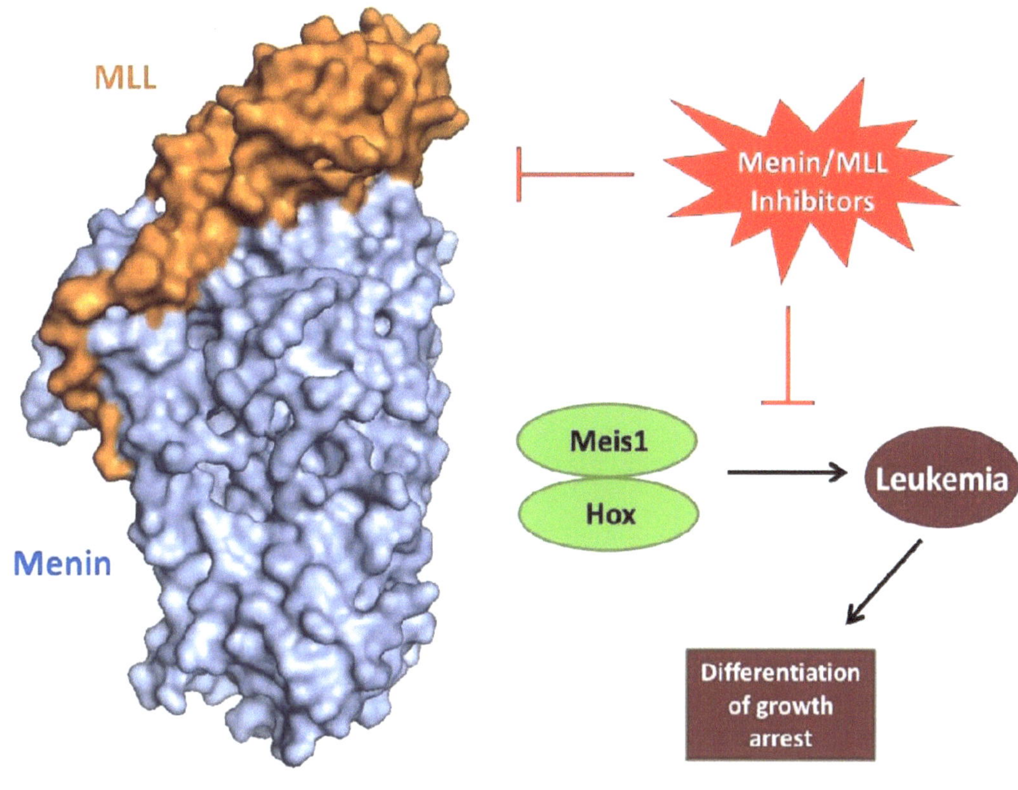

Fig. (27))

Interaction of Menin/MLL and its inhibition with small molecules.

Menin is related with the promoter regions of HOX genes (especially Hoxa9) which promotes the immortalization of leukemic cells. Down-regulations of Menin and MLL lead to disruption of HOX gene expression (Fig. 27). Furthermore, menin and MLL regulate the expression of the p27Kip1 and p18Ink4c25 (cyclin-dependent kinase inhibitors (CDKI)) and Meis1. Therefore, inhibition of Menin-MLL interaction provides approach to develop effective therapeutics for treatment of leukemia [9, 100⁻103].

Small-Molecule Inhibitors of the Menin-MLL Interaction

Interaction between Menin and MLL is critical target to design effective therapeutics for treatment of leukemia. Borkin and co-workers designed a series of thienopyrimidine derivative compounds (MI-136, MI-389, MI-463 and MI-503) (Fig. 28) and their inhibition potentials of menin-MLL interaction were evaluated *in vivo* and *in vitro* leukemia models. Among these compounds, MI-463 and MI-503 directly interacted with menin/MLL complex with low-nanomolar binding affinities and inhibited progression of leukemia *in vitro* and *in vivo*. Also, MI-463 and MI-503 exhibited high oral bioavailability and blocked cancer cell proliferation on a mouse model of MLL leukemia [104].

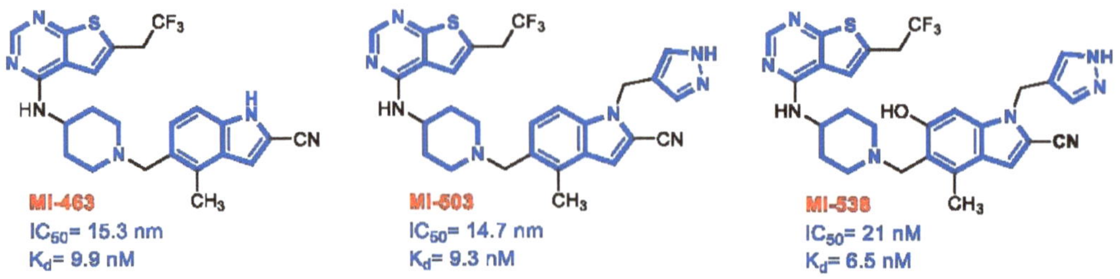

Fig. (28))

Structure of MI-463, MI-503 and MI-538.

Shi *et al.* developed small compounds containing thienopyrimidine scaffold which disrupted menin/MLL interaction and displayed anticancer activities in leukemia cells. One of these compounds, MI-2-2, bond to menin with nanomolar affinities (K_d: 22 nM) and inhibited the menin/MLL interaction. Thus, the cancer cell proliferation was interrupted (IC_{50}: 46 nM) and down-regulation of Hoxa9 expression, and differentiation were determined with MI-2-2 [105].

Hydroxymethylpiperidines had been identified as a synthetically tractable series of inhibitors of the Menin–MLL interactions. SAR studies around compound-18 revealed that around piperidine moiety various alkyl and aromatic groups were tolerated. In this series, compound-11 contains cyclopentyl group (IC50 = 0,39 µM) and compound-12 contains cyclohexyl group (IC50 = 1,7 µM) demonstrated strong and selective activity in MLL leukemia cells. The aminomethylpiperidine compound (MIV-6) (Fig. 29) was synthesized to improve the binding site and specifically block the menin-MLL protein-protein interaction by changing functional group of methylpiperidines. The most pronounced activity increase was obtained after replacing the hydroxyl group with the amino group (IC_{50} = 56 nM) [106].

Fig. (29))

Structure of MIV-6.

CONCLUSION

Recent studies aimed at targeting of PPIs have greatly accelerated to design cancer drugs. p53-MDM2, c-MYC-MAX, Bcl-2/Bcl-xL, Hsp90-Hsp70, β-catenin-TCF4 and Menin-MLL are key PPIs which are involved in almost all steps of the tumorigenesis. Inhibition of these PPIs with small molecules has been an increasingly attractive pharmacological approach for the next generation of target specific cancer drugs. In this regard, numerous compounds were designed, but there are no significant numbers of FDA approved PPIs inhibitors are available in cancer treatment now. Also, drug-like criteria, ADME parameters, and pharmacokinetics properties for PPI inhibitors need to be further investigated. However, more effective PPIs inhibitors will get approval from the FDA, and they will routinely apply to treat various types of cancer in the near future.

CONSENT FOR PUBLICATION

Not applicable.

CONFLICT OF INTEREST

The authors declare no conflict of interest, financial or otherwise.

ACKNOWLEDGEMENTS

Declared none.

REFERENCES

[1]   Pawson T, Nash P. Protein-protein interactions define specificity in signal transduction. Genes Dev 2000; 14(9): 1027-47.[PMID: 10809663]

[2]   Westermarck J, Ivaska J, Corthals GL. Identification of protein interactions involved in cellular signaling. Mol Cell Proteomics 2013; 12(7): 1752-63.[http://dx.doi.org/10.1074/mcp.R113.027771] [PMID: 23481661]

[3]   Warren CFA, Wong-Brown MW, Bowden NA. BCL-2 family isoforms in apoptosis and cancer. Cell Death Dis 2019; 10(3): 177.[http://dx.doi.org/10.1038/s41419-019-1407-6] [PMID: 30792387]

[4]   Chène P. Inhibiting the p53-MDM2 interaction: an important target for cancer therapy. Nat Rev Cancer 2003; 3(2): 102-9.[http://dx.doi.org/10.1038/nrc991] [PMID: 12563309]

[5]   Berg T. Small-molecule modulators of c-Myc/Max and Max/Max interactions. Curr Top Microbiol Immunol 2011; 348: 139-49.[http://dx.doi.org/10.1007/82_2010_90] [PMID: 20680803]

[6]   Moll UM, Petrenko O. The MDM2-p53 interaction. Mol Cancer Res 2003; 1(14): 1001-8.[PMID: 14707283]

[7]   Kale J, Osterlund EJ, Andrews DW. BCL-2 family proteins: changing partners in the dance towards death. Cell Death Differ 2018; 25(1): 65-80.[http://dx.doi.org/10.1038/cdd.2017.186] [PMID: 29149100]

[8]   Poy F, Lepourcelet M, Shivdasani RA, Eck MJ. Structure of a human Tcf4-beta-catenin complex. Nat Struct Biol 2001; 8(12): 1053-7.[http://dx.doi.org/10.1038/nsb720] [PMID: 11713476]

[9]   Cierpicki T, Grembecka J. Challenges and opportunities in targeting the menin-MLL interaction. Future Med Chem 2014; 6(4): 447-62.[http://dx.doi.org/10.4155/fmc.13.214] [PMID: 24635524]

[10]   Tutar L, Tutar Y. Heat shock proteins; an overview. Curr Pharm Biotechnol 2010; 11(2): 216-22.[http://dx.doi.org/10.2174/138920110790909632] [PMID: 20170474]

[11]   Bojadzic D, Buchwald P. Toward Small-Molecule Inhibition of Protein-Protein Interactions: General Aspects and Recent Progress in Targeting Costimulatory and Coinhibitory (Immune Checkpoint) Interactions. Curr Top Med Chem 2018; 18(8): 674-99.[http://dx.doi.org/10.2174/1568026618666180531092503] [PMID: 29848279]

[12]   Cossins BP, Lawson AD. Small Molecule Targeting of Protein-Protein Interactions through Allosteric Modulation of Dynamics. Molecules 2015; 20(9): 16435-45.[http://dx.doi.org/10.3390/molecules200916435] [PMID: 26378508]

[13]   Ni D, Liu N, Sheng C. Allosteric Modulators of Protein-Protein Interactions (PPIs). Adv Exp Med Biol 2019; 1163: 313-34.[http://dx.doi.org/10.1007/978-981-13-8719-7_13] [PMID: 31707709]

[14]   Guo W, Wisniewski JA, Ji H. Hot spot-based design of small-molecule inhibitors for protein-protein interactions. Bioorg Med Chem Lett 2014; 24(11): 2546-54.[http://dx.doi.org/10.1016/j.bmcl.2014.03.095] [PMID: 24751445]

[15]   Cukuroglu E, Engin HB, Gursoy A, Keskin O. Hot spots in protein-protein interfaces: towards drug discovery. Prog Biophys Mol Biol 2014; 116(2-3): 165-73.[http://dx.doi.org/10.1016/j.pbiomolbio.2014.06.003] [PMID: 24997383]

[16]   Morrow JK, Zhang S. Computational prediction of protein hot spot residues. Curr Pharm Des 2012; 18(9): 1255-65.[http://dx.doi.org/10.2174/138161212799436412] [PMID: 22316154]

[17]   Ibarra AA, Bartlett GJ, Hegedüs Z, *et al.* Predicting and Experimentally Validating Hot-Spot Residues at Protein-Protein Interfaces. ACS Chem Biol 2019; 14(10): 2252-63.[http://dx.doi.org/10.1021/acschembio.9b00560] [PMID: 31525028]

[18]   Beckerman R, Prives C. Transcriptional regulation by p53. Cold Spring Harb Perspect Biol 2010; 2(8): a000935.[http://dx.doi.org/10.1101/cshperspect.a000935] [PMID: 20679336]

[19]   Zilfou JT, Lowe SW. Tumor suppressive functions of p53. Cold Spring Harb Perspect Biol 2009; 1(5): a001883.[http://dx.doi.org/10.1101/cshperspect.a001883] [PMID: 20066118]

[20]   Chen J. The Cell-Cycle Arrest and Apoptotic Functions of p53 in Tumor Initiation and Progression. Cold Spring Harb Perspect Med 2016; 6(3): a026104.[http://dx.doi.org/10.1101/cshperspect.a026104] [PMID:

26931810]

[21] Zhao Y, Yu H, Hu W. The regulation of MDM2 oncogene and its impact on human cancers. Acta Biochim Biophys Sin (Shanghai) 2014; 46(3): 180-9.[http://dx.doi.org/10.1093/abbs/gmt147] [PMID: 24389645]

[22] Freedman DA, Wu L, Levine AJ. Functions of the MDM2 oncoprotein. Cell Mol Life Sci 1999; 55(1): 96-107.[http://dx.doi.org/10.1007/s000180050273] [PMID: 10065155]

[23] Iwakuma T, Lozano G. MDM2, an introduction. Mol Cancer Res 2003; 1(14): 993-1000.[PMID: 14707282]

[24] Nag S, Qin J, Srivenugopal KS, Wang M, Zhang R. The MDM2-p53 pathway revisited. J Biomed Res 2013; 27(4): 254-71.[PMID: 23885265]

[25] Khoury K, Dömling A. P53 mdm2 inhibitors. Curr Pharm Des 2012; 18(30): 4668-78.[http://dx.doi.org/10.2174/138161212802651580] [PMID: 22650254]

[26] Shangary S, Wang S. Small-molecule inhibitors of the MDM2-p53 protein-protein interaction to reactivate p53 function: a novel approach for cancer therapy. Annu Rev Pharmacol Toxicol 2009; 49: 223-41.[http://dx.doi.org/10.1146/annurev.pharmtox.48.113006.094723] [PMID: 18834305]

[27] Secchiero P, Bosco R, Celeghini C, Zauli G. Recent advances in the therapeutic perspectives of Nutlin-3. Curr Pharm Des 2011; 17(6): 569-77.[http://dx.doi.org/10.2174/138161211795222586] [PMID: 21391907]

[28] Shen H, Maki CG. Pharmacologic activation of p53 by small-molecule MDM2 antagonists. Curr Pharm Des 2011; 17(6): 560-8.[http://dx.doi.org/10.2174/138161211795222603] [PMID: 21391906]

[29] Ding Q, Zhang Z, Liu JJ, et al. Discovery of RG7388, a potent and selective p53-MDM2 inhibitor in clinical development. J Med Chem 2013; 56(14): 5979-83.[http://dx.doi.org/10.1021/jm400487c] [PMID: 23808545]

[30] Tisato V, Voltan R, Gonelli A, Secchiero P, Zauli G. MDM2/X inhibitors under clinical evaluation: perspectives for the management of hematological malignancies and pediatric cancer. J Hematol Oncol 2017; 10(1): 133.[http://dx.doi.org/10.1186/s13045-017-0500-5] [PMID: 28673313]

[31] Andreeff M, Kelly KR, Yee K, et al. Results of the Phase I Trial of RG7112, a Small-Molecule MDM2 Antagonist in Leukemia. Clin Cancer Res 2016; 22(4): 868-76.[http://dx.doi.org/10.1158/1078-0432.CCR-15-0481] [PMID: 26459177]

[32] Vu B, Wovkulich P, Pizzolato G, et al. Discovery of RG7112: A Small-Molecule MDM2 Inhibitor in Clinical Development. ACS Med Chem Lett 2013; 4(5): 466-9.[http://dx.doi.org/10.1021/ml4000657] [PMID: 24900694]

[33] Higgins B, Glenn K, Walz A, et al. Preclinical optimization of MDM2 antagonist scheduling for cancer treatment by using a model-based approach. Clin Cancer Res 2014; 20(14): 3742-52.[http://dx.doi.org/10.1158/1078-0432.CCR-14-0460] [PMID: 24812409]

[34] https://clinicaltrials.gov/ct2/results?cond=&term=RG7388&cntry=&state=&city=&dist=

[35] Jung J, Lee JS, Dickson MA, et al. TP53 mutations emerge with HDM2 inhibitor SAR405838 treatment in de-differentiated liposarcoma. Nat Commun 2016; 7: 12609.[http://dx.doi.org/10.1038/ncomms12609] [PMID: 27576846]

[36] de Weger VA, de Jonge M, Langenberg MHG, et al. A phase I study of the HDM2 antagonist SAR405838 combined with the MEK inhibitor pimasertib in patients with advanced solid tumours. Br J Cancer 2019; 120(3): 286-93.[http://dx.doi.org/10.1038/s41416-018-0355-8] [PMID: 30585255]

[37] Hoffman-Luca CG, Yang CY, Lu J, et al. Significant Differences in the Development of Acquired Resistance to the MDM2 Inhibitor SAR405838 between In Vitro and In Vivo Drug Treatment. PLoS One 2015; 10(6): e0128807.[http://dx.doi.org/10.1371/journal.pone.0128807] [PMID: 26070072]

[38] Holzer P, Masuya K, Furet P, et al. Discovery of a Dihydroisoquinolinone Derivative (NVP-CGM097): A Highly Potent and Selective MDM2 Inhibitor Undergoing Phase 1 Clinical Trials in p53wt Tumors. J Med Chem 2015; 58(16): 6348-58.[http://dx.doi.org/10.1021/acs.jmedchem.5b00810] [PMID: 26181851]

[39] Ravandi F, Gojo I, Patnaik MM, et al. A phase I trial of the human double minute 2 inhibitor (MK-8242) in patients with refractory/recurrent acute myelogenous leukemia (AML). Leuk Res 2016; 48: 92-100.[http://dx.doi.org/10.1016/j.leukres.2016.07.004] [PMID: 27544076]

[40] Wagner AJ, Banerji U, Mahipal A, et al. Phase I Trial of the Human Double Minute 2 Inhibitor MK-8242 in Patients With Advanced Solid Tumors. J Clin Oncol 2017; 35(12): 1304-11.[http://dx.doi.org/10.1200/JCO.2016.70.7117] [PMID: 28240971]

[41] Rew Y, Sun D. Discovery of a small molecule MDM2 inhibitor (AMG 232) for treating cancer. J Med Chem 2014; 57(15): 6332-41.[http://dx.doi.org/10.1021/jm500627s] [PMID: 24967612]

[42] Canon J, Osgood T, Olson SH, et al. The MDM2 Inhibitor AMG 232 Demonstrates Robust Antitumor Efficacy and Potentiates the Activity of p53-Inducing Cytotoxic Agents. Mol Cancer Ther 2015; 14(3): 649-58.[http://dx.doi.org/10.1158/1535-7163.MCT-14-0710] [PMID: 25567130]

[43]   https://clinicaltrials.gov/ct2/results?cond=&term=AMG-232&cntry=&state=&city=&dist=

[44]   Nair SK, Burley SK. Structural aspects of interactions within the Myc/Max/Mad network. Curr Top Microbiol Immunol 2006; 302: 123-43.[http://dx.doi.org/10.1007/3-540-32952-8_5] [PMID: 16620027]

[45]   Miller DM, Thomas SD, Islam A, Muench D, Sedoris K. c-Myc and cancer metabolism. Clin Cancer Res 2012; 18(20): 5546-53.[http://dx.doi.org/10.1158/1078-0432.CCR-12-0977] [PMID: 23071356]

[46]   Hoffman B, Liebermann DA. Apoptotic signaling by c-MYC. Oncogene 2008; 27(50): 6462-72.[http://dx.doi.org/10.1038/onc.2008.312] [PMID: 18955973]

[47]   Gomez-Roman N, Grandori C, Eisenman RN, White RJ. Direct activation of RNA polymerase III transcription by c-Myc. Nature 2003; 421(6920): 290-4.[http://dx.doi.org/10.1038/nature01327] [PMID: 12529648]

[48]   Berg T, Cohen SB, Desharnais J, et al. Small-molecule antagonists of Myc/Max dimerization inhibit Myc-induced transformation of chicken embryo fibroblasts. Proc Natl Acad Sci USA 2002; 99(6): 3830-5.[http://dx.doi.org/10.1073/pnas.062036999] [PMID: 11891322]

[49]   Lu X, Vogt PK, Boger DL, Lunec J. Disruption of the MYC transcriptional function by a small-molecule antagonist of MYC/MAX dimerization. Oncol Rep 2008; 19(3): 825-30.[http://dx.doi.org/10.3892/or.19.3.825] [PMID: 18288422]

[50]   Yin X, Giap C, Lazo JS, Prochownik EV. Low molecular weight inhibitors of Myc-Max interaction and function. Oncogene 2003; 22(40): 6151-9.[http://dx.doi.org/10.1038/sj.onc.1206641] [PMID: 13679853]

[51]   Wang H, Hammoudeh DI, Follis AV, et al. Improved low molecular weight Myc-Max inhibitors. Mol Cancer Ther 2007; 6(9): 2399-408.[http://dx.doi.org/10.1158/1535-7163.MCT-07-0005] [PMID: 17876039]

[52]   Guo J, Parise RA, Joseph E, et al. Efficacy, pharmacokinetics, tisssue distribution, and metabolism of the Myc-Max disruptor, 10058-F4 [Z,E]-5-[4-ethylbenzylidine]-2-thioxothiazolidin-4-one, in mice. Cancer Chemother Pharmacol 2009; 63(4): 615-25.[http://dx.doi.org/10.1007/s00280-008-0774-y] [PMID: 18509642]

[53]   Kiessling A, Sperl B, Hollis A, Eick D, Berg T. Selective inhibition of c-Myc/Max dimerization and DNA binding by small molecules. Chem Biol 2006; 13(7): 745-51.[http://dx.doi.org/10.1016/j.chembiol.2006.05.011] [PMID: 16873022]

[54]   Xu Y, Shi J, Yamamoto N, Moss JA, Vogt PK, Janda KD. A credit-card library approach for disrupting protein-protein interactions. Bioorg Med Chem 2006; 14(8): 2660-73.[http://dx.doi.org/10.1016/j.bmc.2005.11.052] [PMID: 16384710]

[55]   Han H, Jain AD, Truica MI, et al. Small-Molecule MYC Inhibitors Suppress Tumor Growth and Enhance Immunotherapy. Cancer Cell 2019; 36(5): 483-497.e15.[http://dx.doi.org/10.1016/j.ccell.2019.10.001] [PMID: 31679823]

[56]   Castell A, Yan Q, Fawkner K, et al. A selective high affinity MYC-binding compound inhibits MYC:MAX interaction and MYC-dependent tumor cell proliferation. Sci Rep 2018; 8(1): 10064.[http://dx.doi.org/10.1038/s41598-018-28107-4] [PMID: 29968736]

[57]   Reed JC. Bcl-2 on the brink of breakthroughs in cancer treatment. Cell Death Differ 2018; 25(1): 3-6.[http://dx.doi.org/10.1038/cdd.2017.188] [PMID: 29227986]

[58]   Kim R. Unknotting the roles of Bcl-2 and Bcl-xL in cell death. Biochem Biophys Res Commun 2005; 333(2): 336-43.[http://dx.doi.org/10.1016/j.bbrc.2005.04.161] [PMID: 15922292]

[59]   Janumyan YM, Sansam CG, Chattopadhyay A, et al. Bcl-xL/Bcl-2 coordinately regulates apoptosis, cell cycle arrest and cell cycle entry. EMBO J 2003; 22(20): 5459-70.[http://dx.doi.org/10.1093/emboj/cdg533] [PMID: 14532118]

[60]   Shamas-Din A, Kale J, Leber B, Andrews DW. Mechanisms of action of Bcl-2 family proteins. Cold Spring Harb Perspect Biol 2013; 5(4): a008714.[http://dx.doi.org/10.1101/cshperspect.a008714] [PMID: 23545417]

[61]   Kirsch DG, Doseff A, Chau BN, et al. Caspase-3-dependent cleavage of Bcl-2 promotes release of cytochrome c. J Biol Chem 1999; 274(30): 21155-61.[http://dx.doi.org/10.1074/jbc.274.30.21155] [PMID: 10409669]

[62]   Thomas S, Quinn BA, Das SK, et al. Targeting the Bcl-2 family for cancer therapy. Expert Opin Ther Targets 2013; 17(1): 61-75.[http://dx.doi.org/10.1517/14728222.2013.733001] [PMID: 23173842]

[63]   Kirkin V, Joos S, Zörnig M. The role of Bcl-2 family members in tumorigenesis. Biochim Biophys Acta 2004; 1644(2-3): 229-49.[http://dx.doi.org/10.1016/j.bbamcr.2003.08.009] [PMID: 14996506]

[64]   Wilson WH, O'Connor OA, Czuczman MS, et al. Navitoclax, a targeted high-affinity inhibitor of BCL-2, in lymphoid malignancies: a phase 1 dose-escalation study of safety, pharmacokinetics, pharmacodynamics, and antitumour activity. Lancet Oncol 2010; 11(12): 1149-59.[http://dx.doi.org/10.1016/S1470-2045(10)70261-8]

[PMID: 21094089]

[65] Tse C, Shoemaker AR, Adickes J, *et al.* ABT-263: a potent and orally bioavailable Bcl-2 family inhibitor. Cancer Res 2008; 68(9): 3421-8.[http://dx.doi.org/10.1158/0008-5472.CAN-07-5836] [PMID: 18451170]

[66] Vogler M, Dinsdale D, Dyer MJ, Cohen GM. Bcl-2 inhibitors: small molecules with a big impact on cancer therapy. Cell Death Differ 2009; 16(3): 360-7.[http://dx.doi.org/10.1038/cdd.2008.137] [PMID: 18806758]

[67] Kakkola L, Denisova OV, Tynell J, *et al.* Anticancer compound ABT-263 accelerates apoptosis in virus-infected cells and imbalances cytokine production and lowers survival rates of infected mice. Cell Death Dis 2013; 4: e742.[http://dx.doi.org/10.1038/cddis.2013.267] [PMID: 23887633]

[68] Souers AJ, Leverson JD, Boghaert ER, *et al.* ABT-199, a potent and selective BCL-2 inhibitor, achieves antitumor activity while sparing platelets. Nat Med 2013; 19(2): 202-8.[http://dx.doi.org/10.1038/nm.3048] [PMID: 23291630]

[69] Sleebs BE, Czabotar PE, Fairbrother WJ, *et al.* Quinazoline sulfonamides as dual binders of the proteins B-cell lymphoma 2 and B-cell lymphoma extra long with potent proapoptotic cell-based activity. J Med Chem 2011; 54(6): 1914-26.[http://dx.doi.org/10.1021/jm101596e] [PMID: 21366295]

[70] García CP, Videla Richardson GA, Dimopoulos NA, *et al.* Human Pluripotent Stem Cells and Derived Neuroprogenitors Display Differential Degrees of Susceptibility to BH3 Mimetics ABT-263, WEHI-539 and ABT-199. PLoS One 2016; 11(3): e0152607.[http://dx.doi.org/10.1371/journal.pone.0152607] [PMID: 27030982]

[71] Zhou H, Aguilar A, Chen J, *et al.* Structure-based design of potent Bcl-2/Bcl-xL inhibitors with strong *in vivo* antitumor activity. J Med Chem 2012; 55(13): 6149-61.[http://dx.doi.org/10.1021/jm300608w] [PMID: 22747598]

[72] Bai L, Chen J, McEachern D, *et al.* BM-1197: a novel and specific Bcl-2/Bcl-xL inhibitor inducing complete and long-lasting tumor regression *in vivo.* PLoS One 2014; 9(6): e99404.[http://dx.doi.org/10.1371/journal.pone.0099404] [PMID: 24901320]

[73] Bruncko M, Oost TK, Belli BA, *et al.* Studies leading to potent, dual inhibitors of Bcl-2 and Bcl-xL. J Med Chem 2007; 50(4): 641-62.[http://dx.doi.org/10.1021/jm061152t] [PMID: 17256834]

[74] Chatterjee S, Burns TF. Targeting Heat Shock Proteins in Cancer: A Promising Therapeutic Approach. Int J Mol Sci 2017; 18(9): 1978.[http://dx.doi.org/10.3390/ijms18091978] [PMID: 28914774]

[75] Kumar S, Stokes J, III, Singh UP, *et al.* Targeting Hsp70: A possible therapy for cancer. Cancer Lett 2016; 374(1): 156-66.[http://dx.doi.org/10.1016/j.canlet.2016.01.056] [PMID: 26898980]

[76] Özgür A, Tutar Y. Heat Shock Protein 90 Inhibition in Cancer Drug Discovery: From Chemistry to Futural Clinical Applications. Anticancer Agents Med Chem 2016; 16(3): 280-90.[http://dx.doi.org/10.2174/1871520615666150821093747] [PMID: 26295332]

[77] Saibil H. Chaperone machines for protein folding, unfolding and disaggregation. Nat Rev Mol Cell Biol 2013; 14(10): 630-42.[http://dx.doi.org/10.1038/nrm3658] [PMID: 24026055]

[78] Morán Luengo T, Mayer MP, Rüdiger SGD. The Hsp70-Hsp90 Chaperone Cascade in Protein Folding. Trends Cell Biol 2019; 29(2): 164-77.[http://dx.doi.org/10.1016/j.tcb.2018.10.004] [PMID: 30502916]

[79] Elo MA, Kaarniranta K, Helminen HJ, Lammi MJ. Hsp90 inhibitor geldanamycin increases hsp70 mRNA stabilisation but fails to activate HSF1 in cells exposed to hydrostatic pressure. Biochim Biophys Acta 2005; 1743(1-2): 115-9.[http://dx.doi.org/10.1016/j.bbamcr.2004.09.004] [PMID: 15777846]

[80] Powers MV, Clarke PA, Workman P. Death by chaperone: HSP90, HSP70 or both? Cell Cycle 2009; 8(4): 518-26.[http://dx.doi.org/10.4161/cc.8.4.7583] [PMID: 19197160]

[81] Shrestha L, Bolaender A, Patel HJ, Taldone T. Heat Shock Protein (HSP) Drug Discovery and Development: Targeting Heat Shock Proteins in Disease. Curr Top Med Chem 2016; 16(25): 2753-64.[http://dx.doi.org/10.2174/1568026616666160413141911] [PMID: 27072696]

[82] Koca İ, Gümüş M, Özgür A, Dişli A, Tutar Y. A Novel Approach to Inhibit Heat Shock Response as Anticancer Strategy by Coumarine Compounds Containing Thiazole Skeleton. Anticancer Agents Med Chem 2015; 15(7): 916-30.[http://dx.doi.org/10.2174/1871520615666150407155623] [PMID: 25846761]

[83] Gümus M, Ozgur A, Tutar L, Disli A, Koca I, Tutar Y. Design, Synthesis, and Evaluation of Heat Shock Protein 90 Inhibitors in Human Breast Cancer and Its Metastasis. Curr Pharm Biotechnol 2016; 17(14): 1231-45.[http://dx.doi.org/10.2174/1389201017666161031105815] [PMID: 27804852]

[84] Koca İ, Özgür A, Er M, Gümüş M, Açikalin Coşkun K, Tutar Y. Design and synthesis of pyrimidinyl acyl thioureas as novel Hsp90 inhibitors in invasive ductal breast cancer and its bone metastasis. Eur J Med Chem 2016; 122: 280-90.[http://dx.doi.org/10.1016/j.ejmech.2016.06.032] [PMID: 27376491]

[85] Colvin TA, Gabai VL, Gong J, *et al.* Hsp70-Bag3 interactions regulate cancer-related signaling networks.

Cancer Res 2014; 74(17): 4731-40.[http://dx.doi.org/10.1158/0008-5472.CAN-14-0747] [PMID: 24994713]

[86]   De Marco M, Basile A, Iorio V, *et al.* Role of BAG3 in cancer progression: A therapeutic opportunity. Semin Cell Dev Biol 2018; 78: 85-92.[http://dx.doi.org/10.1016/j.semcdb.2017.08.049] [PMID: 28864347]

[87]   Li X, Colvin T, Rauch JN, *et al.* Validation of the Hsp70-Bag3 protein-protein interaction as a potential therapeutic target in cancer. Mol Cancer Ther 2015; 14(3): 642-8.[http://dx.doi.org/10.1158/1535-7163.MCT-14-0650] [PMID: 25564440]

[88]   Li T, Jiang HL, Tong YG, Lu JJ. Targeting the Hsp90-Cdc37-client protein interaction to disrupt Hsp90 chaperone machinery. J Hematol Oncol 2018; 11(1): 59.[http://dx.doi.org/10.1186/s13045-018-0602-8] [PMID: 29699578]

[89]   Smith JR, Workman P. Targeting CDC37: an alternative, kinase-directed strategy for disruption of oncogenic chaperoning. Cell Cycle 2009; 8(3): 362-72.[http://dx.doi.org/10.4161/cc.8.3.7531] [PMID: 19177013]

[90]   Wang L, Zhang L, Li L, *et al.* Small-molecule inhibitor targeting the Hsp90-Cdc37 protein-protein interaction in colorectal cancer. Sci Adv 2019; 5(9): eaax2277.[http://dx.doi.org/10.1126/sciadv.aax2277] [PMID: 31555737]

[91]   Jung YS, Park JI. Wnt signaling in cancer: therapeutic targeting of Wnt signaling beyond β-catenin and the destruction complex. Exp Mol Med 2020; 52(2): 183-91.[http://dx.doi.org/10.1038/s12276-020-0380-6] [PMID: 32037398]

[92]   Kimelman D, Xu W. beta-catenin destruction complex: insights and questions from a structural perspective. Oncogene 2006; 25(57): 7482-91.[http://dx.doi.org/10.1038/sj.onc.1210055] [PMID: 17143292]

[93]   Shin SH, Lim DY, Reddy K, *et al.* A Small Molecule Inhibitor of the β-Catenin-TCF4 Interaction Suppresses Colorectal Cancer Growth *In Vitro* and *In Vivo.* EBioMedicine 2017; 25: 22-31.[http://dx.doi.org/10.1016/j.ebiom.2017.09.029] [PMID: 29033371]

[94]   Hsu HT, Liu PC, Ku SY, *et al.* Beta-catenin control of T-cell transcription factor 4 (Tcf4) importation from the cytoplasm to the nucleus contributes to Tcf4-mediated transcription in 293 cells. Biochem Biophys Res Commun 2006; 343(3): 893-8.[http://dx.doi.org/10.1016/j.bbrc.2006.02.193] [PMID: 16564030]

[95]   Shang S, Hua F, Hu ZW. The regulation of β-catenin activity and function in cancer: therapeutic opportunities. Oncotarget 2017; 8(20): 33972-89.[http://dx.doi.org/10.18632/oncotarget.15687] [PMID: 28430641]

[96]   Lepourcelet M, Chen YN, France DS, *et al.* Small-molecule antagonists of the oncogenic Tcf/beta-catenin protein complex. Cancer Cell 2004; 5(1): 91-102.[http://dx.doi.org/10.1016/S1535-6108(03)00334-9] [PMID: 14749129]

[97]   Gonsalves FC, Klein K, Carson BB, *et al.* An RNAi-based chemical genetic screen identifies three small-molecule inhibitors of the Wnt/wingless signaling pathway. Proc Natl Acad Sci USA 2011; 108(15): 5954-63.[http://dx.doi.org/10.1073/pnas.1017496108] [PMID: 21393571]

[98]   Wang W, Liu H, Wang S, Hao X, Li L. A diterpenoid derivative 15-oxospiramilactone inhibits Wnt/β-catenin signaling and colon cancer cell tumorigenesis. Cell Res 2011; 21(5): 730-40.[http://dx.doi.org/10.1038/cr.2011.30] [PMID: 21321609]

[99]   Jang GB, Hong IS, Kim RJ, *et al.* Wnt/β-Catenin Small-Molecule Inhibitor CWP232228 Preferentially Inhibits the Growth of Breast Cancer Stem-like Cells. Cancer Res 2015; 75(8): 1691-702.[http://dx.doi.org/10.1158/0008-5472.CAN-14-2041] [PMID: 25660951]

[100]   Brzezinka K, Nevedomskaya E, Lesche R, *et al.* Characterization of the Menin-MLL Interaction as Therapeutic Cancer Target. Cancers (Basel) 2020; 12(1): 201.[http://dx.doi.org/10.3390/cancers12010201] [PMID: 31947537]

[101]   Matkar S, Thiel A, Hua X. Menin: a scaffold protein that controls gene expression and cell signaling. Trends Biochem Sci 2013; 38(8): 394-402.[http://dx.doi.org/10.1016/j.tibs.2013.05.005] [PMID: 23850066]

[102]   Chen YX, Yan J, Keeshan K, *et al.* The tumor suppressor menin regulates hematopoiesis and myeloid transformation by influencing Hox gene expression. Proc Natl Acad Sci USA 2006; 103(4): 1018-23.[http://dx.doi.org/10.1073/pnas.0510347103] [PMID: 16415155]

[103]   Milne TA, Hughes CM, Lloyd R, *et al.* Menin and MLL cooperatively regulate expression of cyclin-dependent kinase inhibitors. Proc Natl Acad Sci USA 2005; 102(3): 749-54.[http://dx.doi.org/10.1073/pnas.0408836102] [PMID: 15640349]

[104]   Borkin D, He S, Miao H, *et al.* Pharmacologic inhibition of the Menin-MLL interaction blocks progression of MLL leukemia *in vivo.* Cancer Cell 2015; 27(4): 589-602.[http://dx.doi.org/10.1016/j.ccell.2015.02.016] [PMID: 25817203]

[105]   Shi A, Murai MJ, He S, *et al.* Structural insights into inhibition of the bivalent menin-MLL interaction by small molecules in leukemia. Blood 2012; 120(23): 4461-9.[http://dx.doi.org/10.1182/blood-2012-05-

429274] [PMID: 22936661]

[106
]   He S, Senter TJ, Pollock J, *et al.* High-affinity small-molecule inhibitors of the menin-mixed lineage leukemia (MLL) interaction closely mimic a natural protein-protein interaction. J Med Chem 2014; 57(4): 1543-56.[http://dx.doi.org/10.1021/jm401868d] [PMID: 24472025]

Efficacy of Hepatic Arterial Infusion Chemotherapy (HAIC) for Advanced Hepatocellular Carcinoma

Kei Moriya

, Tadashi Namisaki, Hitoshi Yoshiji

Department of Gastroenterology and Hepatology, Nara Medical University, Address: 840 Shijo-cho, Kashihara, Nara 634-8522, Japan

Abstract

As per the latest data of the International Agency for Research on Cancer, more than 8 million individuals die annually owing to the exacerbation of a given neoplasm, and the total number of annual deaths due to hepatocellular carcinoma (HCC) is 0.78 million, the second-highest of all cancer-related deaths. HCC has a very poor prognosis, reflected by the fact that the incidence-to-mortality ratio of HCC has been estimated to be more than 90%. Liver cancer is generally diagnosed only in the advanced clinical stage because HCC tends to be clinically silent during the early stages. With regard to HCC management, transarterial chemoembolization (TACE) and hepatic arterial infusion chemotherapy (HAIC), as well as molecularly targeted agents such as sorafenib and lenvatinib, have shown promising benefits for advanced HCC. However, even though the Barcelona Clinic Liver Cancer staging system has been widely accepted, controversies still exist regarding the best choice for the management of HCC in individual cases. In this chapter, we infer that HAIC treatment is not inferior to molecularly targeted therapies for the treatment of advanced HCC—particularly in case of intravascular invasion in both compensated and decompensated cirrhotic patients. Furthermore, the rate of adverse events leading to discontinuation of antitumor treatment appears relatively low.

Given the hepatic function reserve preservation afforded by HAIC chemotherapy, we suggest that HAIC should be considered as an alternative strategy even for advanced-HCC patients with decompensated cirrhosis, who do not respond to TACE.

Keywords: 5-fluorouracil, Advanced stage, Chemotherapy, Child–Pugh classification, Cisplatin, Hepatic arterial infusion, Hepatic functional reserve, Hepatocellular carcinoma, Lenvatinib, Molecularly targeted therapies, Overall survival, Portal invasion, Progression-free survival, Reservoir, Sorafenib.

* **Corresponding author Kei Moriya:** Department of Gastroenterology and Hepatology, Nara Medical University, Address: 840 Shijo-cho, Kashihara, Nara 634-8522, Japan; Tel: +81-744-22-3051; Fax: +81-744-24-7122; E-mail: moriyak@naramed-u.ac.jp

INTRODUCTION

Liver cancer is the sixth most commonly diagnosed cancer and the fourth leading cause of cancer-related death in the world []. In 2015, there were approximately 854,000 new liver cancer cases and compared with an estimated 810,000 liver cancer-related deaths annually, the ratio between incidence and the annual number of deaths is the second highest of all cancer-related deaths []. Hence, liver cancer is a highly fatal disease, with an incidence-to-mortality ratio approaching 1 []. Recent advances in diagnostic imaging techniques and various treatment methods have steadily improved the prognosis of patients with hepatocellular carcinoma (HCC) []; however, at the same time, these various options make the treatment of HCC difficult for clinicians to understand. This might be due to the complexity of various factors preempting a simple classification of the disease.

In this chapter, I would like to explain the advantages as well as the cautions in the case of selecting HAIC as a treatment of HCC. Additionally, HAIC combination therapy with molecularly targeted drugs or surgical resection and new derivation of modified HAIC are also described.

The Best Choice for Managing Advanced Hepatocellular Carcinoma

The major histology underlying primary liver cancer is HCC, the incidence of which remains highest in Asian countries (specifically in the East and southeast Asia) and in Italy []. Japan and Italy, for example, both have an aging population, and relatively many patients with HCC have comorbidities such as diabetes mellitus, hypertension, cardiac disease, cerebrovascular disease, chronic renal failure, or chronic obstructive pulmonary disease. Therefore, when choosing the most appropriate treatment for an individual case from among the various treatment options available, it is necessary to first evaluate the comorbidities and performance status of the patient, followed by an assessment of hepatic functional reserve (HFR). In general, many diabetic patients with cirrhosis have reduced hepatic insulin sensitivity and often require insulin due to marked postprandial hyperglycemia. Patients with long-lasting and/or poorly controlled diabetes mellitus are more likely to develop cardiovascular problems such as heart disease and cerebrovascular disease, as well as chronic renal failure. The degree of tumor progression is assessed only after these evaluations. With the exception of patients previously treated for HCC followed by subsequent routine imaging, it is not uncommon for patients with HCC to have advanced HCC by the time they visit a medical institution due to the general lack of symptoms in the initial stage [].

HCC with vascular invasion is relatively common [], and since HCC with portal vein invasion (Vp) is associated with a relatively high rate of distant metastases [], it is necessary to identify any distant metastases in these cases. In addition, whether the HCC is affecting both lobes or is confined to only one of these may be a criterion for considering surgical treatment. The degree of Vp may also be a criterion for considering arterial embolization.

The Barcelona Clinic Liver Cancer (BCLC) classification, which has been widely applied to evaluating the extent of tumor progression in HCC, has been included in the HCC treatment guidelines developed by the European Association for the Study of the Liver and the American Association for the Study of the Liver Disease [,]. According to this classification, patients with Vp-HCC are classified as advanced-stage HCC (stage C) and are recommended to receive molecularly targeted therapies such as sorafenib and lenvatinib. On the other hand, no randomized study comparing hepatic arterial infusion chemotherapy (HAIC) with the standard of care or no medical treatment has been published, and so no evidence of its benefit or issues with side effects specific to the reservoir system (*e.g.*, vasculitis, peptic ulcers due to arterial occlusion, reservoir infections, and reservoir obstruction) has been reported to date. Subsequently, there has been no recommendation of HAIC to a patient with Vp-HCC as a standard of care in these guidelines. In addition, HAIC is not considered the standard of care in the consensus guidelines of the Asia-Pacific Association for the Study of the Liver (APASL) []. On the other hand, according to the treatment algorithm included in the clinical practice guidelines for HCC 2017 proposed by the Japanese Society of Hepatology, transarterial chemoembolization (TACE), hepatic resection, HAIC, and molecularly targeted therapies are recommended for advanced-HCC cases in patients with Child-Pugh class A of the HFR and vascular involvement, but without distant metastasis [].

It is generally difficult to detect pathological vascular invasion (Vp1) using diagnostic imaging such as computed tomography (CT) and magnetic resonance imaging (MRI), and it is likely that in some cases where very large numbers of HCCs are identified in the liver, at least some of them will exhibit Vp1. In fact, treatment guidelines based on the BCLC classification state that the treatment strategy for "four or more and up to Vp1-HCC" is transcatheter arterial chemoembolization (TACE), molecularly targeted therapies, or best supportive care (BSC), and this strategy diverges significantly from the strategy applied in Japan, which is based on consensus-based HCC treatment algorithms. In fact, the indications for TACE are wide, and if the tumor is sufficiently hypervascular, treatment can be performed, as long as the vessels nourishing the tumor can be sorted out manually, and TACE can be used to treat portal vein tumor thrombi as small as Vp1 without any problems. That is why no clear criteria for the indications for TACE have been provided regarding upper treatment limits for tumor size or the number of tumors, and current guidelines in Western and Asian countries, including Japan, place TACE as the standard of care for intrahepatic HCC that is not amenable to resection and local treatment ["]. However, even after successful embolization of targeted tumor vessels, we often experience cases refractory to TACE in daily practice, such as cases in which embolization does not continue until imaging evaluation a few months later or in which multiple new lesions are present. Specifically, TACE can be performed in patients with more than four tumors or tumors larger than 7 cm in diameter, but the early recurrence can be expected. Therefore, if these patients do not respond to TACE, the definition of "TACE failure" proposed by Kudo *et al.* should be carefully interpreted []. TACE failure/refractoriness is defined as: (1) Intrahepatic lesion i) Two or more consecutive ineffective responses seen within the treated tumors (viable lesions > 50%), even after changing the chemotherapeutic agents and/or reanalysis of feeding artery on response evaluation CT/MRI after 1–3 months following adequately performed selective TACE, ii) Two or more consecutive progressions in the liver (including an increase in the number of tumors compared with that before the previous TACE procedure), even after changing the chemotherapeutic agents and/or reanalysis of feeding artery on response evaluation CT/MRI after 1–3 months following adequately performed selective TACE, (2) Continuous elevation of tumor markers immediately after TACE despite observation of transient minor reduction, (3) Development of vascular invasion, and (4) Extrahepatic spread. If patients meet any of these criteria for TACE failure/refractoriness, physicians may need to consider other therapies or combinations of therapies, such as HAIC, in addition to the option of molecularly targeted therapies, although there is certainly no firm evidence for this recommendation. Specifically, there is already evidence that adherence to repeated TACE is detrimental to the HFR. Arizumi *et al.* found that the Child–Pugh score worsened over time in the TACE continuation group compared with the sorafenib group who underwent treatment conversion to sorafenib []. Ogasawara *et al.* reported that the time from TACE refractory point to Child–Pugh class C was significantly shorter in the TACE continuation group than in the sorafenib group who underwent treatment conversion to sorafenib (29.8 months in the sorafenib group *vs.* 17.0 months in the TACE group, P = 0.030) [].

Thus, taking the definition of TACE refractoriness into account, HAIC would be selected in cases to which TACE treatment would be hardly responding, such as a multiple-tumor case or a very large tumor case. In these cases, there is an overlap with regard to the targets for treatment between molecularly targeted therapies and HAIC. However, an acceptable suggestion would be to select a molecularly targeted agent first if the HFR is Child–Pugh class A, because these molecularly targeted agents are difficult to administer to Child–Pugh class B patients. Then, if there is no response to these molecularly targeted agents, it might prove useful to switch to HAIC. HAIC may be the treatment of choice for patients with Child–Pugh class B HFR at the beginning of the treatment. To our knowledge, no randomized control trial (RCT) directly comparing HAIC with molecularly targeted therapies has been published. Nevertheless, a couple of clinical studies comparing the outcomes of sorafenib and HAIC treatment in patients who did not respond to TACE have been published; however, none of these identified superiorities of HAIC []. Still, Fukubayashi *et al.* performed a retrospective analysis of data on 72 patients with advanced HCC treated with sorafenib and 128 patients treated with HAIC. The clinical backgrounds of the patients had been fully matched by propensity scores. It was shown that although there was no significant difference in overall survival (OS), there was a slightly better progression-free survival when using HAIC, and there was a significant increase in OS with HAIC in patients with Vp-HCC, in patients without extrahepatic lesions, and in patients with Vp-HCC but no extrahepatic lesions [].

What is Hepatic Arterial Infusion Chemotherapy (HAIC)?

HAIC has been widely used in Japan for the treatment of advanced HCC unsuitable for systemic chemotherapy with cytotoxic agents due to decreased HFR or concomitant pancytopenia. By local administration of a small amount of anticancer drug, high concentrations of the drug can be administered to the hepatic tumors, which can be expected to have a relatively high antitumor effect and to minimize systemic invasion. Since some cytotoxic agents are metabolized in the liver, reduced side effects in other organs are expected by such local administration. HAIC has the advantage of being useful for local tumor control and is used as an effective tool for advanced HCC with vascular invasion in countries such as Japan and South Korea. However, any existing survival benefit of HAIC therapy remains to be demonstrated. HAIC comprises two different modalities; one is the "one-shot arterial infusion" approach, applying Selzinger's method, and the other is "continuous arterial infusion," which takes advantage of a subcutaneous reservoir system. Both of these methods involve direct injection of an antitumor agent through the hepatic artery into a tumor nutrient vessel, but the former is mainly concentration-dependent and the latter is time-dependent.

Cisplatin (CDDP) is a platinum complex compound that binds to intracellular DNA strands through passive diffusion and active transport, inhibiting DNA synthesis, and subsequent cell division, thereby exerting a cytotoxic effect (apoptosis). Its antitumor effects are concentration-dependent and can be classified as fast-acting and slow-acting. CDDP has been shown to be effective against a number of cancer types and several studies have reported on the efficacy against HCC [].

Unlike anthracyclines, which are excreted from bile, these drugs are not metabolized by cytochrome P450s and are mainly excreted in the urine, making them easier to administer to cirrhotic patients with reduced HFR. As for another platinum anticancer drug, miliplatin has been approved in Japan for the treatment of HCC with chemolipiodolization. The increased lipid solubility of the CDDP-release ligand and the high affinity of the oil-based contrast medium for lipiodol allows it to stay in the tumor for a longer period of time, resulting in a sustained release of the drug [].

5-fluorouracil (5-FU) is mostly used for continuous arterial infusion because of its concentration-dependent and time-dependent effects. However, because of the low efficacy of single-agent use, combination therapy with selected drugs has been used as a modulator based on the idea of biochemical modulation. Low dose 5-FU and CDDP arterial infusion therapy (low dose FP therapy) and 5-FU arterial infusion with interferon therapy (FAIT therapy) are typical examples of such combination therapies; however, because interferon is very expensive, the latter has not been used widely. The characteristics and outcomes of each treatment method are described below. The response rate (complete response [CR] + partial response [PR]) to multiple agents is generally 30%–40% in combination with HAIC, and 20%–30% for cisplatin used as a single agent, and patients who responded to HAIC have had a longer prognosis than those who did not []. HAIC is considered a treatment used to elicit a clear response, and if only a partial response is achieved, it can be converted to other radical therapies such as surgical resection and radiofrequency ablation to achieve a more significant response.

Incidentally, HFR is an important prognostic factor for life expectancy in cirrhotic patients []. Terashima *et al.* compared the influence of HAIC and sorafenib treatment on HFR after 1 and 3 months in Child–Pugh class A patients and reported that the use of HAIC resulted in a significantly better preservation of HFR at both points [].

In a retrospective study, Saeki *et al.* reported that among cirrhotic patients scored as Child–Pugh class A before first HAIC, 5.6% (1 of 18) of the responders and 20.8% (10 of 48) of the non-responders fell into Child–Pugh class B after the first HAIC. Meanwhile, among patients scored initially as Child–Pugh class B, 27.8% (5 out of 18) of the responders improved to Child–Pugh class A, with 9.5% (4 out of 42) of the non-responders improving to Child–Pugh class A after completion of one course of chemotherapy; however, 11.9% (5 out of 42) of the non-responders fell into Child–Pugh class C [].

Thus, HAIC is relatively well tolerated even in Child–Pugh class B cases, and HAIC should also be considered for Child–Pugh class B patients, as treatment response is well expected to improve liver function, especially in cases of poor HFR due to advanced-HCC progression. However, in case of copious numbers of HCC in both hepatic lobes (so-called diffuse HCC) or in case of strong arterial-portal shunt formation at the lesion of vascular invasion, HCCs are generally considered less likely to respond to HAIC.

One-shot HAIC and its Clinical Outcome for HCC

In Japan, the usefulness of CDDP [] and miriplatin [] for one-shot HAIC during angiography has been evaluated and is now covered by medical insurance.

The first-pass kinetics of CDDP by HAIC provides approximately 48.4% (range, 34.2% to 55%) of HCC uptake, which is more than 10 times higher than the local concentration of anticancer agents administered routinely by the venous route [], and this selective high-concentration infusion into the hepatic arteries results in high effectiveness. Previously, only a low-concentration solution (10 mg/20 mL) of CDDP was available. However, in 2004, a fine-powdered formulation of CDDP (DDP-H) was introduced, which allows the concentration of the drug to be adjusted for use in HAIC and enables the concentration-dependent cytotoxic effects of CDDP to be more efficiently achieved. DDP-H (50 mg/1V) is dissolved in 35 mL of saline solution and then administered over a period of approximately 30 min. The base dose is 65 mg/m^2, adjusted for tumor size and volume, and the treatment is repeated every 4–6 weeks. In the case of miriplatin (70 mg/1V), a highly concentrated dilution (20 mg/mL) is made by dissolving it in 3.5 mL of lysate and then transfer it through the microcatheter for HAIC to the cancer-bearing area in the same way as with CDDP. The maximum dose is 120 mg/body, and it is infused according to tumor volume and administered at intervals of at least 4 weeks. The advantages of one-shot HAIC are that it does not require indwelling catheters, the procedure is simple, and there are few complications. In approximately 20% of the cases, there is a running variant of the hepatic artery (such as the right hepatic artery separating from the superior mesenteric artery or the left hepatic artery separating from the left gastric artery); in such cases, unifying the hepatic artery is necessary, which is performed by modifying intrahepatic circulation using coil embolization.

In a Phase-2 study of 80 patients, Yoshikawa *et al.* reported a response rate of 33.8%, a 1-year survival rate of 67.5%, and a 2-year survival rate of 50.8% []. Hatanaka *et al.* reviewed the outcomes of 123 patients with advanced HCC who underwent HAIC with DDP-H and found that the cumulative survival rate was significantly better ($P < 0.05$) in the responders (CR + PR) than in the non-responders (stable disease [SD] + progressive disease [PD]) and median survival time (MST) for the responders (23.8 months) was significantly longer than that for non-responders (10.6 months) []. In a retrospective study of 84 patients, Iwasa *et al.* reported a response rate of 3.6% (CR, 1.2% [1 out of 84]; PR, 2.4% [2 out of 84], an OS of 7.1 months, and 1-year survival of 27% []. Moriya *et al.* reviewed the outcomes of advanced-HCC patients with compensated cirrhosis who underwent HAIC every 8 weeks with an explicit awareness of the importance of preserving HFR []. They demonstrated a 38% response rate and an MST of 19 months, with no significant decrease in HFR during the treatment period. Even in cases of HAIC failure, the majority of the patients were able to receive another round of treatment. Moriya *et al.* also reported on other treatment outcomes in advanced-HCC patients with Child–Pugh class B status []. Even in these vulnerable patients, a 21% response rate was observed; moreover, the MST was 14 months, and successful post-treatment could be achieved for 13%, with no loss of HFR by HAIC treatment repeated by 8-week intervals. Thus, HAIC is unlikely to have a negative effect on HFR and has the advantage of not limiting post-treatment options in the event of treatment failure. In both compensated and uncompensated cirrhosis cases, no significant renal dysfunction attributable to DDP-H was observed during the duration of treatment. In addition, it was recently reported that DDP-H can be administered with lipiodol or embolic agents, with modest adverse effects and good clinical outcomes [,]. The response rate of HAIC with DDP-H ranges between 3.6% and 38.0% [, ̄,].

Meanwhile, Nagahama *et al.* reported a response rate of 9.3% in HCC patients treated with intravenous systemic CDDP chemotherapy []. Additionally, Court *et al.* observed an average accumulation of 48.4% (34.2%–55.4%) in tumors after HAIC, using radiolabeled CDDP []. In light of these results, it is hoped that HAIC will continue to be effective in the future; unfortunately however, the results reported by each institution vary, and no large-scale RCT that has validated the benefit to OS has been published. Under these circumstances, Ikeda *et al.* sought to explore the efficacy of DDP-H HAIC in 106 cases of advanced HCC (Vp-HCC, 53.7%; Child–Pugh class A, 90.6%) by adding DDP-H HAIC to sorafenib monotherapy. A randomized Phase-2 study was performed to investigate the effect of combining the two drugs. The OS was 8.7 months in the sorafenib monotherapy group and 10.6 months in the combined therapy group (hazard ratio, 0.60 [0.38–0.96], P = 0.031), achieving the endpoint of the Phase-2 study. This result suggests that DDP-H HAIC has a positive effect on OS [].

Miriplatin is an agent with a slow-release effect on tumors due to its high affinity for the carrier lipiodol. Moreover, it tends to have a significantly shorter local time to progression (TTP) (3.2 months *vs.* 15.1 months, P = 0.0293) and a lower rate of complete tumor necrosis (P = 0.058) compared with epirubicin, which has traditionally been used predominantly for TACE treatment []. In a Phase-3 RCT of unresectable advanced HCC, Ikeda *et al.* found that miriplatin was no longer superior with regard to OS []. Meanwhile, in an RCT comprising 198 patients with unresectable HCC treated with TACE, Kubota *et al.* found that although the response rate (79% *vs.* 77%, P = 0.862) and adverse-event rate (37% *vs.* 46%) were similar in the miriplatin and epirubicin groups, the median TTP (7.6 months *vs.* 5.9 months, P = 0.021) was significantly prolonged in the miriplatin group []. In addition, basic research in rats has shown that vascular injury caused by miriplatin was significantly less severe than that caused by epirubicin and comparable with that of the control group []. The low intravascular toxicity may be a major advantage because of the repetitive nature of HAIC as well as TACE treatment, and the efficacy of miriplatin, a platinum-based agent similar to CDDP, should be evaluated for more cases. Matsumoto *et al.* used repeated TACE with miriplatin administered for three or more sessions and found that the initial and final treatment sessions could be performed with no major impairment of liver or kidney function, and the incidence of other adverse events was similar, suggesting that the treatment could be safely repeated [].

Some clinicians may be concerned about the use of molecularly targeted agents such as sorafenib and lenvatinib following HAIC in patients with Child–Pugh class A due to deterioration of HFR. However, Saeki *et al.* suggested that the response to one-shot HAIC can be predicted two weeks after implementation [], because the mean half-life of des-gamma-carboxy prothrombin (DCP) (3.2 days) as well as alpha-fetoprotein (AFP) (6.0 days) is quite brief []. Exacerbation of liver damage is less likely to occur if treatment is changed at this time. Hence, the future challenge is to identify a simple factor that can more accurately predict the efficacy of one-shot HAIC in order to avoid unnecessary treatment at an earlier stage.

Reservoir Systems for Chemotherapy

Setting of Reservoir Systems

The most common route for reservoir implantation is the femoral artery, and the reservoir is often implanted in the subcutaneous space of the right lower quadrant of the abdomen. The subclavian and brachial arteries are also used in some cases. Usually, the gastroduodenal artery coil method is used for catheter placement. The tip of the catheter is secured to the gastroduodenal artery with a coil, and the catheter is placed so that the anticancer drug flows through the anterior lateral foramen to the intrinsic hepatic artery. If this artery is breached, the other hepatic arteries are embolized to unify with the original native hepatic artery. Embolization does not result in hepatic ischemia because of the presence of a traffic branch between the hepatic arteries and portal blood flow. Embolization of the right gastric artery and other vascular branches to the gastrointestinal tract, if identified, is necessary to prevent complications of drug leakage to the gastrointestinal tract. In addition to this, the right diaphragmatic artery and the right superior adrenal artery, which feed the HCC, should be combined with permanent embolization, preferably with a metal coil. In general, the reservoir is fixed subcutaneously and ready for use within 3–4 days after implantation. In case of hypoalbuminemia due to cirrhosis, the patient should be monitored for wound healing for about one week before taking the reservoir into use. When administering 5-FU with an infuser, the viscosity of 5-FU should be taken into account when selecting the type of infuser.

Management of Reservoir System and its Related Adverse Events

Because of the arterial pressure on the reservoir system, it is necessary to flush the reservoir system with a heparin solution every 2–3 weeks to prevent obstruction. During flushing, any resistance, pain, and swelling should be observed. The position of the catheter should be confirmed periodically by X-ray or CT for the evaluation of treatment efficacy. The side effects specific to reservoir HAIC include complications related to the implantation of the reservoir system, such as hematoma, wound infection, and dehiscence at the site of implantation, catheter dislocation or breakage, system obstruction, gastrointestinal ulceration, vascular disease, liver damage, and stroke. These complications require early detection and treatment since the patient may not be able to continue treatment if the treatment is delayed. Specifically, hematomas include inadequate hemostasis of the wound and bleeding at the arterial puncture site when the catheter is replaced with an indwelling catheter from a sheath, the latter of which can be prevented by using a 3-Fr sheath initially. To avoid catheter dislocation, the catheter should be stabilized by inserting the tip of the catheter into the gastroduodenal artery (GDA) and embolizing the GDA with a coil. Continuation of HAIC for > 6 months may result in vascular damage such as aneurysms and vascular occlusion; therefore, it is recommended that the reservoir be removed within 6 months, if the patient is in remission. In addition, prophylactic antiplatelet medication is required, as implantation of the reservoir through the upper arm or subclavian artery may result in cerebral infarction.

Reservoir HAIC Regimen and Clinical Outcome for HCC

The concept is that the CDDP acts as a modulator to enhance the effect of the effector 5-FU. This treatment regimen uses a reservoir to provide repetitive or continuous dosing and the method of Ando *et al.* which was reported early on is the method most often used. In this method, CDDP at a dose of 10 mg/body is administered over one hour, followed by 250 mg 5-FU/body over 5 hours. This is followed by four cycles of five consecutive days of infusion and two days of rest, each cycle lasting seven days. After treatment, continued treatment is considered based on the antitumor effect observed, and a 48% response rate has been reported []. Park *et al.* reported a response rate of 22% in patients with advanced HCC treated by a slightly modified CDDP and 5-FU regimen []. Okuda *et al.* demonstrated a response rate of 71% and a 5-year survival rate of 45.7% []. Ueshima *et al.* reported a response rate of 38.5% and an OS of 15.9 months []. In addition, there has been a study in which a total of 1,250–2,500 mg of 5-FU was arterially infused by an infuser over a 5-day period for 24 hours, with a one-hour infusion of CDDP in between []. In this treatment, prophylactic hydration for nephrotoxicity is not necessary because of the small CDDP dose. In addition, Nagamatsu *et al.* performed chemolipiodolization of DDP-H (50 mg/1V) by mixing it with 5–10 mL of lipiodol and administered it to the patients with portal invasion of Vp2 (invasion into the secondary order branch of the portal vein) to Vp4 (invasion into the main trunk/contralateral branch of the portal vein). In 51 patients with advanced HCC, 10 patients (10.9%) were in complete remission, 34 patients (66.7%) in partial remission, and 5 patients (9.8%) remained unchanged three months after the beginning of treatment according to the RECIST criteria, resulting in a disease control rate of 86.3% []. Furthermore, the long-term prognosis was 37.1% for complete and partial response patients (n = 44) with a 3-year survival rate of 37.1%, and the 24 patients who were able to achieve a complete response with additional treatment reported a 3-year survival rate of 53.7%.

These results suggest that the response rate to LFP therapy is around 30%–40% and MST is around 10–15 months, although the tumor background of the treated advanced cases of HCCs differs to some extent. However, these are the results of a single-arm study, and although the response rate is relatively high, it has not been demonstrated whether HAIC actually improves patient's prognosis.

Based on the results of the Phase-2 study, which showed that sorafenib plus one-shot HAIC could be expected to have a positive effect on OS, Kudo *et al.* performed a Phase-3 SILIUS study to evaluate the additional effect of LFP-HAIC in combination with sorafenib [].

Two hundred and six advanced-HCC patients with Child-Pugh scores ≤ 7 who were not eligible for surgical resection/local ablation/TACE were randomly and evenly allocated into a sorafenib plus LFP-HAIC group or a sorafenib monotherapy group. In this study, the primary endpoint of MST was 11.8 months in the LFP-HAIC combination group and 11.5 months in the sorafenib monotherapy group (HR, 1.01 [95% CI, 0.74–1.37]; P = 0.955 [log-rank test]), demonstrating that LFP-HAIC provided no additional effect on the patients. Still, in the patients with Vp4-HCC, the MST was 11.4 months in the LFP-HAIC combined group and 6.5 months in the sorafenib monotherapy group (HR, 0.493 [95% CI, 0.240–1.014]; P = 0.050 [log-rank test]), suggesting a trend toward longer OS in the LFP-HAIC combined group. The median TTP was 5.3 months in the LFP-HAIC combined group and 3.5 months in the sorafenib monotherapy group (P = 0.004 [log-rank test]), demonstrating that adding HAIC is effective for elongation of TTP. The response rates were 36.3% and 17.5% in the LFP-HAIC and sorafenib monotherapy groups, respectively (P = 0.002: Mann–Whitney U test).

Thus, one-shot HAIC and LFP-HAIC, although effective for local control, have not been widely accepted due to the lack of evidence of improved prognosis. However, as shown in the SILIUS trial, there is still a possibility that they may be effective in cases of severe vascular invasion, and if a response is achieved, an extended OS may be observed. Even if new molecularly targeted agents and immune checkpoint inhibitors become available in the clinical setting, they are not expected to eliminate or significantly reduce vascular invasion, so HAIC could be used for the treatment of HCC patients with vascular invasion, albeit on certain indications only.

Evaluation of the Curative Effect of HAIC and its Prognostic Value

In a recent study, the evaluation of HAIC efficacy was determined one month after treatment based on the Response Evaluation Criteria in Cancer of the Liver 2019 proposed by the Japan Society of Hepatology, with contrast-enhanced CT scan and blood tumor markers (alpha-fetoprotein [AFP], DCP, and the Lens culinaris agglutinin-reactive fraction of AFP [L3-AFP]) [].

However, in cases where it is considered difficult to wait for a month after one-shot HAIC due to a large tumor diameter or a high tumor growth rate, it may be possible to evaluate the effect of HAIC on tumor necrosis using these indicators only two weeks after treatment.

In addition to tumor vascular invasion and the presence of extrahepatic metastases [], factors contributing to a poor treatment response include neutrophil: lymphocyte ratio (NLR) ≥ 2.87 [], serum vascular endothelial growth factor (VEGF) ≥ 100 pg/mL [], HCV antibody negativity and platelet levels ≥ 150,000 [], and DCP reduction <20% after 2 weeks of HAIC [].

Poor prognostic factors include an increase in the number and size of tumors [], vascular invasion [,], and extrahepatic metastasis [, ,], as well as poor HFR [, , , ⁻], poor ECOG performance status (PS) [,], TACE failure [,], high AFP levels [, ,], a reduction in tumor markers (AFP, DCP) < 20% after two weeks of HAIC [], high levels of inflammatory

markers (NLR, CRP) [], low levels of serum transferrin [], high levels of serum VEGF [], and positive serum HBs antigen [].

As previously mentioned, HFR is an important prognostic factor in the treatment of HCC, and Kudo *et al.* already reported that the prognosis of patients with advanced HCC treated with sorafenib can be clearly stratified by HFR []. In addition, Hatooka *et al.* recently reported that the life expectancy of patients with advanced HCC treated with HAIC is clearly associated with HFR [].

A comparison of the outcomes of HAIC in patients with extrahepatic metastasis and patients representing uncomplicated cases showed that patients with extrahepatic metastasis had a significantly poorer prognosis with regard to life expectancy than patients with the uncomplicated disease [].

Which Type of HAIC Would be Useful?

For LFP-HAIC, 5-FU (250 mg/body) is administered over 5 hours following the administration of CDDP (10 mg/body), based on the hypothesis that CDDP enhances the effects of the effector 5-FU as a modulator. This is followed by four cycles of five consecutive days of infusion followed by two days of rest, each cycle lasting for seven days. In principle, no hydration is needed, and the response rate is approximate 30%–40%, with an MST of 10–15 months.

One-shot HAIC can use DDP-H, which can be injected selectively into the hepatic artery at high concentrations for high therapeutic efficacy and does not require catheter placement, making the procedure less complicated.

Meanwhile, a considerable amount of CDDP (65 mg/m^2) is administered over a short period of time, and so hydration is essential to avoid kidney damage. Response rates vary substantially but are generally slightly lower than LFP-HAIC, ranging from 3.6% to 38.0% [, ¯,]. It is difficult to recommend one over the other because, as mentioned above, each has its own advantages and disadvantages; the choice of a more practical treatment method, taking into account the characteristics of each institution where HAIC is performed, is more realistic from the perspective of successfully avoiding therapeutic adverse effects.

When to use HAIC Combination Therapy with Molecularly Targeted Drugs or Surgical Resection for Advanced HCC with Major Ductal Invasions

Advanced cases of HCC with vascular invasion have the potential to involve the portal vein, hepatic vein, and bile duct, of which Vp is most commonly seen, followed by the invasion of the hepatic vein and bile duct []. In other words, Vp is one of the characteristics of HCC. HCC generally develops in a cirrhotic liver, whether induced by viral or non-viral causes. Therefore, quite a few cases with HCC are associated with portal hypertension. In patients with portal hypertension, rupture of esophagogastric varices is a serious condition that can cause hypovolemic shock, leading to liver failure, and consequently, death. This means that the presence of Vp is an important factor to consider when considering treatment options, since Vp-HCC can lead to more pronounced portal hypertension due to the blockage of portal blood flow, which can result in exacerbation of esophagogastric varices and ascitic fluid retention. To date, the efficacy of surgical resection for Vp-HCC has only been demonstrated to a limited extent, and the BCLC classification does not recommend surgical resection as such.

Meanwhile, a couple of reports on HAIC and HAIC combined with radiotherapy demonstrating the efficacy of HAIC have been published [,], and the combination of HAIC and surgical resection has been reported to promote long-term survival [¯]. Indeed, molecularly targeted agents such as sorafenib and lenvatinib represent the standard of care worldwide for advanced HCC of BCLC classification stage C, including Vp-HCC; however, in these cases, complications, such as decreased intrahepatic portal blood flow and development of portal hypertension, may be observed. In addition, imaging analyses such as perfusion CT and enhanced ultrasonography have been used to document a decrease in parenchymal hepatic blood flow following the administration of molecularly targeted agents [,]. Molecularly targeted agents have several unique characteristics: their main therapeutic effect is to inhibit tumor growth, they are metabolized by glucuronidation in the liver and therefore cannot be safely used in patients with a Child–Pugh Score ≥ 8, and it takes some time to determine whether they are effective or not and before they show efficacy.

In light of these considerations, it may be difficult to maintain long-term use of molecularly targeted therapies, which are aimed at controlling tumor activity (*i.e.*, long-lasting SD), in the treatment of vascular-invasive HCC such as Vp. In fact, the prognosis of Vp-HCC is very poor, and conditions in which esophagogastric varices rupture in Vp3 (invasion into the first order branch of the portal vein)/Vp4-HCC are highly fatal []. According to previous reports, the efficacy rate of HAIC for Vp-HCC is reportedly 30%–50% [, , , ¯], but the antitumor effect can be predicted to some extent by a decrease in tumor markers after treatment. In many cases of treatment response, Vp reduction may also improve portal hypertension, and in clinical practice, it has been safely used in patients with Child–Pugh class B HFR []. In addition to these, there are several other reports where HAIC was administered only in cases of vascular invasion; Obi *et al.* reported the outcome of FAIT therapy in 116 advanced-HCC cases of Vp3/4, with a vascular invasion of the main portal vein trunk or primary branch. The report showed a response rate of 52% and an MST of 6.9 months in patients with lower HFR (only 6% of patients were Child–Pugh class A), which was significantly better than that of historical background-matched, untreated patients [].Similarly, Nagano *et al.* reported a response rate of 39.2% and an MST of 9.0 months for 102 patients with Vp3/4-HCC, including 37% with Child-Pugh class A patients, following FAIT therapy []. Nouso *et al.* used propensity score-matched analysis of LFP-HAIC and BSC cases selected from a nationwide multi-center survey of patients in Japan. That sub-analysis yielded a HR of 0.40 (0.32–0.49) and an MST of 7.9 months for Vp3/4-HCC *vs.* no treatment []. Thus, although no evidence has been provided by acknowledged study designs, such as RCTs, on HAIC treatment for advanced HCC with major vascular invasion, HAIC undoubtedly provides a certain therapeutic benefit. Song *et al.* published a clinical study comparing the outcome of sorafenib and HAIC in patients with Vp-HCC for which the BCLC class of recommended treatments for advanced HCC included molecularly targeted agents []. They observed a significantly better disease control rate in the HAIC group (*P* < 0.001), but the objective response rate did not differ significantly (*P* = 0.214). The MST was significantly better in the HAIC group (7.1 months *vs.* 5.5 months in the sorafenib group, *P* = 0.011) and the median TTP was also significantly longer in the HAIC group (3.3 months *vs.* 2.1 months in the sorafenib group, *P* = 0.034), indicating that HAIC is more effective than sorafenib for Vp-HCC.

Based on the overall results of these studies, and in light of the fact that the benefit of sorafenib upon radical therapy could not be confirmed in the STORM study, the strategy for the treatment of unresectable HCC with gross vascular invasion is to initiate treatment with (1) HAIC and (2) molecularly targeted agents, in that order, and if it is determined that gross curative resection can be safely achieved, conversion to surgical resection is considered to be ideal. However, since early postoperative recurrence is inevitable in Vp3/4-HCC, even if hepatic resection can be performed safely, adjuvant therapy must be introduced as early as possible after surgery to prevent recurrence and ensure long-term survival. Kojima *et al.* found that 66 patients with Vp3/4-HCC managed from 2001 to 2010 were treated with surgical resection. Introducing LFP-HAIC with resection and, if the postoperative course was good, LFP-HAIC for two to three weeks postoperatively and every two weeks thereafter for six months, resulted in a longer recurrence-free period (12.4 months *vs.* 6.2 months, $P = 0.043$) and a longer MST in the combined postoperative HAIC group than in the non-combined group (33.2 months *vs.* 21.5 months, $P = 0.044$) [].

In other words, molecularly targeted therapies are the current global standard of care for advanced HCC, with tumor vascular invasion as the first choice of treatment. In addition to the fact that the outcomes for these tumors are very poor, HAICs, which are the treatment of choice in regions such as Japan and South Korea, offer acceptable outcomes compared with molecularly targeted therapies, and the optimal treatment should be determined on an individual basis. Various clinical trials involving molecularly targeted therapies and HAIC for advanced HCC are currently underway, and it is hoped that evidence on their effect alone and in combination will be established in the near future.

A New Derivation of Modified HAIC

Iron, the largest population of inorganic minerals in animals, is essential for cellular metabolism under normal conditions, but it is more required in cancerous conditions due to enhanced DNA synthesis, and iron metabolism is highly active in cancer. Free iron that cannot bind to transferrin is called non-transferrin-bound iron (NTBI) under iron-rich conditions. Normally, trivalent iron ions are present, but as the number of trivalent iron ions increases, the number of equilibrated divalent iron ions also increases. Divalent iron ions generate hydroxyl radicals *via* the Fenton reaction and become the main reactive oxygen species (ROS), which are responsible for iron toxicity, and ROS enrichment leads to cellular damage, fibrosis, DNA damage, and carcinogenesis. In fact, ROS has been reported to be a poor prognostic factor in HCC cases [], and HCCs with low transferrin levels are associated with more NTBI in the blood compared HCCs with high transferrin levels, which results in more ROS being produced. The fact that transferrin is an iron chelator by nature and is responsible for iron level regulation is consistent with reports that low transferrin levels are a significant predictor of poor prognosis []. Incidentally, chelated iron has an antitumor effect in various cancer types, including HCC [,]. Iron chelators firstly deactivate the cell cycle (G1/S phase) of cancer cells, suppress PI3K/AKT/mTOR signaling and Ras/Raf/MEK/ERK signaling, and promote JNK/P38 pathways in cancer cells. Next, upregulation of the metastasis suppressor gene NDRG1 (N-myc downstream-regulated gene 1) is thought to suppress epithelial-mesenchymal transition and metastasis by suppressing the TGFβ/Wnt pathway. Another possibility is the induction of autophagy []. Yamasaki *et al.* used HAIC with deferoxamine (DFO), an iron-chelating agent, and reported its usefulness for the first time in the world []. The authors administered 10–80 mg/kg of DFO by continuous hepatic infusion for 24 hours, three times a week, every other day, to 10 patients with advanced HCCs (males/females = 6/4; mean age, 64 years, HCV/HBV/others = 7/2/1; tumor stage II/IV,A/IV,B = 1,2,7; Child–Pugh class A/B/C = 3/5/2) who had proven HAIC-refractory, with a response rate of 20% (partial response, 2; stable disease,3; progressive disease, 5 [ECOG evaluation]), and a 1-year survival rate of 20%. In that study, four non-serious cases of interstitial pneumonia (Grade 2 in two cases and Grade 3 in the two remaining cases) and one case of renal dysfunction (Grade 2) were also observed.

In a subsequent study, the authors suggested that HCC patients with low transferrin levels may develop a poor response to HAIC and have a poor prognosis []. In this sense, it makes sense to administer artificial iron chelators to patients with general HAIC failure. Some cases of interstitial pneumonia have been reported, and although the safety of the drug should be carefully evaluated before it can be put into practice, it is a very interesting finding.

Which is Better, HAIC, or Molecularly Targeted Agents?

To date, HAIC, which has been used mainly in Japan and South Korea, has not been prospectively compared with sorafenib, placebo, or no treatment, but in real-world clinical practice, tumor shrinkage has indeed been documented [,]. In addition, patients with tumor shrinkage have shown a marked improvement in prognosis, and it can be argued that there is a significant difference in prognosis depending on whether or not HAIC is effective in each case [,]. Although there is limited evidence of HAIC treatment being associated with prolonged life expectancy, and although the treatment requires a safe reservoir implantation technique and is somewhat complicated when it comes to managing the side effects associated with the reservoir, tumor shrinkage is seen in approximately 30% of cases. Moreover, subsequent additional treatment offers a promising long-term prognosis. Therefore, more than 10 years after the evidence for sorafenib was published, HAIC continues to be used for advanced HCC confined to the liver. The outcome of HCC treatment in Japan and South Korea is very good compared with Europe and North America; for instance, the age-standardized 5-year survival rate of HCC in the United States is about 17.4%, while the one in Japan is substantially higher, 30.1% []. Multiple factors are presumed to be responsible for this, including careful screening for viral hepatitis, local percutaneous therapy such as radiofrequency ablation, post-treatment course management, and super-selective TACE; however, the use of HAIC for advanced HCC may also contribute to a major extent.

Meanwhile, molecularly targeted agents have a low response rate. Still, they confer a high rate of disease control, and, above all, there is strong evidence of prolonged life expectancy associated with treatment response. In addition, although the adverse effects of molecularly targeted agents must be managed, the fact that these agents are administered orally and can be easily administered is a major advantage. Thus, there are probably quite a few cases of HCC where the choice between HAIC and molecularly targeted agents is not straight-forward; in such cases, the treatment option should be matched with individual patient characteristics.

In principle, patients with an HFR of Child–Pugh class A are considered candidates for treatment with molecularly targeted agents, including sorafenib, and for some Child–Pugh class B patients (Child–Pugh score $\leq$ 7), the treatment may also be considered safe. In a subgroup analysis in the SHARP trial, the HR for patients with major vascular involvement was 0.68 (95% CI, 0.49–0.93), compared with 0.74 (95% CI, 0.54–1.00) for patients with no vascular involvement; *i.e.*, a lower HR and an upper limit of 95% CI of less than 1.0 were observed in those with major vascular invasion. This suggests that sorafenib may be more effective in patients with major vascular invasion. Subsequent Asia-Pacific studies have shown that sorafenib is more effective in patients with no vascular invasion. In the sub-analysis in the SHARP study, in addition to the above results, a HR of 0.77 (95% CI, 0.60–0.99) for either major vascular involvement or extrahepatic disease, and a HR of 0.52 (95% CI, 0.32–0.85) for neither major vascular involvement nor extrahepatic disease, were identified. In the absence of major vascular involvement and extrahepatic lesions, sorafenib may be interpreted as being more effective []. In a sub-analysis of the Asia-Pacific study, a HR of 0.75 (95% CI, 0.54–1.05) was reported in the presence of either major vascular involvement or extrahepatic disease, and a HR of 0.45 (95% CI, 0.19–1.06) was observed in the absence of major vascular involvement and extrahepatic disease. Similar to the sub-analysis of the SHARP study, a clearer therapeutic effect of sorafenib has been reported in the absence of extrahepatic disease and major vascular involvement [].

Concerning lenvatinib, its non-inferiority to sorafenib in advanced-HCC treatment was demonstrated in the REFLECT trial []; no sub-analysis on the presence or absence of vascular involvement has been reported at this time, and further analyses are expected.

In addition, the results of a global, multi-center, open-label Phase-3 study of 501 patients with unresectable HCC who had not received systemic treatment were recently disclosed []. In this trial, Finn *et al.* reported that the OS and PFS in patients receiving a combination of atezolizumab (an anti-PD-L1 antibody) and bevacizumab (an anti-VEGF monoclonal antibody) were both significantly prolonged compared with those in the sorafenib monotherapy group, with the former group's hazard ratio for disease progression or death relative to the latter being 0.59 (95% CI, 0.47–0.76; P < 0.001). Therefore, it will be very interesting to see the outcome of HCC treatment with immune checkpoint inhibitors and molecularly targeted therapies in the future.

Meanwhile, with regard to HAIC, there are only a couple of studies involving single-arm Phase-2 equivalent clinical trials with up to approximately 100 patients with advanced HCC. These trials have primarily targeted patients ineligible for local therapy, TACE, and surgical resection; these include not only Vp-HCC but also cases of multiple intrahepatic metastasis, making simple comparisons of the outcomes of molecularly targeted therapies and HAIC difficult. In fact, HAIC for Vp-HCC has been used in many cases of reduced HFR, including Child–Pugh class B patients. However, there are several reports showing that HAIC provides a survival advantage equivalent to or better than that of sorafenib. Overall, these facts suggest that HAIC may be superior to molecularly targeted agents for Vp-HCC, and that molecularly targeted agents may be superior for patients with extrahepatic metastasis.

With regard to HFR, HAIC is the first treatment of choice for patients with major vascular involvement in the Child–Pugh class A category. However, if these patients do not have esophagogastric varices associated with portal hypertension, molecularly targeted agents may be also considered. Patients with localized advanced HCC, such as in cases of vascular involvement, except for major lesion of the portal vein, can be eligible for both molecularly targeted agents and HAIC. If tumor exacerbation occurs after prior therapy, patients can be switched to HAIC. Recently, it has been suggested that second and third-line treatment after failure of first-line chemotherapy might result in OS in patients with colorectal cancer and lung cancer. For this reason, the duration of these treatments is considered to be important for post-progression survival (PPS), and it is considered practical to aim for prolongation of PPS by switching treatment methods of HCC [].

Although HAIC is likely to be the main treatment option for Vp-HCC patients with HFR of Child–Pugh class B, molecularly targeted agents may be used for HCC patients with a Child–Pugh score ≤ 7 in the absence of vascular involvement.

There seems to be consensus that molecularly targeted agents are inappropriate for patients with Child–Pugh class C. On the other hand, there is no reason to choose HAIC only in cases where a reduction of HFR is suspected to be due to tumor vascular invasion; it is possible to select HAIC in anticipation of improved HFR after tumor shrinkage.

SUMMARY

In this chapter, indications for the use of HAIC in various treatments of advanced-stage HCC were reviewed, and practical implementation methods, as well as complications to be aware of, were discussed. In addition to the outcomes of HAIC, how to use and combine HAIC with molecularly targeted therapies were discussed. Furthermore, new developments within HAIC treatment, including the recent positive results of employing the HAIC regimen using the iron chelator DFO, as well as the scope for incorporating surgery into HAIC were outlined. It is hoped that the further accumulation of research data on the use of various therapies for advanced HCC, such as HAIC and molecularly targeted agents, will sufficiently inform treatment strategies aiming to significantly prolong life expectancy in patients with advanced HCC.

CONSENT FOR PUBLICATION

Not Applicable.

CONFLICT OF INTEREST

The author declares no conflict of interest, financial or otherwise.

ACKNOWLEDGEMENTS

Declared none.

REFERENCES

[1]   GBD 2015 mortality and causes of death collaboratorsGlobal, regional, and national life expectancy, all-cause mortality, and cause-specific mortality for 249 causes of death, 1980-2015: a systematic analysis for the Global Burden of Disease Study 2015. Lancet 2016; 388(10053): 1459-544.[http://dx.doi.org/10.1016/S0140-6736(16)31012-1] [PMID: 27733281]

[2]   Akinyemiju T, Abera S, Ahmed M, et al. The Burden of Primary Liver Cancer and Underlying Etiologies From 1990 to 2015 at the Global, Regional, and National Level: Results From the Global Burden of Disease Study 2015. JAMA Oncol 2017; 3(12): 1683-91.[http://dx.doi.org/10.1001/jamaoncol.2017.3055] [PMID:

28983565]

[3] Singal AG, Lampertico P, Nahon P. Epidemiology and surveillance for hepatocellular carcinoma: New trends. J Hepatol 2020; 72(2): 250-61.[http://dx.doi.org/10.1016/j.jhep.2019.08.025] [PMID: 31954490]

[4] Hasegawa K, Kokudo N, Makuuchi M, *et al.* Comparison of resection and ablation for hepatocellular carcinoma: a cohort study based on a Japanese nationwide survey. J Hepatol 2013; 58(4): 724-9.[http://dx.doi.org/10.1016/j.jhep.2012.11.009] [PMID: 23178708]

[5] Shiina S, Tateishi R, Arano T, *et al.* Radiofrequency ablation for hepatocellular carcinoma: 10-year outcome and prognostic factors. Am J Gastroenterol 2012; 107(4): 569-77.[http://dx.doi.org/10.1038/ajg.2011.425] [PMID: 22158026]

[6] Takayasu K, Arii S, Kudo M, *et al.* Superselective transarterial chemoembolization for hepatocellular carcinoma. Validation of treatment algorithm proposed by Japanese guidelines. J Hepatol 2012; 56(4): 886-92.[http://dx.doi.org/10.1016/j.jhep.2011.10.021] [PMID: 22173160]

[7] Llovet JM, Ricci S, Mazzaferro V, *et al.* Sorafenib in advanced hepatocellular carcinoma. N Engl J Med 2008; 359(4): 378-90.[http://dx.doi.org/10.1056/NEJMoa0708857] [PMID: 18650514]

[8] Petrick JL, Florio AA, Znaor A, *et al.* International trends in hepatocellular carcinoma incidence, 1978-2012. Int J Cancer 2020; 147(2): 317-30.[http://dx.doi.org/10.1002/ijc.32723] [PMID: 31597196]

[9] Zhong JH, Peng NF, You XM, *et al.* Tumor stage and primary treatment of hepatocellular carcinoma at a large tertiary hospital in China: A real-world study. Oncotarget 2017; 8(11): 18296-302.[http://dx.doi.org/10.18632/oncotarget.15433] [PMID: 28407686]

[10] Quirk M, Kim YH, Saab S, Lee EW. Management of hepatocellular carcinoma with portal vein thrombosis. World J Gastroenterol 2015; 21(12): 3462-71.[http://dx.doi.org/10.3748/wjg.v21.i12.3462] [PMID: 25834310]

[11] Electronic address: easloffice@easloffice.eu; European Association for the Study of the Liver. EASL Clinical Practice Guidelines: Management of hepatocellular carcinoma. J Hepatol 2018; 69(1): 182-236.[http://dx.doi.org/10.1016/j.jhep.2018.03.019] [PMID: 29628281]

[12] Heimbach JK, Kulik LM, Finn RS, *et al.* AASLD guidelines for the treatment of hepatocellular carcinoma. Hepatology 2018; 67(1): 358-80.[http://dx.doi.org/10.1002/hep.29086] [PMID: 28130846]

[13] Omata M, Cheng AL, Kokudo N, *et al.* Asia-Pacific clinical practice guidelines on the management of hepatocellular carcinoma: a 2017 update. Hepatol Int 2017; 11(4): 317-70.[http://dx.doi.org/10.1007/s12072-017-9799-9] [PMID: 28620797]

[14] Kokudo N, Takemura N, Hasegawa K, *et al.* Clinical practice guidelines for hepatocellular carcinoma: The Japan Society of Hepatology 2017 (4th JSH-HCC guidelines) 2019 update. Hepatol Res 2019; 49(10): 1109-13.[http://dx.doi.org/10.1111/hepr.13411] [PMID: 31336394]

[15] Kudo M, Matsui O, Izumi N, *et al.* JSH Consensus-Based Clinical Practice Guidelines for the Management of Hepatocellular Carcinoma: 2014 Update by the Liver Cancer Study Group of Japan. Liver Cancer 2014; 3(3-4): 458-68.[http://dx.doi.org/10.1159/000343875] [PMID: 26280007]

[16] EASL-EORTC clinical practice guidelines: management of hepatocellular carcinoma. J Hepatol 2012; 56(4): 908-43.[http://dx.doi.org/10.1016/j.jhep.2011.12.001] [PMID: 22424438]

[17] Arizumi T, Ueshima K, Minami T, *et al.* Effectiveness of Sorafenib in Patients with Transcatheter Arterial Chemoembolization (TACE) Refractory and Intermediate-Stage Hepatocellular Carcinoma. Liver Cancer 2015; 4(4): 253-62.[http://dx.doi.org/10.1159/000367743] [PMID: 26734579]

[18] Ogasawara S, Chiba T, Ooka Y, *et al.* Efficacy of sorafenib in intermediate-stage hepatocellular carcinoma patients refractory to transarterial chemoembolization. Oncology 2014; 87(6): 330-41.[http://dx.doi.org/10.1159/000365993] [PMID: 25227534]

[19] Ikeda M, Mitsunaga S, Shimizu S, *et al.* Efficacy of sorafenib in patients with hepatocellular carcinoma refractory to transcatheter arterial chemoembolization. J Gastroenterol 2014; 49(5): 932-40.[http://dx.doi.org/10.1007/s00535-013-0853-7] [PMID: 23793266]

[20] Kondo M, Morimoto M, Ishii T, *et al.* Hepatic arterial infusion chemotherapy with cisplatin and sorafenib in hepatocellular carcinoma patients unresponsive to transarterial chemoembolization: a propensity score-based weighting. J Dig Dis 2015; 16(3): 143-51.[http://dx.doi.org/10.1111/1751-2980.12221] [PMID: 25495751]

[21] Hatooka M, Kawaoka T, Aikata H, *et al.* Comparison of Outcome of Hepatic Arterial Infusion Chemotherapy and Sorafenib in Patients with Hepatocellular Carcinoma Refractory to Transcatheter Arterial Chemoembolization. Anticancer Res 2016; 36(7): 3523-9.[PMID: 27354618]

[22] Fukubayashi K, Tanaka M, Izumi K, *et al.* Evaluation of sorafenib treatment and hepatic arterial infusion chemotherapy for advanced hepatocellular carcinoma: a comparative study using the propensity score matching method. Cancer Med 2015; 4(8): 1214-23.[http://dx.doi.org/10.1002/cam4.476] [PMID: 26044168]

[23] Kajanti M, Rissanen P, Virkkunen P, Franssila K, Mäntylä M. Regional intra-arterial infusion of cisplatin in primary hepatocellular carcinoma. A phase II study. Cancer 1986; 58(11): 2386-8.[http://dx.doi.org/10.1002/1097-0142(19861201)58:11<2386::AID-CNCR2820581105>3.0.CO;2-G] [PMID: 3021314]

[24] Abe R, Akiyoshi T, Koba F, Tsuji H, Baba T. 'Two-route chemotherapy' using intra-arterial cisplatin and intravenous sodium thiosulfate, its neutralizing agent, for hepatic malignancies. Eur J Cancer Clin Oncol 1988; 24(10): 1671-4.[http://dx.doi.org/10.1016/0277-5379(88)90061-2] [PMID: 2850191]

[25] Court WS, Order SE, Siegel JA, et al. Remission and survival following monthly intraarterial cisplatinum in nonresectable hepatoma. Cancer Invest 2002; 20(5-6): 613-25.[http://dx.doi.org/10.1081/CNV-120002486] [PMID: 12197216]

[26] Maeda M, Uchida NA, Sasaki T. Liposoluble platinum(II) complexes with antitumor activity. Jpn J Cancer Res 1986; 77(6): 523-5.[PMID: 3015851]

[27] Kishimoto S, Noguchi T, Yamaoka T, Fukushima S, Takeuchi Y. In vitro release of SM-11355, cis[(((1R,2R)-1,2-cyclohexanediamine-N,N′)bis(myristato)] platinum(II) suspended in lipiodol. Biol Pharm Bull 2000; 23(5): 637-40.[http://dx.doi.org/10.1248/bpb.23.637] [PMID: 10823679]

[28] Kishimoto S, Miyazawa K, Fukushima S, Takeuchi Y. In vitro antitumor activity, intracellular accumulation, and DNA adduct formation of cis-[((1R,2R)-1,2-cyclohexanediamine-N,N′)bis(myristato)] platinum (II) suspended in lipiodol. Jpn J Cancer Res 2000; 91(1): 99-104.[http://dx.doi.org/10.1111/j.1349-7006.2000.tb00865.x] [PMID: 10744050]

[29] Yoshikawa M, Ono N, Yodono H, Ichida T, Nakamura H. Phase II study of hepatic arterial infusion of a fine-powder formulation of cisplatin for advanced hepatocellular carcinoma. Hepatol Res 2008; 38(5): 474-83.[http://dx.doi.org/10.1111/j.1872-034X.2008.00338.x] [PMID: 18430093]

[30] Ando E, Tanaka M, Yamashita F, et al. Hepatic arterial infusion chemotherapy for advanced hepatocellular carcinoma with portal vein tumor thrombosis: analysis of 48 cases. Cancer 2002; 95(3): 588-95.[http://dx.doi.org/10.1002/cncr.10694] [PMID: 12209752]

[31] Miyaki D, Aikata H, Honda Y, et al. Hepatic arterial infusion chemotherapy for advanced hepatocellular carcinoma according to Child-Pugh classification. J Gastroenterol Hepatol 2012; 27(12): 1850-7.[http://dx.doi.org/10.1111/j.1440-1746.2012.07276.x] [PMID: 23020312]

[32] Yamasaki T, Kimura T, Kurokawa F, et al. Prognostic factors in patients with advanced hepatocellular carcinoma receiving hepatic arterial infusion chemotherapy. J Gastroenterol 2005; 40(1): 70-8.[http://dx.doi.org/10.1007/s00535-004-1494-7] [PMID: 15692792]

[33] Terashima T, Yamashita T, Arai K, et al. Beneficial Effect of Maintaining Hepatic Reserve during Chemotherapy on the Outcomes of Patients with Hepatocellular Carcinoma. Liver Cancer 2017; 6(3): 236-49.[http://dx.doi.org/10.1159/000472262] [PMID: 28626734]

[34] Saeki I, Yamasaki T, Maeda M, et al. Evaluation of the "assessment for continuous treatment with hepatic arterial infusion chemotherapy" scoring system in patients with advanced hepatocellular carcinoma. Hepatol Res 2018; 48(3): E87-97.[http://dx.doi.org/10.1111/hepr.12932] [PMID: 28656680]

[35] Okusaka T, Kasugai H, Ishii H, et al. A randomized phase II trial of intra-arterial chemotherapy using SM-11355 (Miriplatin) for hepatocellular carcinoma. Invest New Drugs 2012; 30(5): 2015-25.[http://dx.doi.org/10.1007/s10637-011-9776-4] [PMID: 22187203]

[36] Stewart DJ, Benjamin RS, Zimmerman S, et al. Clinical pharmacology of intraarterial cis-diamminedichloroplatinum(II). Cancer Res 1983; 43(2): 917-20.[PMID: 6681533]

[37] Hatanaka T, Kakizaki S, Ueno T, Takeuchi S, Takizawa D, Katakai K. Transarterial infusion chemotherapy using fine-powder cisplatin in patients with advanced hepatocellular carcinoma. Gan To Kagaku Ryoho 2014; 41(2): 205-9.[PMID: 24743198]

[38] Iwasa S, Ikeda M, Okusaka T, et al. Transcatheter arterial infusion chemotherapy with a fine-powder formulation of cisplatin for advanced hepatocellular carcinoma refractory to transcatheter arterial chemoembolization. Jpn J Clin Oncol 2011; 41(6): 770-5.[http://dx.doi.org/10.1093/jjco/hyr037] [PMID: 21459893]

[39] Moriya K, Namisaki T, Sato S, et al. Efficacy of bi-monthly hepatic arterial infusion chemotherapy for advanced hepatocellular carcinoma. J Gastrointest Oncol 2018; 9(4): 741-9.[http://dx.doi.org/10.21037/jgo.2018.03.13] [PMID: 30151271]

[40] Moriya K, Namisaki T, Sato S, et al. Bi-monthly hepatic arterial infusion chemotherapy as a novel strategy for advanced hepatocellular carcinoma in decompensated cirrhotic patients. Clin Mol Hepatol 2019; 25(4): 381-9.[http://dx.doi.org/10.3350/cmh.2019.0037] [PMID: 31405269]

[41] Moriguchi M, Takayama T, Nakamura M, et al. Phase I/II study of a fine-powder formulation of cisplatin for

transcatheter arterial chemoembolization in hepatocellular carcinoma. Hepatol Res 2010; 40(4): 369-75.[http://dx.doi.org/10.1111/j.1872-034X.2009.00606.x] [PMID: 20070392]

[42] Yamashita Y, Taketomi A, Itoh S, *et al*. Phase I/II study of the lipiodolization using DDP-H (CDDP powder; IA-call(®)) in patients with unresectable hepatocellular carcinoma. Cancer Chemother Pharmacol 2010; 65(2): 301-7.[http://dx.doi.org/10.1007/s00280-009-1034-5] [PMID: 19495755]

[43] Kondo M, Morimoto M, Numata K, Nozaki A, Tanaka K. Hepatic arterial infusion therapy with a fine powder formulation of cisplatin for advanced hepatocellular carcinoma with portal vein tumor thrombosis. Jpn J Clin Oncol 2011; 41(1): 69-75.[http://dx.doi.org/10.1093/jjco/hyq145] [PMID: 20688778]

[44] Nagahama H, Okada S, Okusaka T, *et al*. Predictive factors for tumor response to systemic chemotherapy in patients with hepatocellular carcinoma. Jpn J Clin Oncol 1997; 27(5): 321-4.[http://dx.doi.org/10.1093/jjco/27.5.321] [PMID: 9390209]

[45] Ikeda M, Shimizu S, Sato T, *et al*. Sorafenib plus hepatic arterial infusion chemotherapy with cisplatin *versus* sorafenib for advanced hepatocellular carcinoma: randomized phase II trial. Ann Oncol 2016; 27(11): 2090-6.[http://dx.doi.org/10.1093/annonc/mdw323] [PMID: 27573564]

[46] Shirono T, Iwamoto H, Niizeki T, *et al*. Epirubicin is More Effective than Miriplatin in Balloon-Occluded Transcatheter Arterial Chemoembolization for Hepatocellular Carcinoma. Oncology 2019; 96(2): 79-86.[http://dx.doi.org/10.1159/000492822] [PMID: 30293080]

[47] Ikeda M, Kudo M, Aikata H, *et al*. Transarterial chemoembolization with miriplatin *vs*. epirubicin for unresectable hepatocellular carcinoma: a phase III randomized trial. J Gastroenterol 2018; 53(2): 281-90.[http://dx.doi.org/10.1007/s00535-017-1374-6] [PMID: 28766016]

[48] Kubota K, Hidaka H, Nakazawa T, *et al*. Prospective, randomized, controlled study of the efficacy of transcatheter arterial chemoembolization with miriplatin for hepatocellular carcinoma. Hepatol Res 2018; 48(3): E98-E106.[http://dx.doi.org/10.1111/hepr.12933] [PMID: 28656607]

[49] Kishimoto S, Aoki H, Suzuki R, Inoue M, Fukushima S. Angiographic Evaluation of Vascular Damage in Rat Liver After Administration of Epirubicin or Miriplatin. Anticancer Res 2018; 38(1): 247-51.[PMID: 29277779]

[50] Matsumoto T, Ichikawa H, Imai J, *et al*. Feasibility and Safety of Repeated Transarterial Chemoembolization Using Miriplatin-Lipiodol Suspension for Hepatocellular Carcinoma. Anticancer Res 2017; 37(6): 3183-7.[PMID: 28551662]

[51] Saeki I, Yamasaki T, Tanabe N, *et al*. A new therapeutic assessment score for advanced hepatocellular carcinoma patients receiving hepatic arterial infusion chemotherapy. PLoS One 2015; 10(5)e0126649[http://dx.doi.org/10.1371/journal.pone.0126649] [PMID: 25992784]

[52] Kishi K, Sonomura T, Mitsuzane K, *et al*. Time courses of PIVKA-II and AFP levels after hepatic artery embolization and hepatic artery infusion against hepatocellular carcinoma: relation between the time course and tumor necrosis. Radiat Med 1992; 10(5): 189-95.[PMID: 1279748]

[53] Park JY, Ahn SH, Yoon YJ, *et al*. Repetitive short-course hepatic arterial infusion chemotherapy with high-dose 5-fluorouracil and cisplatin in patients with advanced hepatocellular carcinoma. Cancer 2007; 110(1): 129-37.[http://dx.doi.org/10.1002/cncr.22759] [PMID: 17508408]

[54] Okuda K, Tanaka M, Shibata J, *et al*. Hepatic arterial infusion chemotherapy with continuous low dose administration of cisplatin and 5-fluorouracil for multiple recurrence of hepatocellular carcinoma after surgical treatment. Oncol Rep 1999; 6(3): 587-91.[http://dx.doi.org/10.3892/or.6.3.587] [PMID: 10203596]

[55] Ueshima K, Kudo M, Takita M, *et al*. Hepatic arterial infusion chemotherapy using low-dose 5-fluorouracil and cisplatin for advanced hepatocellular carcinoma. Oncology 2010; 78 (Suppl. 1): 148-53.[http://dx.doi.org/10.1159/000315244] [PMID: 20616598]

[56] Kanayama M, Nagai H, Sumino Y. Influence of the etiology of liver cirrhosis on the response to combined intra-arterial chemotherapy in patients with advanced hepatocellular carcinoma. Cancer Chemother Pharmacol 2009; 64(1): 109-14.[http://dx.doi.org/10.1007/s00280-008-0851-2] [PMID: 18979100]

[57] Nagamatsu H, Hiraki M, Mizukami N, *et al*. Intra-arterial therapy with cisplatin suspension in lipiodol and 5-fluorouracil for hepatocellular carcinoma with portal vein tumour thrombosis. Aliment Pharmacol Ther 2010; 32(4): 543-50.[http://dx.doi.org/10.1111/j.1365-2036.2010.04379.x] [PMID: 20500734]

[58] Kudo M, Ueshima K, Yokosuka O, *et al*. Sorafenib plus low-dose cisplatin and fluorouracil hepatic arterial infusion chemotherapy *versus* sorafenib alone in patients with advanced hepatocellular carcinoma (SILIUS): a randomised, open label, phase 3 trial. Lancet Gastroenterol Hepatol 2018; 3(6): 424-32.[http://dx.doi.org/10.1016/S2468-1253(18)30078-5] [PMID: 29631810]

[59] Kudo M, Ikeda M, Ueshima K, *et al*. Response Evaluation Criteria in Cancer of the Liver version 5 (RECICL 2019 revised version). Hepatol Res 2019; 49(9): 981-9.[http://dx.doi.org/10.1111/hepr.13394] [PMID:

31231916]

[60]   Terashima T, Yamashita T, Iida N, *et al.* Blood neutrophil to lymphocyte ratio as a predictor in patients with advanced hepatocellular carcinoma treated with hepatic arterial infusion chemotherapy. Hepatol Res 2015; 45(9): 949-59.[http://dx.doi.org/10.1111/hepr.12436] [PMID: 25319848]

[61]   Niizeki T, Sumie S, Torimura T, *et al.* Serum vascular endothelial growth factor as a predictor of response and survival in patients with advanced hepatocellular carcinoma undergoing hepatic arterial infusion chemotherapy. J Gastroenterol 2012; 47(6): 686-95.[http://dx.doi.org/10.1007/s00535-012-0555-6] [PMID: 22382631]

[62]   Nouso K, Miyahara K, Uchida D, *et al.* Effect of hepatic arterial infusion chemotherapy of 5-fluorouracil and cisplatin for advanced hepatocellular carcinoma in the Nationwide Survey of Primary Liver Cancer in Japan. Br J Cancer 2013; 109(7): 1904-7.[http://dx.doi.org/10.1038/bjc.2013.542] [PMID: 24008659]

[63]   Obi S, Yoshida H, Toune R, *et al.* Combination therapy of intraarterial 5-fluorouracil and systemic interferon-alpha for advanced hepatocellular carcinoma with portal venous invasion. Cancer 2006; 106(9): 1990-7.[http://dx.doi.org/10.1002/cncr.21832] [PMID: 16565970]

[64]   Zaitsu J, Yamasaki T, Saeki I, *et al.* Serum transferrin as a predictor of prognosis for hepatic arterial infusion chemotherapy in advanced hepatocellular carcinoma. Hepatol Res 2014; 44(5): 481-90.[http://dx.doi.org/10.1111/hepr.12141] [PMID: 23607437]

[65]   Kawaoka T, Aikata H, Hyogo H, *et al.* Comparison of hepatic arterial infusion chemotherapy *versus* sorafenib monotherapy in patients with advanced hepatocellular carcinoma. J Dig Dis 2015; 16(9): 505-12.[http://dx.doi.org/10.1111/1751-2980.12267] [PMID: 26121102]

[66]   Kirikoshi H, Yoneda M, Mawatari H, *et al.* Is hepatic arterial infusion chemotherapy effective treatment for advanced hepatocellular carcinoma resistant to transarterial chemoembolization? World J Gastroenterol 2012; 18(16): 1933-9.[http://dx.doi.org/10.3748/wjg.v18.i16.1933] [PMID: 22563174]

[67]   Kudo M, Ikeda M, Takayama T, *et al.* Safety and efficacy of sorafenib in Japanese patients with hepatocellular carcinoma in clinical practice: a subgroup analysis of GIDEON. J Gastroenterol 2016; 51(12): 1150-60.[http://dx.doi.org/10.1007/s00535-016-1204-2] [PMID: 27106231]

[68]   Hatooka M, Kawaoka T, Aikata H, *et al.* Hepatic arterial infusion chemotherapy followed by sorafenib in patients with advanced hepatocellular carcinoma (HICS 55): an open label, non-comparative, phase II trial. BMC Cancer 2018; 18(1): 633.[http://dx.doi.org/10.1186/s12885-018-4519-y] [PMID: 29866075]

[69]   Katamura Y, Aikata H, Kimura Y, *et al.* Intra-arterial 5-fluorouracil/interferon combination therapy for hepatocellular carcinoma with portal vein tumor thrombosis and extrahepatic metastases. J Gastroenterol Hepatol 2010; 25(6): 1117-22.[http://dx.doi.org/10.1111/j.1440-1746.2009.06110.x] [PMID: 20074168]

[70]   Ikai I, Arii S, Kojiro M, *et al.* Reevaluation of prognostic factors for survival after liver resection in patients with hepatocellular carcinoma in a Japanese nationwide survey. Cancer 2004; 101(4): 796-802.[http://dx.doi.org/10.1002/cncr.20426] [PMID: 15305412]

[71]   Song DS, Song MJ, Bae SH, *et al.* A comparative study between sorafenib and hepatic arterial infusion chemotherapy for advanced hepatocellular carcinoma with portal vein tumor thrombosis. J Gastroenterol 2015; 50(4): 445-54.[http://dx.doi.org/10.1007/s00535-014-0978-3] [PMID: 25027973]

[72]   Kodama K, Kawaoka T, Aikata H, *et al.* Comparison of Outcome of Hepatic Arterial Infusion Chemotherapy Combined with Radiotherapy and Sorafenib for Advanced Hepatocellular Carcinoma Patients with Major Portal Vein Tumor Thrombosis. Oncology 2018; 94(4): 215-22.[http://dx.doi.org/10.1159/000486483] [PMID: 29428943]

[73]   Sakamoto K, Nagano H. Surgical treatment for advanced hepatocellular carcinoma with portal vein tumor thrombus. Hepatol Res 2017; 47(10): 957-62.[http://dx.doi.org/10.1111/hepr.12923] [PMID: 28618075]

[74]   Nagano H, Kobayashi S, Marubashi S, *et al.* Combined IFN-α and 5-FU treatment as a postoperative adjuvant following surgery for hepatocellular carcinoma with portal venous tumor thrombus. Exp Ther Med 2013; 5(1): 3-10.[http://dx.doi.org/10.3892/etm.2012.736] [PMID: 23251233]

[75]   Nagano H, Miyamoto A, Wada H, *et al.* Interferon-alpha and 5-fluorouracil combination therapy after palliative hepatic resection in patients with advanced hepatocellular carcinoma, portal venous tumor thrombus in the major trunk, and multiple nodules. Cancer 2007; 110(11): 2493-501.[http://dx.doi.org/10.1002/cncr.23033] [PMID: 17941012]

[76]   Kamiyama T, Nakanishi K, Yokoo H, *et al.* Efficacy of preoperative radiotherapy to portal vein tumor thrombus in the main trunk or first branch in patients with hepatocellular carcinoma. Int J Clin Oncol 2007; 12(5): 363-8.[http://dx.doi.org/10.1007/s10147-007-0701-y] [PMID: 17929118]

[77]   Hidaka H, Nakazawa T, Kaneko T, *et al.* Portal hemodynamic effects of sorafenib in patients with advanced hepatocellular carcinoma: a prospective cohort study. J Gastroenterol 2012; 47(9): 1030-

5.[http://dx.doi.org/10.1007/s00535-012-0563-6] [PMID: 22402773]

[78] Hidaka H, Uojima H, Nakazawa T, *et al.* Portal hemodynamic effects of lenvatinib in patients with advanced hepatocellular carcinoma: A prospective cohort study. Hepatol Res 2020; 50(9): 1083-90. [Online ahead of print.].[http://dx.doi.org/10.1111/hepr.13531] [PMID: 32515895]

[79] Kodama H, Aikata H, Murakami E, *et al.* Clinical outcome of esophageal varices after hepatic arterial infusion chemotherapy for advanced hepatocellular carcinoma with major portal vein tumor thrombus. Hepatol Res 2011; 41(11): 1046-56.[http://dx.doi.org/10.1111/j.1872-034X.2011.00857.x] [PMID: 22032677]

[80] Sakon M, Nagano H, Dono K, *et al.* Combined intraarterial 5-fluorouracil and subcutaneous interferon-alpha therapy for advanced hepatocellular carcinoma with tumor thrombi in the major portal branches. Cancer 2002; 94(2): 435-42.[http://dx.doi.org/10.1002/cncr.10246] [PMID: 11900229]

[81] Ota H, Nagano H, Sakon M, *et al.* Treatment of hepatocellular carcinoma with major portal vein thrombosis by combined therapy with subcutaneous interferon-alpha and intra-arterial 5-fluorouracil; role of type 1 interferon receptor expression. Br J Cancer 2005; 93(5): 557-64.[http://dx.doi.org/10.1038/sj.bjc.6602742] [PMID: 16106266]

[82] Uka K, Aikata H, Takaki S, *et al.* Clinical features and prognosis of patients with extrahepatic metastases from hepatocellular carcinoma. World J Gastroenterol 2007; 13(3): 414-20.[http://dx.doi.org/10.3748/wjg.v13.i3.414] [PMID: 17230611]

[83] Yamashita T, Arai K, Sunagozaka H, *et al.* Randomized, phase II study comparing interferon combined with hepatic arterial infusion of fluorouracil plus cisplatin and fluorouracil alone in patients with advanced hepatocellular carcinoma. Oncology 2011; 81(5-6): 281-90.[http://dx.doi.org/10.1159/000334439] [PMID: 22133996]

[84] Yamasaki T, Sakaida I. Hepatic arterial infusion chemotherapy for advanced hepatocellular carcinoma and future treatments for the poor responders. Hepatol Res 2012; 42(4): 340-8.[http://dx.doi.org/10.1111/j.1872-034X.2011.00938.x] [PMID: 22151009]

[85] Terashima T, Yamashita T, Arai K, *et al.* Response to chemotherapy improves hepatic reserve for patients with hepatocellular carcinoma and Child-Pugh B cirrhosis. Cancer Sci 2016; 107(9): 1263-9.[http://dx.doi.org/10.1111/cas.12992] [PMID: 27315783]

[86] Nagano H, Wada H, Kobayashi S, *et al.* Long-term outcome of combined interferon-α and 5-fluorouracil treatment for advanced hepatocellular carcinoma with major portal vein thrombosis. Oncology 2011; 80(1-2): 63-9.[http://dx.doi.org/10.1159/000328281] [PMID: 21659784]

[87] Kojima H, Hatano E, Taura K, Seo S, Yasuchika K, Uemoto S. Hepatic Resection for Hepatocellular Carcinoma with Tumor Thrombus in the Major Portal Vein. Dig Surg 2015; 32(6): 413-20.[http://dx.doi.org/10.1159/000437375] [PMID: 26316188]

[88] Chen S, Ling Q, Yu K, *et al.* Dual oxidase 1: A predictive tool for the prognosis of hepatocellular carcinoma patients. Oncol Rep 2016; 35(6): 3198-208.[http://dx.doi.org/10.3892/or.2016.4745] [PMID: 27108801]

[89] Lui GY, Kovacevic Z, Richardson V, Merlot AM, Kalinowski DS, Richardson DR. Targeting cancer by binding iron: Dissecting cellular signaling pathways. Oncotarget 2015; 6(22): 18748-79.[http://dx.doi.org/10.18632/oncotarget.4349] [PMID: 26125440]

[90] Bogdan AR, Miyazawa M, Hashimoto K, Tsuji Y. Regulators of Iron Homeostasis: New Players in Metabolism, Cell Death, and Disease. Trends Biochem Sci 2016; 41(3): 274-86.[http://dx.doi.org/10.1016/j.tibs.2015.11.012] [PMID: 26725301]

[91] Yamasaki T, Terai S, Sakaida I. Deferoxamine for advanced hepatocellular carcinoma. N Engl J Med 2011; 365(6): 576-8.[http://dx.doi.org/10.1056/NEJMc1105726] [PMID: 21830988]

[92] Yamasaki T, Saeki I, Sakaida I. Efficacy of iron chelator deferoxamine for hepatic arterial infusion chemotherapy in advanced hepatocellular carcinoma patients refractory to current treatments. Hepatol Int 2014; 8 (Suppl. 2): 492-8.[http://dx.doi.org/10.1007/s12072-013-9515-3] [PMID: 26201330]

[93] Sano S, Nakata S, Wada S, *et al.* Pathological complete response by advanced hepatocellular carcinoma with massive macrovascular invasion to hepatic arterial infusion chemotherapy: a case report. World J Surg Oncol 2019; 17(1): 229.[http://dx.doi.org/10.1186/s12957-019-1772-8] [PMID: 31878937]

[94] Ogawa K, Kamimura K, Watanabe Y, *et al.* Effect of double platinum agents, combination of miriplatin-transarterial oily chemoembolization and cisplatin-hepatic arterial infusion chemotherapy, in patients with hepatocellular carcinoma: Report of two cases. World J Clin Cases 2017; 5(6): 238-46.[http://dx.doi.org/10.12998/wjcc.v5.i6.238] [PMID: 28685137]

[95] Sung PS, Yang K, Bae SH, *et al.* Reduction of Intrahepatic Tumour by Hepatic Arterial Infusion Chemotherapy Prolongs Survival in Hepatocellular Carcinoma. Anticancer Res 2019; 39(7): 3909-

16.[http://dx.doi.org/10.21873/anticanres.13542] [PMID: 31262920]

[96]   Wada H, Nagano H, Noda T, *et al*. Complete remission of hepatocellular carcinoma with portal vein tumor thrombus and lymph node metastases by arterial infusion of 5-fluorouracil and interferon-alpha combination therapy following hepatic resection. J Gastroenterol 2007; 42(6): 501-6.[http://dx.doi.org/10.1007/s00535-007-2028-x] [PMID: 17671767]

[97]   Allemani C, Matsuda T, Di Carlo V, *et al*. Global surveillance of trends in cancer survival 2000-14 (CONCORD-3): analysis of individual records for 37 513 025 patients diagnosed with one of 18 cancers from 322 population-based registries in 71 countries. Lancet 2018; 391(10125): 1023-75.[http://dx.doi.org/10.1016/S0140-6736(17)33326-3] [PMID: 29395269]

[98]   Bruix J, Raoul JL, Sherman M, *et al*. Efficacy and safety of sorafenib in patients with advanced hepatocellular carcinoma: subanalyses of a phase III trial. J Hepatol 2012; 57(4): 821-9.[http://dx.doi.org/10.1016/j.jhep.2012.06.014] [PMID: 22727733]

[99]   Cheng AL, Guan Z, Chen Z, *et al*. Efficacy and safety of sorafenib in patients with advanced hepatocellular carcinoma according to baseline status: subset analyses of the phase III Sorafenib Asia-Pacific trial. Eur J Cancer 2012; 48(10): 1452-65.[http://dx.doi.org/10.1016/j.ejca.2011.12.006] [PMID: 22240282]

[100] Kudo M, Finn RS, Qin S, *et al*. Lenvatinib *versus* sorafenib in first-line treatment of patients with unresectable hepatocellular carcinoma: a randomised phase 3 non-inferiority trial. Lancet 2018; 391(10126): 1163-73.[http://dx.doi.org/10.1016/S0140-6736(18)30207-1] [PMID: 29433850]

[101] Finn RS, Qin S, Ikeda M, *et al*. Atezolizumab plus Bevacizumab in Unresectable Hepatocellular Carcinoma. N Engl J Med 2020; 382(20): 1894-905.[http://dx.doi.org/10.1056/NEJMoa1915745] [PMID: 32402160]

[102] Terashima T, Yamashita T, Arai K, *et al*. Feasibility and efficacy of hepatic arterial infusion chemotherapy for advanced hepatocellular carcinoma after sorafenib. Hepatol Res 2014; 44(12): 1179-85.[http://dx.doi.org/10.1111/hepr.12266] [PMID: 24171787]

Targeting Cancer Stem Cells: Implications in Health and Disease

Roshia Ali[1, 2, *], Hilal Ahmad Mir[2], Rabia Hamid[3], Sahar Saleem Bhat[4], Firdous A. Khanday[2]

[1] Department of Biochemistry, University of Kashmir, Srinagar, Jammu and Kashmir-190006, India

[2] Department of Biotechnology, University of Kashmir, Srinagar, Jammu and Kashmir-190006, India

[3] Department of Nanotechnology, University of Kashmir, Srinagar, Jammu and Kashmir-190006, India

[4] Division of Biotechnology, SKUAST-K, FVSc& AH, Shuhama, Srinagar, Jammu and Kashmir, India

Abstract

Cancer is a serious global health concern as it accounts for about 9.6 million deaths worldwide. Despite striking breakthroughs made in understanding, prevention, and treatment of cancer, the mortality rate is still high and no permanent cure has been found. The major concern is the lack of effective therapies against advanced metastasis. Thus, there is a dire need to implement new treatment approaches to combat this dreadful disease. Cancer stem cells (CSCs), being critical players of tumors can be the potential target for therapy. Currently, cancer stem cell therapy is gaining much attention from researchers because of its ability to target the CSCs, which are responsible for tumor initiation, progression, metastasis, therapeutic resistance, and recurrence. While most conventional treatment strategies target fast-growing tumor cells, CSCs may remain in the latent stage for extended periods thereby escaping the traditional therapies and leading to treatment resistance. Hence, specific targeting of the tumor-initiating cells has become the heart of cancer research, aiming at the complete elimination of malignancies. Major strategies against CSCs include targeting surface CSC biomarkers, blockage of self-renewal signaling pathways (Wnt, Nanog,

Hippo/YAP, Notch, PTEN, Hedgehog, and/or STAT3), genetic targeting of CSCs, cell therapy, RNA interference utilizing miRNAs. Based on this concept, the present chapter summarizes the current strategies and the lead molecules which have found their route to preclinical and clinical studies. Since the evolution of clinical trials targeting CSCs holds a sanguine promise of affecting cancer medicine. This chapter will further throw light on rapid advancement made in this field, shortcomings faced in targeting CSCs, and several critical issues that are yet to be resolved.

Keywords: Apoptosis, Angiogenesis, Cancer recurrence, Cancer stem cells, CSC biomarkers, CSC niche, CSC origin, Differentiation, Immunotherapy, Metastasis, Mutation, Oncogenic signaling, Plasticity, Self renewal, Stemness, Targeted therapy, Transformation, Treatment resistance, Tumorigenesis, VSELs.

* **Corresponding author Roshia Ali:** Department of Biochemistry, University of Kashmir, Srinagar, Jammu and Kashmir-190006 & Department of Biotechnology, University of Kashmir, Srinagar, Jammu and Kashmir-190006, India; Tel: 9018514288; E-mail: sheikhroshia@gmail.com

INTRODUCTION

Cancer remains one of the major public health concerns, with approximately 18.1 million cases and 9.6 million cancer-related deaths worldwide [1]. Despite substantial advancements in the diagnosis and therapeutics, metastatic dissemination, cancer recurrence, and drug resistance continues to be a major clinical concern. Cancer stem cells (CSCs) are immortal tumor-initiating cells characterized by exclusive abilities of self-renewal and multi-lineage differentiation that drive tumor growth and heterogeneity [2]. The stemness phenotype of these CSCs is a consequence of genetic mutations or abnormal epigenetic changes. The exact origin of CSC has been abstruse and cell of origin for tumor initiation varies across different cancer types. The cell of origin of CSC may arise from somatic cells, partially differentiated progenitors, or differentiated cells that acquire self-renewal and differentiation properties through various mechanisms [3, 4]. CSCs may also arise from normal noncancerous stem cells that acquire malignant phenotype over time through transformation and reprogramming [5]. CSCs are known to reside in a specialized microenvironment referred to as the niche, which is composed of diverse cell types that promote CSC survival and ameliorate their stemness phenotype. CSCs are considered to be a major cause of cancer therapy failure due to their resistance to current conventional therapeutics, resulting in tumor relapse and eventually metastasis [6]. Moreover, in recent times CSC based targeted therapies have proven to be beneficial in suppressing tumor development in various pre-clinical and clinical studies [7]. A thorough understanding of the CSC biology is crucial for developing novel cancer diagnostic and therapeutic strategies. CSC based therapeutics are aimed at interfering with the functions of surface markers, drug efflux transporters, stemness pathways, epigenetic regulators and oncogenic signaling pathways. Besides, immunotherapeutics and differentiation therapies have also been established to target CSCs. In this chapter, we have summarized the biological characteristics of CSCs, the role of the niche in CSCs, current therapeutic approaches to target CSCs, and the lead molecules that have found their route to preclinical and clinical studies.

STEM Cells

Stem cells are a small subset of undetermined cells in the human body characterized by remarkable self-renewal capability with perpetual multilineage potential [8]. These non-specialized cells strikingly differ in their capacity to differentiate into different cell lineages and based on their multilineage potential they can be hierarchically classified into totipotent, pluripotent, multipotent and unipotent. Totipotent stem cells are most versatile, having the highest differentiation potential. The embryonic totipotent cells differentiate into pluripotent embryonic stem cells which further differentiate into multipotent adult stem cells. However, with each differentiation the potency and phenotypic plasticity of embryonic stem cells gets restricted. Embryonic stem cells (ESCs) are pluripotent cell lines derived from the undifferentiated inner cell mass of blastocyst-stage early mammalian embryo. ESCs are unique in their ability to renew themselves indefinitely in a pluripotent state and retain the extraordinary potential to differentiate virtually into all the cell types of an adult organism, thereby, producing a diverse range of specialized cell types with varying phenotypes. These peculiar features make them a promising source of cells for regenerative and transplantation medicine, cell replacement therapy, basic biological research, compound screening for drug development, and in understanding developmental biology and gene function in adult organism [9⁻11]. Although ESCs offer enormous potential and hope for new innovative therapies in the treatment of a variety of diseases and debilities, however, the clinical application of these cells raises numerous ethical and safety concerns that limit their exploitation in cell-based therapeutics and research. In addition to ESCs, the tissues of our body are known to harbor diverse stem cell populations that have gradually evolved from ESCs and migrated to different organs or tissues during the course of development with the definite purpose to recoup tissue repair and homeostasis. These specialized stem cells are referred to as Adult stem cells or tissue-specific stem cells. In contrast to ESCs, adult stem cells are multipotent cells having the capacity to generate only several differentiated lineages for the specific tissues wherein they reside. Stem cells are known to interact with the dynamic physiological system that primarily governs the outcome of developmental morphogenetic events and organismal stress, as these cells have a crucial role in tissue generation, maintenance and repair. The stem cell niche is the specialized anatomic location where stem cells both reside and receive stimuli that provide an idiosyncratic microenvironment for the stem cell functioning as well as determine their fate. The behavior of stem cells in the niche is stringently regulated by a milieu of biochemical factors that ensure proper stem cell functioning [12ˉ15]. Thus, stem cell niche is a basic unit of tissue physiology, having great anatomical as well as functional importance, integrating signals that orchestrate response of stem cells to the needs of organisms. The cell-cell and cell-matrix interaction of stem cells stimulate diverse signaling pathways that activate and/or repress transcription programs that maintain stem cells either in a dormant state or induce self renewal and/or differentiation in them. Under normal physiological conditions, a striking balance exists between stem cells self-renewal and generation of differentiated progenitor cells to maintain tissue homeostasis. Stem cells employ various strategies to regulate the dynamism between self-renewal and progeny production. One such strategy employed by stem cells to accomplish the above described tasks is asymmetric cell division, wherein each stem cell divides asymmetrically to generate one stem cell and one progenitor cell. Stem cells may also self renew symmetrically to produce two daughter stem cells or differentiate symmetrically to produce two progenitor cells and the balance between symmetric and asymmetric modes is tightly controlled by microenvironmental signals to maintain appropriate numbers of stem cells and progenitor cells (Fig. 1). Since stem cell niches primarily dictate stem cell fate governing the balance between stemness and differentiation; alterations in the niche by genetic or environmental factors could influence stem cell functionality and may contribute to the development of many cancers.

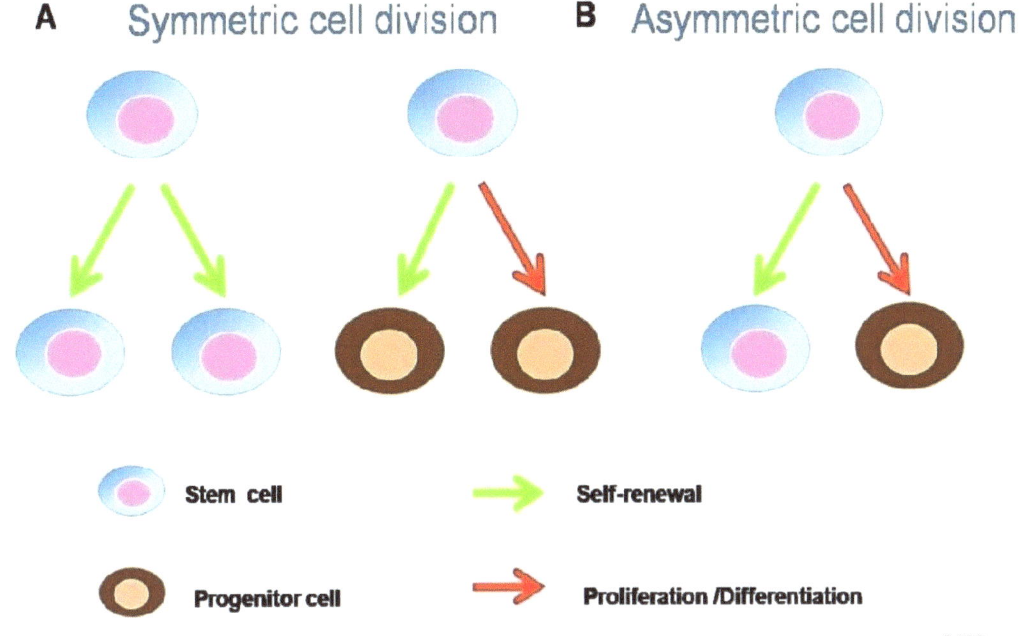

Fig. (1))

Symmetric and Asymmetric modes of cell division in stem cells.

CANCER STEM CELLS

Cancer stem cells or tumor-initiating/propagating cells are distinct populations of tumorigenic cells present within heterogeneous tumor mass stem endowed with stem cell-like phenotype and are characterized by four distinct features: (a) self-renewal (b) differentiation (c) tumorigenicity (d) specific surface markers. CSCs are dynamic entities undergoing a reversible transition between their differentiated and stem cell-like states due to their intrinsic phenotypic plasticity. These quiescent slow-cycling tumor propagating cells harbor distinctive pluripotent capacities giving rise to new stem cells either through asymmetric or symmetric divisions, ultimately leading to tumor formation. CSCs have been demonstrated in multiple human malignancies and are thought to mediate tumorigenesis, metastasis, recurrence and conventional therapy resistance *via* their self-renewal, proliferation, differentiation, and immune evasion abilities [16-22]. The stemness phenotype of CSCs is primarily governed by several signaling pathways, including Wnt/β-catenin, Hedgehog (Hh), PI3K/Akt/mTOR, transforming growth factor-β (TGF-β), polycomb group B lymphoma Mo-MLV insertion region 1 homolog (BMI1), and Notch (notch1-4/DLL/JAG) signaling pathways [23-27]. In addition to this, CSCs have been shown to have suppressive immunomodulatory properties like that of normal stem cells and are endowed with drug-resistant phenotype. Various factors are known to attribute to the inherent drug resistance mechanisms and stem cell-like tumor phenotype of CSCs These include cellular quiescence, environmental niche, dysregulation of growth and developmental signaling pathways, elevated expression of anti-apoptotic proteins, enhanced activity of DNA damage repair enzymes, epigenetic reprogramming, higher expression of multidrug transporter family genes and alteration of cellular metabolism [28⁻37]. Therefore, development of strategies targeting CSCs *via* specific surface CSC biomarkers, drug transporters, blockage of self-renewal signaling pathways or their components, genetic targeting of CSCs and destroying their tumor microenvironment holds hope for improvement of clinical outcome of patients with cancer, especially for patients with metastatic disease (Fig. 2).

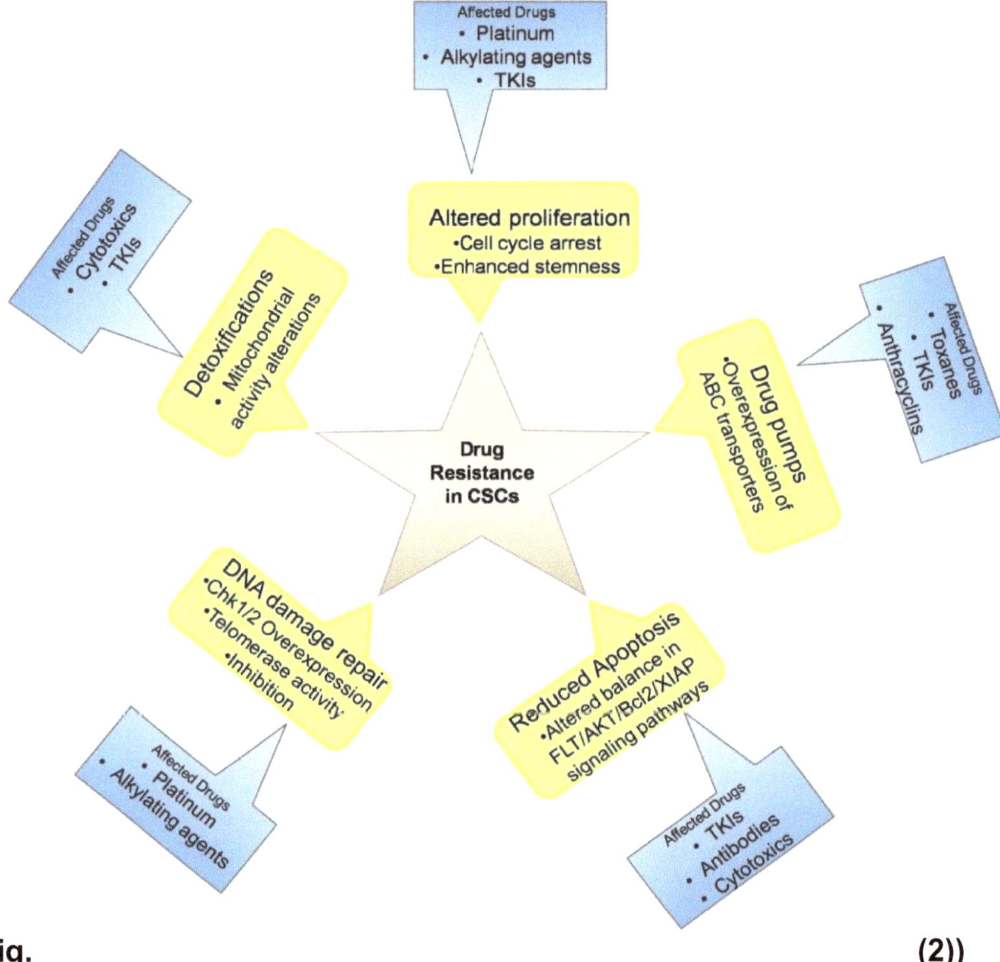

Fig. (2))

Mechanisms employed by CSCs contributing towards therapeutic resistance.

The origin of CSCs is still controversial as multiple hypotheses suggesting the potential origin of CSCs have been put forth. One of the hypotheses explaining CSCs origin states that CSCs arise from non-stem cancer cells (NSCCs) present within the tumor mass. NSCCs have limited proliferative potential but they constitute the bulk of tumor mass. These non-stem cells may acquire several types of mutations that might aid in gaining stemness potential [3, 4]. The stemness properties of a cell are governed by various stemness- related signaling pathways which might be dysregulated in NSCCs due to genetic and epigenetic modifications. In this context Yanger *et al.*, posited that CSCs may arise from NSCCs by the activation of several pathways involved in pluripotency and self-renewal like Wnt/β-catenin, Jagged2-Notch and Hh [38]. Accordingly in another study, inactivation of the Hippo pathway was found to be sufficient to de-differentiate NSCCs into cells with CSC like phenotype [39]. Mounting evidence suggests that several microenvironmental factors modulate stemness contributing to CSC differentiation and transformation thereby fostering tumorigenesis. For instance, production of proinflammatory cytokines (Tumor Necrosis Factor [TNF], interleukin-1 [IL-1] and interleukin-6 [IL-6]) by CSC, which activate transcription factors like nuclear factor Kappa-β (NF-κβ) and STAT3, have been reported to impart to stem cell-like tumor phenotype in non-stem cancer cells [40⁻45]. Endothelial cells in the tumor microenvironment have also been found to increase stemness phenotype in cancer cells by up-regulating self-renewal and differentiation signaling pathways (Wnt, Sonic Hedgehog (SHh), nitric oxide and Notch) that in turn enhances stemness-related markers (OCT4, SOX2, OLIG2 and BMI1) thereby facilitating reprogramming of non-stem cancer cell to CSC [46, 47]. Moreover, up-regulation of hypoxia-inducible factors (HIF1α and HIF2α) in tumor microenvironment caused increased expression of Notch-1, CD117, EMT-specific genes like SNAIL, SLUG, TWIST, and N-Cadherin that further induces dedifferentiation of non-stem cancer cells promoting stemness and metastasis [48, 49]. According to recent studies, aberrant epigenetic alterations of tumor suppressor genes and/or differentiation-related genes can also contribute to the transition of NSCCs to CSCs [50]. Dysregulation of polycomb protein levels have been closely linked with the establishment of cancer stem cells. Various subunits of polycomb-repressor complex 2 (PRC2) like enhancer of zeste homolog 2 (EZH2) and suppressor of zeste 12 homolog (SUZ12) have been reported to be overexpressed in a variety of different tumors contributing to stemness properties in these cells [51, 52]. An alternative hypothesis for the origin of CSCs suggests that the CSCs arise from the normal stem cells or progenitor cells that acquire malignant phenotype over time through transformation and reprogramming. Stem cell self-renewal and differentiated related pathways are stringently regulated in somatic stem cells under normal physiological conditions [53, 54]. However, aberrance in any of these pathways in adult stem cells can contribute to the generation of CSCs [5]. Furthermore, alterations in stem cell niche or mutations in proto-oncogenes and/or tumor suppressor genes can also induce the transformation of somatic stem cells into CSCs [55]. In a study, Tomasetti & Vogelstein have shown that random mutations can occur in the normal stem cells during DNA replication, which can transform these normal stem cells to CSCs [56]. Another study demonstrated that alterations in stromal signaling and inflammation conditions in adult stem cells facilitate their transformation to epithelial cancers [4]. Recent evidence indicates very small embryonic/epiblast-like stem cells (VSELs) as a possible origin of CSCs which are having properties similar to that of pluripotent stem cells [57⁻59].

CSC NICHE - CROSS TALK BETWEEN CSC AND TUMOR MICROENVIRONMENT

CSCs are known to reside in specialized regions within the tumor microenvironment (TME) known as CSC niche that has been strongly associated with the maintenance of CSC function and biology. The CSC state in the TME is dynamic which can be acquired or lost in response to perturbations in the CSC microenvironment [60]. In addition to maintaining CSC phenotypic plasticity, the CSC niche also contributes to stemness phenotype, tumor initiation, immune evasion, therapy resistance and metastasis [61⁻63]. The CSC niche comprises of a heterogeneous population of cancer cells along with resident tumor stroma, secreted factors and extracellular matrix proteins. Tumor stroma is a group of non-cancer cells consisting of stromal cells like Tumor-associated endothelial cells, cancer-associated fibroblast (CAFs), mesenchymal stromal cells (MSCs), immune cells like tumor-associated macrophages (TAMs), lymphocytes,, T-regulatory cells (Treg cells), adipocytes and myeloid-derived suppressor cells (MDSCs). The elements of the niche are in close association with tumor cells contributing to tumorigenesis [64, 65]. This interaction can be facilitated by various soluble factors (ECM proteins, growth factors, pro-tumor cytokines/chemokines, lipids and exosomes) present in the CSC niche.

The hypoxia of the TME plays a pivotal role in the formation and maintenance of CSC nurtures CSCs in their undifferentiated stem-like state, enhances their doubling rate and induces expression of CSC specific biomarkers. Increasing evidences have indicated towards the importance of HIFs in the regulation stem cell properties. HIF-1α and HIF-2α functioned in cancer cell proliferation and survival in glioblastoma and promoted self-renewal capability and stemness of CSCs by activating cell survival pathways [66, 67].

Tumor-associated endothelial cells are vital elements of the CSC niche that serve as building blocks for tumor-associated blood vasculature. Besides accelerating the formation of tumor vasculature niche, these endothelial cells are involved in modulating cancer cell properties promoting their invasive and migratory capabilities. Vascular endothelial growth factor (VEGF) is a crucial factor that drives tumor angiogenesis; however clinical outcomes of anti-

VEGF monotherapy in patients with solid tumors has been largely negative and is of limited utility [68, 69]. Endothelial cells exhibit alteration in cellular signaling in response to various tumor-derived signals, chemotherapy and environmental metabolic stress. Recent evidence suggests that Chemotherapy downregulates the expression of IGFBP7 in tumor-associated endothelial cells and stimulates expression of FGF4 in IGF1R+ tumor stem cells where they initiate FGF4-FGFR1-ETS2 angiocrine cascade, converting naïve tumor cells into chemoresistant tumor stem cells, thereby enhancing their invasiveness and progression [70]. Furthermore, increased expression of IL-6, NO, and factors linked to Notch and Wnt signaling pathway has been reported in endothelial cells in response to tumor cell-derived signals and metabolic stress [71-73].

Cancer-associated fibroblasts (CAFs) are one major stromal cell type of TME that fosters cancer cell growth enhances extracellular matrix production and promotes angiogenesis. Moreover, multiple studies have demonstrated that CAFs recruit immune suppressive cells into TME that facilitate immune evasion and activate cancer immunotherapy resistance [74, 75]. Overwhelming evidences have pointed towards the role of CAFs in maintenance of the CSC niche through their secretion of unique cytokine (IL-6, CXCL-12, *etc.*) and growth factors (vascular endothelial growth factor [VEGF], platelet-derived growth factor [PDGF] and hepatocyte growth factor [HGF]). The interplay between proinflammatory cytokines and growth factors modulates cancer cell phenotype. For instance, HGF produces by CAFs stemness properties in colon cells *via* induction of Wnt and Notch pathways [76]. Through the secretion of IL-6 and HGF, CAFs from hepatocellular carcinoma (HCC) were shown to promote the CSC phenotype in HCC cells [77]. A recent study also demonstrated that CD10$^+$ GPR77$^+$ double-positive CAF subtype enhances chemo-resistance and cancer stemness through increased production of IL-6, IL-8 and CA-5 [78].

Mesenchymal stem cells (MSCs) are self-renewing, multipotent stromal cells that have been demonstrated to have a multifaceted role in tumorigenesis exacerbating cancer cell proliferation, invasion, and metastasis, fostering angiogenesis, and promoting immunosuppressive TME [79, 80]. According to a study, induction of GREM1 expression by MSCs stimulates colon tumorigenesis and enhances stemness in cancer cells [81]. MSCs also dysregulated Micro RNA expression (miR-199a) in breast cancers and suppressed FOXP2 expression imparting stem cell characteristics to tumor cells [79]. MSCs secrete a myriad of molecules, such as chemokines, cytokines and growth factors that are known to act in a paracrine manner on their respective receptors present on the surface of cancer cells in tumor milieu, thus regulating cancer growth and progression. For instance, MSCs have been shown to enhance cancer cell proliferation in various cancer cell models *via* paracrine action of chemokines, like CXCL1, CXCL2 or CXCL12/SDF-1 [82,

[83]. Similarly, MSCs promote cancer stemness in context to several cancers through the induction of NF-κB pathway by secreting CXCL12, IL6, and IL8 [84‑86]. Furthermore, MSC-derived growth factors such as epidermal growth factor (EGF) have been shown to stimulate tumor progression in breast cancer [87].

TME is known to harbor multitudinous immune cells of the innate and adaptive immune systems known as tumor-infiltrating immune cells. These immune cells infiltrate TME in response to a plethora of chemotactic cytokines and chemokines produced by cancer cells. TAMs are critical components of TME that have been shown to support tumor stemness, tumor growth, suppress antitumor immunity and promote tumor angiogenesis and metastasis through their production of growth factors, cytokines and chemokines [88]. Moreover, these tumor-infiltrating macrophages drive immune suppression by facilitating the recruitment of TREG cells in TME and triggering the release of inhibitory immune checkpoint proteins in these cells [89, 90].

Tumor-derived exosomes are nano-sized membrane vesicles that have been recognized as multifaceted regulators of cancer development. Clinical analysis has revealed that tumor cells released higher levels of exosomes into the microenvironment than normal cells. The exosomes released by cancer cells harbor molecules derived from cancer that alters TME thereby promoting angiogenesis, facilitating immune evasion, inducing differentiation of fibroblasts into tumor-related fibroblasts, and initiating metastatic cascade. For example, CSC derived exosomes are known to contain various angiogenic factors that promote vascular growth. According to a recent study, glioblastoma stem-like cells release the pro-angiogenic factor VEGF-A *via* exosomes [91]. Another study found that glioma stem cells promote the angiogenic behavior of endothelial cells by secreting miR-21 containing exosomes that facilitate angiogenic switch *via* miR-21/VEGF/VEGFR2 signaling pathway [92]. CSC derived exosomes also enable tumor cells to evade immune surveillance. Domenis *et al.* showed that glioma stem cell-derived exosomes transformed the phenotype of monocytic cells into monocytic myeloid-derived suppressor cells thereby suppressing T-cell immune response [93]. Exosomes regulate oncogenesis and tumor development by facilitating signaling crosstalk between CSCs and normal stem cells [94]. They also modulate the growth of CSCs by targeting specific signaling pathways (Wnt, Notch, Hippo, Hh and NF-κβ) [95, 96]. CSC enhances cell proliferation and self-renewal potential through crosstalk between exosomal signaling and TME [97]. Moreover, the study has shown that CSC derived exosomes induce signal transduction pathways in breast cancer cells that promote their stemness phenotype [98].

CSC BIOMARKERS

CSC expresses a unique repertoire of surface biomarkers that distinguishes them from other tumor cells or normal stem cells. These cell surface macromolecules aid in the identification and isolation of CSCs in various human cancers using flow cytometry or magnetic sorting. The CSCs were first identified in acute myeloid leukemia (AML) in which the leukemia stem cells (LSCs) were found to display a $CD34^+$ $CD38^-$ surface marker phenotype [99]. When transplanted into non-obese diabetic/severe combined immunodeficiency (NOD/SCID) mice, the $CD34^+$ $CD38^-$ subpopulation was shown to be highly capable of engrafting leukemia in recipient mice whereas, the major subset of AML cells with $CD34^+$ $CD38^+$ phenotype was not effective in regenerating same leukemia [100]. Subsequently, LSCs were characterized by a combination of surface markers that were used for their identification. For example, LSCs displayed $CD34^+$, $CD38^-$, $CD71^-$, $CD90^-$, $CD117^-$, HLA-DR$^-$ and $CD123^+$ phenotype. Although some of these LSCs markers are present on normal hematopoietic stem cells ($CD34^+$, $CD38^-$, $CD71^-$, and HLA-DR$^-$) three of them are uniquely present on the surface of LSCs ($CD90^-$, $CD117^-$, and $CD123^+$) [101]. Besides leukemia, CSCs were also identified in solid tumors including breast and brain cancer [21, 102]. In solid tumors, the CSCs were first identified in breast cancer where a distinct subpopulation of breast cancer cells was found to express ESA$^+$ $CD44^+$ $CD24^-$ phenotype and these breast cancer stem cells were capable of inducing tumorigenesis in immunodeficient NOD/SCID mice [21]. Furthermore, another study demonstrated the importance of brain cancer cells with CD133 phenotype in tumorigenesis and these cancer cells were able to generate tumors in NOD/SCID mice [103]. Later several studies showed the presence of CSCs population in various tumor types including melanoma, colon, pancreas, liver, lung, prostate and glioblastoma [19, 20, 104, 105]. There is a huge array of markers such as CD90, CD133, CD117, CD166, CD44, IL-6R, CD24, CD29, CD166, CD177, epithelial-specific antigen (ESA), epithelial cell adhesion molecule (EpCAM), leucine-rich repeat-containing G-protein coupled receptor 5 (Lgr5), chemokines receptor 4 (CXCR4), aldehyde dehydrogenase1 (ALDH1), alpha-fetoprotein (AFP), nestin, stage-specific embryonic antigen 4 (SSEA4) that have been used alone or in combination to identify or isolate CSCs from different tumors. CSCs are known to exhibit heterogeneous expression patterns of surface biomarkers that are usually tissue-specific as well as tumor subtype-specific. For instance, breast CSCs are characterized by presence of $CD44^+$, $CD24^-$ and ALDH$^+$; colon, brain and lung CSCs by $CD133^+$; leukemia CSCs by $CD34^+$ $CD8^-$; liver CSCs by $CD90^+$; head and neck CSCs by $CD44^+$; pancreatic CSCs by $CD44^+$ $CD24^+$ ESA$^+$ biomarkers

[106, 107]. The phenotypes of CSC markers according to the cancer types are summarized in Table 1.

Table 1 **Phenotypes of CSC markers in various cancers.**

S. No.	Tumor Type	Phenotype of CSC Markers	References
1.	Leukemia	CD34$^+$, CD38$^-$,CD47$^+$,CD96$^+$, CD117$^-$, HLA-DR-CD71$^-$, CCL-1$^+$, CD123$^+$, CD90$^-$	[100, 101, 108]
2.	Breast	ESA$^+$, CD133$^+$, CD44$^+$, CD24$^-$, ALDH-1, EpCAM$^+$	[21, 106, 109, 110]
3.	Colon	CD133$^+$, CD44$^+$, CD44v6, CD 166, CD49f$^+$, CD90$^+$, ALDH, ABCG2, CD24$^+$, Lgr5, ESA	[20, 110$^-$112]
4.	Liver	CD133$^+$, CD44$^+$, CD49f$^+$, CD24$^+$, ABCG2, CD90$^+$, CD166$^+$, EpCAM$^+$, ALDH, ESA$^+$	[108, 109, 113, 114]
5.	Gastric	CD133$^+$,CD44$^+$, CD24$^+$	[115$^-$117]
6.	Lung	Sca1, CD34$^+$, CCA, CD133$^+$, CD44$^+$, ABCG2, ALDH, CD87$^+$, SP, CD90$^+$	[115, 118, 119]
7.	Prostate	CD133$^+$, CD44$^+$, α2β1, ABCG2, ALDH	[19, 109, 115, 120]
8.	Pancreatic	CD133$^+$, CD44$^+$, CD24$^+$, ABCG2, ALDH, EpCAM$^+$, CXCR4, ESA	[121$^-$123]
9.	Melanoma	ABCB5$^+$, CD271$^+$,CD20$^+$	[16, 124, 125]
10.	Head and neck	SSEA-1$^+$, CD44$^+$, CD133$^+$	[111, 126, 127]

CD133

CD133 (AC133 or Prominin-1) is a 97 kDa cholesterol-binding pentaspan transmembrane single chain glycoprotein, generally expressed on undifferentiated cells but not in mature endothelial cells [128]. CD133 has been identified as CSC marker with tumorigenic properties. Several studies have suggested CD133 as a prognostic marker in multiple cancer types such as glioblastoma, pancreatic, breast, colon, liver and prostate cancer and it aids in the identification and isolation of CSCs in these tumor types [129$^-$133]. Overwhelming evidences suggest that CD133 expressing CSCs might perpetuate tumor growth and metastasis as they exhibit enhanced self-renewal potential and chemoresistance phenotype than CD133 negative cell population.

When transplanted into immunodeficient NOD-SCID mouse models CD133 positive cancer cells were shown to exhibit the greater capability to regenerate histologically similar tumor mass in comparison to CD133 negative populations. Another study demonstrated that overexpression of CD133 enhanced stemness properties and tumorigenic potential of MIA PaCa-2 pancreatic cells by upregulating expression of various stemness associated genes. CD133 expression also induced epithelial-mesenchymal transition and enhanced invasiveness in these cells by activating NF-κβ pathway [134]. Furthermore, knockdown of CD133 in head and neck cancer-initiating cells (HN-CIC) has been associated with reduced expression of OCT4 and NANOG stemness genes, enhanced epithelial differentiation as well as increased apoptotic capabilities [135]. The crosstalk of CD133 with Wnt/β-catenin and PI3K-Akt signaling pathways is well established that further contributes to cancer cell growth and development [136, 137]. CD133 has also been shown to upregulate the expression of FLICE-like inhibitory protein (FLIP) in CD133-positive cells thereby inhibiting apoptosis [138, 139]. CD133 promotes neovascularisation and angiogenesis by activating the Wnt signaling pathway that in turn increases the expression of proangiogenic factors like VEGF-A and interleukin-8 [140, 141].

CD24

CD24 (Heat stable antigen or nectadrin) is small mucin-like glycosylphosphatidylinositol (GPI)-linked membrane glycoprotein broadly overexpressed in multiple cancer types that functions in cell-cell and cell-matrix interactions [142]. Higher expression levels of CD24 have been reported in various human cancers [143-147]. CD24 has been postulated to be an important marker in tumor prognosis and diagnosis as it promotes tumor cell proliferation, invasion and metastasis [145, 148]. In tumor cells, CD24 interacts with P-selectin, an adhesion receptor present on activated platelets and endothelial cells, thus facilitating the infiltration and metastatic spread of CD24-expressing tumor cells [149-151]. CD24 has been shown to enhance tumorigenicity by promoting adhesion of tumor cells to fibronectin, collagen and lamin [152]. The expression levels of CD24 in invasive breast carcinomas were found to be significantly higher than in precancerous lesions and this increased expression correlated with adverse prognostic parameters [153]. In another study, CD24 expression was found to be an independent prognostic marker for the overall survival in nonsmall cell lung cancer patients [154]. Use of small-interfering RNA silencing and anti-CD24 monoclonal antibody displayed significant inhibition on tumor cell survival and proliferation [155, 156]. Moreover, the tumor size of hepatocellular carcinoma induced by transgenic expression of hepatitis B virus genes was reduced in response to targeted mutations of CD24 genes [157].

CD44

CD44 is a multifunctional transmembrane glycoprotein acting as a receptor for hyaluronic acid and many other extracellular matrix components. CD44 also acts as a cofactor for various growth factors and cytokines thereby regulating numerous functions including cell-matrix adhesion, proliferation, migration, differentiation and cell survival [158]. Recent studies have confirmed the potential use of CD44 as a CSC biomarker, implicated in regulating stemness properties of CSCs. In gastric cancers increased expression of CD44 was associated with promotion of tumorigenesis [159]. Contrastingly, mice lacking CD44 were found to have smaller tumors. Enhanced expression of CD44 was also found to be critical for tumor initiation and progression in glioma mouse models [160]. CD44 also plays a pivotal role in CSC self-renewal, maintenance, chemoresistance and survival by regulating miR-21 and miR-203 expression levels. CD44 associates with hyaluronic acid and extra cellular matrix proteins like osteopontin, activating Nanog-Stat3, Oct4-Sox2-Nanog and c-Src kinase signaling pathways resulting in up-regulation of miR-21 and downregulation of miR-203 [161, 162]. Furthermore, CD44 in combination with CD133 and CD34 was found to promote stemness properties in breast cancers [21]. The splicing variants of CD44 like CD44v3, CD44v5 and CD44v6 have been directly associated with the metastatic and tumorigenic potential of breast cancers [163]. Similarly, these variants were also found to promote the metastatic potential of lung carcinomas [164]. In leukemia, numbers of CD44 splice variants were found to be overexpressed in hematopoietic malignancies. For example, CD44v3, CD44v6, CD44v9and CD44v10 are expressed in bone marrow progenitors, while CD44v3, CD44v6, and CD44v9 are expressed by lymphocytes and monocytes in response to inflammatory cytokines stimulation [165]. Isoform CD44v9 was recently found as a novel marker of cancer stemness in head and neck cancers. CD44v9 functions by increasing intracellular glutathione (GSH) levels resulting in protection from oxidative stress and ROS, which is a distinct feature of CSCs [166]. Since EMT is one of the features for acquiring stemness like properties in tumors, CD44 was found to induce EMT in breast cancers on binding to hyaluronic acid. Blocking the binding of hyaluronic acid to CD44 reduces EMT, metastasis and aggressiveness of breast cancers [167].

ALDH

Aldehyde dehydrogenase is a superfamily consisting of 19 human isozymes which are localized throughout the body, overlapping in their tissue distribution and substrate specificities but differing in their aldehyde metabolizing efficiency [168]. The ALDH is a class of $NAD(P)^+$-dependent enzymes involved in the retinoic acid synthesis, drug resistance and detoxification of various exogenous, and endogenous aldehydes [168]. ALDH has also been portrayed as a potential marker for CSCs. In prostate tumor cells, expression of ALDH was found to be high and was reported to enhance the ability to form spheres and colonies. Furthermore, ALDH1A1 activity and expression were found to correlate with tumor stage, patient survival, metastasis, and tumorigenicity in animal models [169]. ALDH has been also shown to initiate tumor formation in various types of tissues. In cervical SCC or cervical intraepithelial neoplasia (CIN) II-III, a high expression of ALDH was observed. Likewise, ALDH1A1 expression was also found high in plasma samples from the same patients as compared to healthy persons. Increased expression of ALDH was also observed to correlate with lymph nodal metastasis and disease recurrence in invasive SCC patients [170]. Recently, ALDH activation was demonstrated to activate the glycolytic pathway in endometrial CSCs. GLUT1 an important factor for self-renewal and tumor-initiating capacity for glioma CSCs was found to be activated by ALDH thereby helping in maintenance and chemoresistance of CSCs [171]. The study was also supported by the exogenous introduction of ALDH in endometrial cancer cells, enhancing their stemness features. Various studies have reported that tumor cells expressing ALDH surface marker show resistance to a variety of cytotoxic drugs including doxorubicin, cisplatin, decarbazine and cylclophosphamide, *etc* [172, 173]. Besides, ALDH also reduces ROS levels and oxidative damage as a result of protecting cancer cells from ROS-induced oxidative stress [174].

CSCs IN TUMORIGENIC PROCESS

Tumorigenesis is characterized by the gain of malignant properties in normal cells, including dedifferentiation, proliferation, metastasis and evasion of apoptosis *etc*. CSCs act as critical regulators of tumor development, driving initiation, promotion and metastatic stages of cancer. Several studies have found the ability of isolated CSCs to promote tumor growth in immunodeficient mouse [175]. Mechanistically, expression of SOX2 a stemness transcription factor was found to be induced in CSCs, which in turn regulated expression of genes involved in stemness, proliferation, invasion and survival of tumors thereby promoting the initiation and progression of tumor [176]. Under inflammatory conditions, stemness markers like Oct3/4 and CD44v6 were found to be upregulated in inflammation-related urinary bladder cancer [177]. This crosstalk between CSCs and inflammation resulted in tumor development *via* the NF-κβ pathway by inducing DNA damage and expansion of mutated stem cells. Likewise, Oct3/4 and CD133 stemness markers were found to trigger tumor initiation in response to Opisthorchis viverrini induced inflammation [178]. Besides, the interplay of CSCs with MSC also facilitated the initiation and progression of tumors. This interplay was found to promote the stemness of CSCs *via* NF-κβ pathway activation in response to MSC secreted factors including, CXCL12, IL-6 and IL-8 [86]. In breast cancer the same crosstalk triggered CXCL7 release from MSC consequently, inducing the production of a number of cytokines involved in promoting the growth of CSCs [80]. Also, the crosstalk of CSCs and MSC was found to promote tumor angiogenesis, invasion and drug resistance. Under hypoxic conditions, CSCs were found to promote HIF gene-mediated angiogenesis by activating VEGF. Moreover, activated HIF genes also regulated stemness of CSCs by activating TGF-β, Wnt/β-catenin, TNF-α and NF-κβ pathway [179, 180]. MSC and CSCs interaction also encouraged metastasis and growth of cancers *via* ERK1/2 and Wnt/β-catenin pathways [181, 182]. Similarly, endothelial cell crosstalk with CSCs significantly promoted expansion, cell survival and angiogenesis by secreting pro-angiogenic factors including Jagged-1, SHH, IL-6, CXCL1 and CCL21 in various cancers [46, 183-185]. The tumorigenic process is also influenced by surrounding extracellular matrix components (ECM). Several studies have suggested the potential role of ECM in stemness maintenance of CSCs and their differentiation into tumor phenotypes. For example, tenascinan ECM protein and a CSCs biomarker were shown to exhibit a direct correlation with cancer progression and drug resistance in melanoma cells. Interestingly, this protein was also found to initiate the metastatic ability of breast cancers [186]. Epithelial-mesenchymal transition (EMT) a key step in metastasis has been also related to CSCs. Epithelial cells expressing mesenchymal markers have been found to acquire stemness like properties. Furthermore, the ability of glioma CSCs to metastasize has been found to associate with increased epithelial marker MMP-2 and decreased E-cadherin [187]. Accordingly, untransformed immortalized human mammary epithelial cells have been shown to acquire CSC state by expressing EMT markers including FoxC2, N-cadherin and Zeb factors [188].

THERAPEUTIC APPROACHES TO TARGET CSCs - PRECLINICAL AND CLINICAL ROUTE

Traditional and mainstream therapeutic strategies existing against cancer, chemotherapy and radiotherapy, have serious limitations such as systemic or local toxicity and drug resistance that frequently lead to treatment failure and cancer relapse. Besides, these conventional treatment methods target fast-growing tumor cells and fail to eliminate CSCs that may remain in the latent stage for extended periods thereby escaping the traditional therapies and leading to treatment resistance. Several molecular mechanisms are known to operate in CSCs that contribute to resistance to conventional anticancer therapies. Therefore, for the development of high-efficient treatments for cancer therapy that can induce a long-lasting clinical response preventing tumor relapse, traditional therapies should be combined with novel strategies designed specifically to target and eliminate CSCs (Fig. 3).

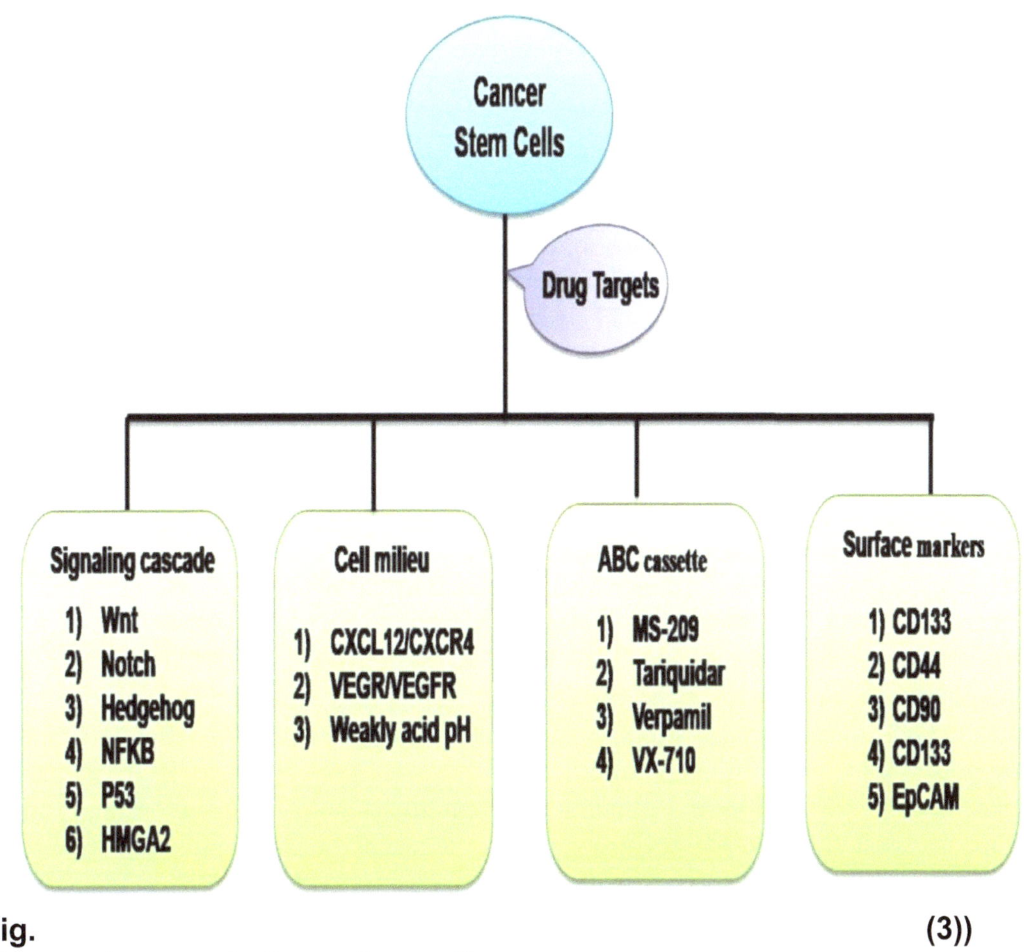

Fig. (3))
Therapeutic targets in Cancer Stem cells.

Targeting Cellular Surface CSC Markers

CSCs in various tumors show increased expression of specific surface markers, such as $CD44^+$ $CD24^-$ $ALDH^+$ in breast CSCs, $CD133^+$ in colon, brain, liver, gastric and lung CSCs; $CD44^+$ $CD24^+$ ESA in pancreatic CSCs. Recent studies have shown that targeting cytotoxic drugs to CSCs by using antibodies against tumor-specific CSC surface markers enhances the efficacy and specificity of existing therapeutic strategies. For instance, CD33 is overexpressed in the majority of AML cells. Researchers have developed antibody-drug conjugate gemtuzumab ozogamicin, a recombinant humanized anti CD33 mouse monoclonal antibody covalently linked to cytotoxic drug calicheamicin, which has been recently approved by FDA for the treatment of CD33$^+$ AML [189-191]. Furthermore, differential expression of CD44, IL-3R and the T-cell immunoglobulin mucin TIM-3 has been reported between normal and CSCs and have been used to specifically target and eradicate leukemia stem cells in patients with AML. Therapeutic targeting using activated monoclonal antibodies against these surface markers remarkable reduced leukemia repopulation in immuno-deficient NOD/SCID mice transplanted with human AML [192, 193]. Similarly, double cortin-like kinase 1 (Dclk1) specifically marks CSCs in the intestine that continuously produces tumor progeny in the polyps of Apc$^{Min/+}$ mice [194, 195]. Lineage abreption of Dclk1+ CSCs resulted in the pronounced retrogression of tumor polyps without impairment to the normal intestine [195]. CD44 marker has demonstrated promising results in preclinical studies. Anti-CD44 antibodies promoted terminal differentiation in AML blasts, decreased metastatic dissemination, as well as retarded tumor growth in solid cancers [164]. CD44 monoclonal antibody conjugated gold nanorods have also been used to target and photo-ablate CSCs in MCF-7 breast cancer [196]. In the clinical setting, antiCD44v6 antibody bivatuzumab labeled with 186re or coupled with microtubule targeting cytotoxic agent mertansine, stabilized heavily pretreated CD44v6$^+$ metastatic breast cancer patients, however, severe dose limiting toxicities occurred. Moreover, immunogenic accumulation of antibody in keratinocytes caused transient and mild skin disorders in 75% of patients and a case of fatal toxic epidermal necrolysis stopped the clinical trial in the early stage [197]. RG7356 is another humanized anti-CD44 monoclonal antibody specifically designed against the constant region of CD44 to inhibit the interaction between CD44 and HA. RG7356 has recently completed Phase 1 clinical trial in patients with solid tumors and the data suggest that CD44 isoform status is a novel predictive biomarker for clinical patient response to treatment with RG7356 [198]. A new humanized CD44 antibody, R05429083, specifically designed to target a glycosylated epitope of CD44 has been shown to effectively target the CSCs as well as nurture the NK cell population in a pre-clinical model of neck squamous cell carcinoma [199]. This humanized CD44 antibody is currently undergoing clinical trials in patients with CD44 expressing metastatic tumors or AML (NCT01358903 and NCT01641250). CD133 is an important CSC marker in many tissues and a CD133 antibody conjugated cytotoxic drugs have shown promising *in vivo* results in hepatocellular and gastric cancer [200]. Recently, bi-specific antibodies, which act by equipping activated T-cells to CD133$^+$ cells have been developed and are currently undergoing clinical trials in a range of cancers (NCT02541370) [201]. Imatinib, a tyrosine kinase inhibitor, specifically targets CD117, BCR/ABL and PDGF receptors and is approved for the treatment of chronic myelogenous leukemia (CML) and metastatic CD117$^+$ gastrointestinal stromal tumors [202, 203]. The results of clinical trials of Imatinib monotherapy in solid cancers were disappointing [204, 205].

However, Imatinib when conjugated with cisplatin selectively targets and eliminates lung CSCs, suggesting that it may have efficacy in combination therapies [206].

Immunotherapeutic Approaches to Targeting CSCs

Emerging literature clearly demonstrates that CSCs exhibit distinct gene expression profiles and express different antigens [207] Therefore, the potential of immunotherapies to specifically target multiple antigens makes them promising approaches to the targeting of heterogenous CSC populations. In a study, CSC-specific CD8$^+$ T cells were generated from human AML stem cells and these activated CD8$^+$ T cells were shown to mediate tumor retrogression in AML transplanted NOD/SCID mice [208]. In another study, CSC-specific CD8$^+$ T cells were generated *in-vitro* by using antigenic peptide from ALDH1A1 and the subsequent adoptive transfer of ALDH1A1-specific CD8$^+$ T cells eliminated ALDH1A1 specific CSCs in xenografts of head and neck squamous cell carcinoma [209, 210]. However, this adoptive immunotherapy approach may lead to resistance as CSCs can evolve strategies to escape the T-cell-mediated attack. CSC from colorectal cancer patients shows weak immunogenicity and higher expression levels of IL-4, resulting in the neutralization of cytotoxic T cells [211]. Another major problem with targeting CSCs with CSC-specific T cells is the clonal evolution of CSC subpopulation that in turn leads to antigen loss and expression of the new antigen. One way to mitigate against antigen loss variants may be the use of professional antigen-presenting cells, such as dendritic cells (DCs) in a CSC-based vaccine approach. CSC-DC vaccine confers significant antitumor immunity in various syngeneic immunocompetent mouse tumor models in comparison to immunization with bulk tumor cells. In this connection, Ning *et al.* demonstrated that ALDH$^+$ primed DC vaccination was significantly more effective at preventing lung metastasis and subcutaneous tumor growth compared to ALDH$^-$ DC vaccination [212]. Furthermore, increasing evidence suggest that CSC based DC vaccination may have an important role in targeting the micrometastatic disease. In the murine mouse tumor model, treatment of primary tumor by radiation therapy alone increased the percentage of CSCs, whereas mice treated with a combination of radiation therapy and CSC-DC vaccine resulted in a significant decrease of CSCs in primary tumors and a reduction in spontaneous metastatic disease [213]. In antigen-specific immunotherapy, DCs have been successfully generated *ex vivo*, loaded with different kinds of cancer antigens and then injected into patients [214]. Clinical studies have shown that DC-based vaccines are safe and can trigger the expansion of circulating CD4$^+$ and CD8$^+$ T cells that are specific for a tumor antigen. Currently, Phase II and Phase III clinical trials are in progress that utilizes a proteome based screen of peripheral blood of cancer patients to develop personalized CSC specific DC vaccination in glioblastoma and brain metastasis from primary tumor sites (NCT01782287, NCT01782274, NCT01759810).

Targeting CSC Metabolism

In normal non transformed cells which are mainly slowly proliferating or quiescent cells, mitochondria are the major subcellular organelle that produces principle source of energy ATP through tricarboxylic acid cycle (TCA) associated with oxidative phosphorylation (OXPHOS). However, highly proliferating cancer cells adapt their cellular metabolism utilizing less efficient glycolysis rather than OXPHOS for energy production to cope with their needs during tumor growth: rapid division and growth rate, rapid ATP production to maintain energy status, enhanced biosynthesis of macromolecules including nucleic acids, lipids and amino acids and stringent regulation of the cellular redox status. In contrast to highly proliferating differentiated bulk tumor cells that rely primarily on glycolysis for energy production, CSCs show a distinct metabolic phenotype that can be either highly glycolytic or OXPHOS based on the tumor type [215]. Increasing evidences suggest that CSCs undergo metabolic reprogramming including mitochondrial respiration and glycolysis in response to microenvironmental signals and genetic background to cater the process of CSC transformation or support the biological processes that facilitate tumor progression [216]. In induced pluripotent stem cells (iIPS), the stem cell reprogramming process has been shown to be associated with metabolic change from OXPHOS to glycolytic programme and this metabolic switching is essential for effective acquisition of pluripotent state. These findings suggest that glycolytic reprogramming and stemness are intricately linked, thereby, revealing the importance of cellular metabolism in regulation of stemness phenotype. Various studies have supported the hypothesis that CSCs are more glycolytic than normal cancer cells. Glucose is an essential metabolite for CSCs like that of normal stem cells that enhances the number of cancer stem cells in cancer cell population. Glucose is known to induce expression of specific genes linked to glucose metabolism pathway (c-Myc, HK-1, HK-2, GLUT-1 and PDK-1) in CSCs that contributes to increase in CSC population [217]. Moreover, the CSC population tends to decline in response to deprivation of glucose or inhibition of glycolysis. Small cell population with stem cell like phenotype from breast cancer, glioblastoma, ovarian cancer, lung cancer and colon cancer were found to rely more on glycolysis than the bulk of differentiated tumor progeny [218⁻220]. CSCs show enhanced glucose uptake, glycolytic enzyme expression, lactate production and ATP content in comparison to non CSCs suggesting importance of glycolytic metabolic reprogramming in CSC maintenance and cancer progression.

Furthermore, several studies have demonstrated that CSCs utilize OXPHOS as preferred process for energy production. Recent evidence has shown that quiescent slow-cycling CSCs in various cancer types including pancreatic ductal adenocarcinoma (PDAC), glioblastoma, lung cancer, breast cancer and hepatocellular carcinoma are less glycolytic and were found to higher ATP concentration in comparison to their differentiated highly proliferating cancer progeny cells and mitochondria function has been found to be critical in regulation of stemness properities of CSCs [221ˉ223]. Therefore, exploring the role of CSC metabolism and the mechanism of the CSCs metabolic plasticity in carcinogenesis has become a major focus in current cancer research and extensive efforts are being made to design effective therapies specifically targeting CSCs metabolic phenotype in clinical setting. Glycolytic enzymes or glucose transporters (lactate dehydrogenase, Pyruvate kinase M2, Hexokinase1-2 and GLUT-2) are considered as major targets for inhibition of glycolysis metabolism. Adaptive metabolic response of CSCs is also a potential target for CSC based cancer therapy. CSCs are known to undergo rapid metabolic transition in response to microenvironmental changes that plays a crucial role in metastasis and resistance. In addition, OXPHOS dependent CSCs can be targeted by impairing mitochondrial energy metabolism.

Targeting Key Signal Pathways

Dysregulation of signaling pathway networks plays an important role in enabling CSCs to resist cancer treatment and to retain their characteristic features. The new treatment strategies targeting key signaling pathways that are involved in the regulation of self-renewal and differentiation of CSCs are under development (Fig. 4). In the Notch signaling pathway two major classes of inhibitors are currently in clinical development: γ-secretase complex inhibitor (GSIs) and monoclonal antibodies against Notch receptors or ligands. In preclinical studies, GSIs when used in combination therapy abated relapse and have demonstrated significant anti-CSC activity in *ex-vivo* derived tumor specimens and breast cancer-derived secondary mammospheres [224]. The early clinical trial data of GSIs showed promising results [225]. For instance, in Phase I clinical trials, gamma-secretase inhibitor BMS-906024 reduced bone marrow blast percentage by 50% in 32% of patients with relapsed T-cell Acute Lymphoblastic Leukemia [226]. However, due to drug-related toxicities, the clinical development of GSIs was hampered. Therapeutic targeting of DLL4, a Notch ligand, has demonstrated good safety and efficacy in preclinical and clinical development. MEDI10639, an anti-DLL4 humanized monoclonal antibody, showed significant reduction of tumor CSCs in preclinical studies. In a phase 1 clinical trial of small-cell lung cancer, MEDI10639 treatment reduced tumor CSC count by 50% in 3 out of 8 patients as well as decreased expression of CSC genes in 3 out of 7 patients (NCT01577745) [227]. Recently the development of OMP-59R5 (tarextumab), anti-Notch2/3 antibody, was reported which alone or together with chemotherapeutic drugs was efficacious in broad spectrum of epithelial cancers [228]. Currently, a large number of inhibitors targeting Hh pathway are under clinical development. Vismodegib, an inhibitor of SMO, is the most clinically advanced Hh targeted therapy which has been approved by FDA for the treatment of locally advanced or metastatic basal cell carcinoma [5]. Inhibitors of targeting Wnt/β-catenin signaling cascade include small molecule inhibitors and biological inhibitors. In clinical studies OMP-18R5, an inhibitor of Frizzled receptor, has shown interesting anti-CSC activity in several advanced tumors [229]. In glioblastoma preclinical models, targeted therapy against STAT3 was shown to reduce the number of glioblastoma brain stem cells [230]. WP1066, a STAT3 inhibitor, is currently undergoing Phase I clinical trial in patients with recurrent malignant glioma or progressive brain metastasis from melanoma (NCT01904123). FAK inhibition has shown promising results in preclinical/ early clinical studies and currently clinical trials are investigating combination therapy for FAK inhibitors. Defacitinib, small molecule FAK inhibitor, has completed Phase I clinical trials in over 300 patients with advanced solid tumors and has shown that the therapy is well tolerated with low adverse effects (NCT02546531) [231]. The preclinical work and the phase I study have led to Phase II clinical trial combining neo adjuvant and adjuvant chemotherapeutic treatment using Pembrolizumab with or without Defacitinib in patients with high risk resectable PDAC (NCT03727880).

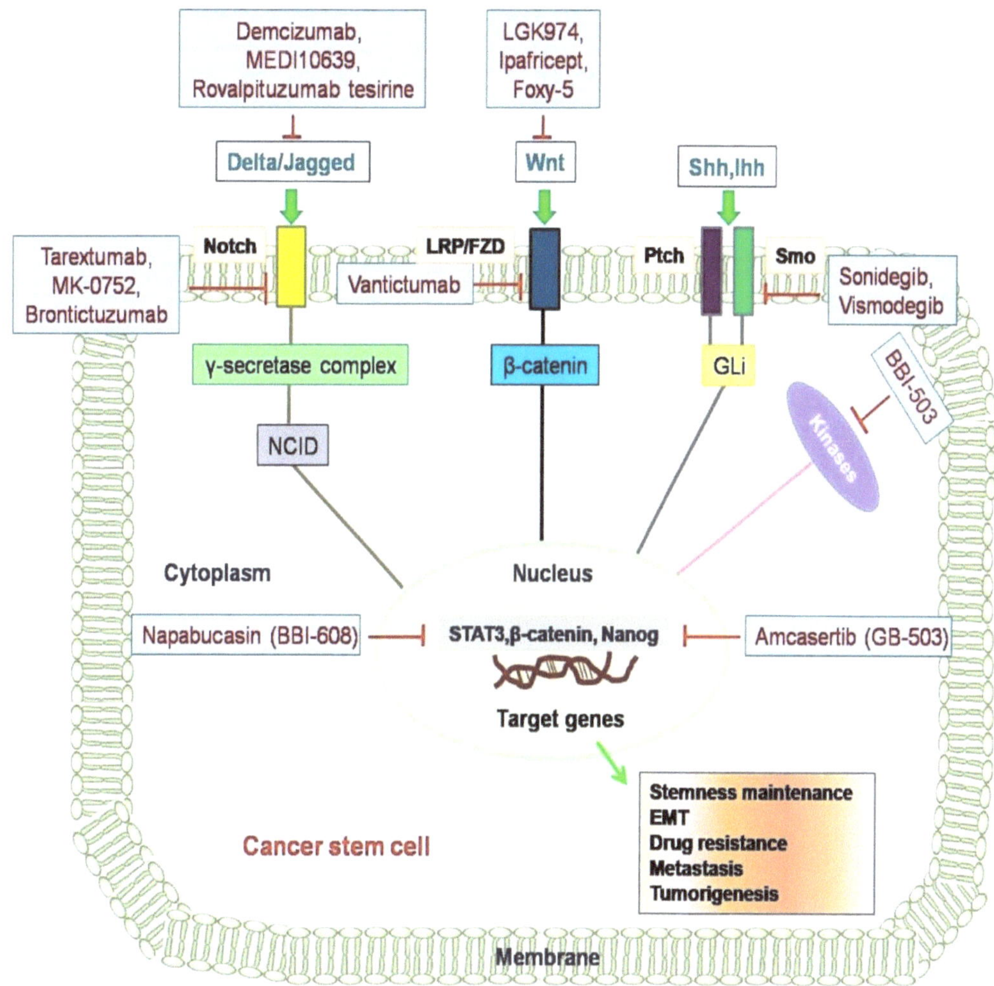

Fig. (4))

Emerging drugs targeting stemness signaling cascades in cancer stem cells.

CONCLUSION AND PERSPECTIVES

Emerging evidence suggests that CSCs are the root cause of cancers and are primarily responsible for cancer therapy failure due to their resistance to current conventional therapeutics, leading to recurrence and metastasis [6]. Therefore, in order to circumvent the limitations of traditional therapies, it is imperative to target CSC selectively. Moreover, in recent times CSC based targeted therapies have shown promising results in clinical research. The cell surface biomarkers have been of great interest in CSC-based drug targeting. However, the lack of specificity and instability restricts the applicability of this strategy to target CSC of specific phenotype only. Despite the fact that various strategies are being investigated to target CSC in preclinical and clinical studies, however, most of these strategies have been worked out only in preclinical settings, and none of them has passed the clinical trials due to non-specificity and toxicity related issues. Thus, further understanding of CSC biology and related mechanisms can pave the way towards development of novel and specific CSC targeting strategies or redesigning of currently existing strategies for efficient targeting of CSC without affecting their normal counter parts.

AUTHOR CONTRIBUTIONS

RA conceptualized the manuscript, carried out the literature review and wrote the manuscript. HM carried out the literature review and wrote a section of manuscript. RA, HM and SSB prepared Figures and table included in manuscript. RH and FAK supervised the writing and edited the manuscript.

CONSENT FOR PUBLICATION

Not Applicable.

CONFLICT OF INTEREST

The authors declare no conflict of interest, financial or otherwise.

ACKNOWLEDGEMENTS

Research funding provided by Council of Scientific & Industrial Research (CSIR), India (No. 09/251(0086)/2017-EMR-I) to Roshia Ali is highly acknowledged.

REFERENCES

[1]   Bray F, Ferlay J, Soerjomataram I, Siegel RL, Torre LA, Jemal A. Global cancer statistics 2018: GLOBOCAN estimates of incidence and mortality worldwide for 36 cancers in 185 countries. CA Cancer J Clin 2018; 68(6): 394-424.[http://dx.doi.org/10.3322/caac.21492] [PMID: 30207593]

[2]   Schatton T, Murphy GF, Frank NY, et al. Identification of cells initiating human melanomas. Nature 2008; 451(7176): 345-9.[http://dx.doi.org/10.1038/nature06489] [PMID: 18202660]

[3]   Escoll M, Gargini R, Cuadrado A, Anton IM, Wandosell F. Mutant p53 oncogenic functions in cancer stem cells are regulated by WIP through YAP/TAZ. Oncogene 2017; 36(25): 3515-27.[http://dx.doi.org/10.1038/onc.2016.518] [PMID: 28166194]

[4]   White AC, Lowry WE. Refining the role for adult stem cells as cancer cells of origin. Trends Cell Biol 2015; 25(1): 11-20.[http://dx.doi.org/10.1016/j.tcb.2014.08.008] [PMID: 25242116]

[5]   Takebe N, Miele L, Harris PJ, et al. Targeting Notch, Hedgehog, and Wnt pathways in cancer stem cells:

clinical update. Nat Rev Clin Oncol 2015; 12(8): 445-64.[http://dx.doi.org/10.1038/nrclinonc.2015.61] [PMID: 25850553]

[6]   Vinogradov S, Wei X. Cancer stem cells and drug resistance: the potential of nanomedicine. Nanomedicine (Lond) 2012; 7(4): 597-615.[http://dx.doi.org/10.2217/nnm.12.22] [PMID: 22471722]

[7]   Bao S, Wu Q, Li Z, *et al.* Targeting cancer stem cells through L1CAM suppresses glioma growth. Cancer Res 2008; 68(15): 6043-8.[http://dx.doi.org/10.1158/0008-5472.CAN-08-1079] [PMID: 18676824]

[8]   Zakrzewski W, Dobrzyński M, Szymonowicz M, Rybak Z. Stem cells: past, present, and future. Stem Cell Res Ther 2019; 10(1): 68.[http://dx.doi.org/10.1186/s13287-019-1165-5] [PMID: 30808416]

[9]   Mountford JC. Human embryonic stem cells: origins, characteristics and potential for regenerative therapy. Transfus Med 2008; 18(1): 1-12.[http://dx.doi.org/10.1111/j.1365-3148.2007.00807.x] [PMID: 18279188]

[10] Péault B, Rudnicki M, Torrente Y, *et al.* Stem and progenitor cells in skeletal muscle development, maintenance, and therapy. Mol Ther 2007; 15(5): 867-77.[http://dx.doi.org/10.1038/mt.sj.6300145] [PMID: 17387336]

[11] Beltrami AP, Barlucchi L, Torella D, *et al.* Adult cardiac stem cells are multipotent and support myocardial regeneration. Cell 2003; 114(6): 763-76.[http://dx.doi.org/10.1016/S0092-8674(03)00687-1] [PMID: 14505575]

[12] Zon LI. Intrinsic and extrinsic control of haematopoietic stem-cell self-renewal. Nature 2008; 453(7193): 306-13.[http://dx.doi.org/10.1038/nature07038] [PMID: 18480811]

[13] Shenghui H, Nakada D, Morrison SJ. Mechanisms of stem cell self-renewal. Annual Review of cell and Developmental 2009; 25: 377-406.[http://dx.doi.org/10.1146/annurev.cellbio.042308.113248]

[14] Molofsky AV, Pardal R, Morrison SJ. Diverse mechanisms regulate stem cell self-renewal. Curr Opin Cell Biol 2004; 16(6): 700-7.[http://dx.doi.org/10.1016/j.ceb.2004.09.004] [PMID: 15530784]

[15] Galan-Caridad JM, Harel S, Arenzana TL, *et al.* Zfx controls the self-renewal of embryonic and hematopoietic stem cells. Cell 2007; 129(2): 345-57.[http://dx.doi.org/10.1016/j.cell.2007.03.014] [PMID: 17448993]

[16] Fang D, Nguyen TK, Leishear K, *et al.* A tumorigenic subpopulation with stem cell properties in melanomas. Cancer Res 2005; 65(20): 9328-37.[http://dx.doi.org/10.1158/0008-5472.CAN-05-1343] [PMID: 16230395]

[17] Piccirillo SG, Reynolds BA, Zanetti N, *et al.* Bone morphogenetic proteins inhibit the tumorigenic potential of human brain tumour-initiating cells. Nature 2006; 444(7120): 761-5.[http://dx.doi.org/10.1038/nature05349] [PMID: 17151667]

[18] Szotek PP, Pieretti-Vanmarcke R, Masiakos PT, *et al.* Ovarian cancer side population defines cells with stem cell-like characteristics and Mullerian Inhibiting Substance responsiveness. Proc Natl Acad Sci USA 2006; 103(30): 11154-9.[http://dx.doi.org/10.1073/pnas.0603672103] [PMID: 16849428]

[19] Collins AT, Berry PA, Hyde C, Stower MJ, Maitland NJ. Prospective identification of tumorigenic prostate cancer stem cells. Cancer Res 2005; 65(23): 10946-51.[http://dx.doi.org/10.1158/0008-5472.CAN-05-2018] [PMID: 16322242]

[20] O'Brien CA, Pollett A, Gallinger S, Dick JE. A human colon cancer cell capable of initiating tumour growth in immunodeficient mice. Nature 2007; 445(7123): 106-10.[http://dx.doi.org/10.1038/nature05372] [PMID: 17122772]

[21] Al-Hajj M, Wicha MS, Benito-Hernandez A, Morrison SJ, Clarke MF. Prospective identification of tumorigenic breast cancer cells. Proc Natl Acad Sci USA 2003; 100(7): 3983-8.[http://dx.doi.org/10.1073/pnas.0530291100] [PMID: 12629218]

[22] Wang D, Plukker JTM, Coppes R. Cancer stem cells with increased metastatic potential as a therapeutic target for esophageal cancer. Seminars in cancer biology 2017.[http://dx.doi.org/10.1016/j.semcancer.2017.03.010]

[23] Mao J, Fan S, Ma W, *et al.* Roles of Wnt/β-catenin signaling in the gastric cancer stem cells proliferation and salinomycin treatment. Cell Death Dis 2014; 5(1): e1039-9.[http://dx.doi.org/10.1038/cddis.2013.515] [PMID: 24481453]

[24] Lee Y, Lee JK, Ahn SH, Lee J, Nam DH. WNT signaling in glioblastoma and therapeutic opportunities. Lab Invest 2016; 96(2): 137-50.[http://dx.doi.org/10.1038/labinvest.2015.140] [PMID: 26641068]

[25] Chen S, Fisher RC, Signs S, *et al.* Inhibition of PI3K/Akt/mTOR signaling in PI3KR2-overexpressing colon cancer stem cells reduces tumor growth due to apoptosis. Oncotarget 2016; 8(31): 50476-88.[http://dx.doi.org/10.18632/oncotarget.9919] [PMID: 28881576]

[26] Wang X, Wang C, Zhang X, *et al.* Bmi-1 regulates stem cell-like properties of gastric cancer cells *via* modulating miRNAs. J Hematol Oncol 2016; 9(1): 90.[http://dx.doi.org/10.1186/s13045-016-0323-9]

[PMID: 27644439]

[27] Aljedai A, Buckle AM, Hiwarkar P, Syed F. Potential role of Notch signalling in CD34+ chronic myeloid leukaemia cells: cross-talk between Notch and BCR-ABL. PLoS One 2015; 10(4)e0123016[http://dx.doi.org/10.1371/journal.pone.0123016] [PMID: 25849484]

[28] Chaffer CL, Brueckmann I, Scheel C, et al. Normal and neoplastic nonstem cells can spontaneously convert to a stem-like state. Proc Natl Acad Sci USA 2011; 108(19): 7950-5.[http://dx.doi.org/10.1073/pnas.1102454108] [PMID: 21498687]

[29] Cabrera MC, Hollingsworth RE, Hurt EM. Cancer stem cell plasticity and tumor hierarchy. World J Stem Cells 2015; 7(1): 27-36.[http://dx.doi.org/10.4252/wjsc.v7.i1.27] [PMID: 25621103]

[30] Borovski T, De Sousa E Melo F, Vermeulen L, Medema JP. Cancer stem cell niche: the place to be. Cancer Res 2011; 71(3): 634-9.[http://dx.doi.org/10.1158/0008-5472.CAN-10-3220] [PMID: 21266356]

[31] Plaks V, Kong N, Werb Z. The cancer stem cell niche: how essential is the niche in regulating stemness of tumor cells? Cell Stem Cell 2015; 16(3): 225-38.[http://dx.doi.org/10.1016/j.stem.2015.02.015] [PMID: 25748930]

[32] Moore N, Lyle S. Quiescent, slow-cycling stem cell populations in cancer: a review of the evidence and discussion of significance 2011.[http://dx.doi.org/10.1155/2011/396076]

[33] Chen W. Cancer stem cell quiescence and plasticity as major challenges in cancer therapy. Stem cells international 2016; 2016

[34] Koch U, Krause M, Baumann M. Cancer stem cells at the crossroads of current cancer therapy failures—radiation oncology perspective.Seminars in cancer biology 2010.[http://dx.doi.org/10.1016/j.semcancer.2010.02.003]

[35] Wainwright EN, Scaffidi P. Epigenetics and cancer stem cells: unleashing, hijacking, and restricting cellular plasticity. Trends Cancer 2017; 3(5): 372-86.[http://dx.doi.org/10.1016/j.trecan.2017.04.004] [PMID: 28718414]

[36] Jiang Y, He Y, Li H, et al. Expressions of putative cancer stem cell markers ABCB1, ABCG2, and CD133 are correlated with the degree of differentiation of gastric cancer. Gastric Cancer 2012; 15(4): 440-50.[http://dx.doi.org/10.1007/s10120-012-0140-y] [PMID: 22395309]

[37] Xie Z-Y, Lv K, Xiong Y, Guo WH. ABCG2-mediated multidrug resistance and tumor-initiating capacity of side population cells from colon cancer. Oncol Res Treat 2014; 37(11): 666-668, 670-672.[http://dx.doi.org/10.1159/000368842] [PMID: 25427584]

[38] Yanger K, Zong Y, Maggs LR, et al. Robust cellular reprogramming occurs spontaneously during liver regeneration. Genes Dev 2013; 27(7): 719-24.[http://dx.doi.org/10.1101/gad.207803.112] [PMID: 23520387]

[39] Yimlamai D, Christodoulou C, Galli GG, et al. Hippo pathway activity influences liver cell fate. Cell 2014; 157(6): 1324-38.[http://dx.doi.org/10.1016/j.cell.2014.03.060] [PMID: 24906150]

[40] Iliopoulos D, Hirsch HA, Wang G, Struhl K. Inducible formation of breast cancer stem cells and their dynamic equilibrium with non-stem cancer cells via IL6 secretion. Proc Natl Acad Sci USA 2011; 108(4): 1397-402.[http://dx.doi.org/10.1073/pnas.1018898108] [PMID: 21220315]

[41] Lau EYT, Ho NPY, Lee TKW. Cancer stem cells and their microenvironment. biology and therapeutic implications. Stem Cells International 2017; 2017[http://dx.doi.org/10.1155/2017/3714190]

[42] Grivennikov SI, Greten FR, Karin M. Immunity, inflammation, and cancer. Cell 2010; 140(6): 883-99.[http://dx.doi.org/10.1016/j.cell.2010.01.025] [PMID: 20303878]

[43] Hanahan D, Weinberg RA. Hallmarks of cancer: the next generation. cell 2011; 144(5): 646-74.[http://dx.doi.org/10.1016/j.cell.2011.02.013]

[44] Liu T. NF-κB signaling in inflammation. Signal Transduct Target Ther 2017; 2(1): 1-9.[http://dx.doi.org/10.1038/sigtrans.2017.23]

[45] Kortylewski M, Xin H, Kujawski M, et al. Regulation of the IL-23 and IL-12 balance by Stat3 signaling in the tumor microenvironment. Cancer Cell 2009; 15(2): 114-23.[http://dx.doi.org/10.1016/j.ccr.2008.12.018] [PMID: 19185846]

[46] Yan GN, Yang L, Lv YF, et al. Endothelial cells promote stem-like phenotype of glioma cells through activating the Hedgehog pathway. J Pathol 2014; 234(1): 11-22.[http://dx.doi.org/10.1002/path.4349] [PMID: 24604164]

[47] Charles N, Ozawa T, Squatrito M, et al. Perivascular nitric oxide activates notch signaling and promotes stem-like character in PDGF-induced glioma cells. Cell Stem Cell 2010; 6(2): 141-52.[http://dx.doi.org/10.1016/j.stem.2010.01.001] [PMID: 20144787]

[48] Jögi A, Øra I, Nilsson H, et al. Hypoxia alters gene expression in human neuroblastoma cells toward an

immature and neural crest-like phenotype. Proc Natl Acad Sci USA 2002; 99(10): 7021-6.[http://dx.doi.org/10.1073/pnas.102660199] [PMID: 12011461]

[49] Xing F, Okuda H, Watabe M, *et al.* Hypoxia-induced Jagged2 promotes breast cancer metastasis and self-renewal of cancer stem-like cells. Oncogene 2011; 30(39): 4075-86.[http://dx.doi.org/10.1038/onc.2011.122] [PMID: 21499308]

[50] Easwaran H, Johnstone SE, Van Neste L, *et al.* A DNA hypermethylation module for the stem/progenitor cell signature of cancer. Genome Res 2012; 22(5): 837-49.[http://dx.doi.org/10.1101/gr.131169.111] [PMID: 22391556]

[51] Patra SK, Deb M, Patra A. Molecular marks for epigenetic identification of developmental and cancer stem cells. Clin Epigenetics 2011; 2(1): 27-53.[http://dx.doi.org/10.1007/s13148-010-0016-0] [PMID: 22704268]

[52] Rizzo S, Hersey JM, Mellor P, *et al.* Ovarian cancer stem cell-like side populations are enriched following chemotherapy and overexpress EZH2. Mol Cancer Ther 2011; 10(2): 325-35.[http://dx.doi.org/10.1158/1535-7163.MCT-10-0788] [PMID: 21216927]

[53] Reya T. Stem cells, cancer, and cancer stem cells. nature 2001; 414(6859): 105-11.

[54] Oh M, Nör JE. The perivascular niche and self-renewal of stem cells. Front Physiol 2015; 6: 367.[http://dx.doi.org/10.3389/fphys.2015.00367] [PMID: 26696901]

[55] Bétous R, Renoud ML, Hoede C, *et al.* Human adipose-derived stem cells expanded under ambient oxygen concentration accumulate oxidative DNA lesions and experience procarcinogenic DNA replication stress. Stem Cells Transl Med 2017; 6(1): 68-76.[http://dx.doi.org/10.5966/sctm.2015-0401] [PMID: 28170194]

[56] Tomasetti C, Vogelstein B. Cancer etiology. Variation in cancer risk among tissues can be explained by the number of stem cell divisions. Science 2015; 347(6217): 78-81.[http://dx.doi.org/10.1126/science.1260825] [PMID: 25554788]

[57] Kucia M, Reca R, Campbell FR, *et al.* A population of very small embryonic-like (VSEL) CXCR4(+)SSEA-1(+)Oct-4+ stem cells identified in adult bone marrow. Leukemia 2006; 20(5): 857-69.[http://dx.doi.org/10.1038/sj.leu.2404171] [PMID: 16498386]

[58] Chang Y-J, Tien KE, Wen CH, Hsieh TB, Hwang SM. Recovery of CD45(-)/Lin(-)/SSEA-4(+) very small embryonic-like stem cells by cord blood bank standard operating procedures. Cytotherapy 2014; 16(4): 560-5.[http://dx.doi.org/10.1016/j.jcyt.2013.10.009] [PMID: 24364909]

[59] Ratajczak MZ, Ratajczak J, Suszynska M, Miller DM, Kucia M, Shin DM. A novel view of the adult stem cell compartment from the perspective of a quiescent population of very small embryonic-like stem cells. Circ Res 2017; 120(1): 166-78.[http://dx.doi.org/10.1161/CIRCRESAHA.116.309362] [PMID: 28057792]

[60] Batlle E, Clevers H. Cancer stem cells revisited. Nat Med 2017; 23(10): 1124-34.[http://dx.doi.org/10.1038/nm.4409] [PMID: 28985214]

[61] Fessler E, Dijkgraaf FE, De Sousa E Melo F, Medema JP. Cancer stem cell dynamics in tumor progression and metastasis: is the microenvironment to blame? Cancer Lett 2013; 341(1): 97-104.[http://dx.doi.org/10.1016/j.canlet.2012.10.015] [PMID: 23089245]

[62] Kreso A, Dick JE. Evolution of the cancer stem cell model. Cell Stem Cell 2014; 14(3): 275-91.[http://dx.doi.org/10.1016/j.stem.2014.02.006] [PMID: 24607403]

[63] Mercurio AM. VEGF/neuropilin signaling in cancer stem cells. Int J Mol Sci 2019; 20(3): 490.[http://dx.doi.org/10.3390/ijms20030490] [PMID: 30678134]

[64] Quail DF, Joyce JA. Microenvironmental regulation of tumor progression and metastasis. Nat Med 2013; 19(11): 1423-37.[http://dx.doi.org/10.1038/nm.3394] [PMID: 24202395]

[65] Hanahan D, Coussens LM. Accessories to the crime: functions of cells recruited to the tumor microenvironment. Cancer Cell 2012; 21(3): 309-22.[http://dx.doi.org/10.1016/j.ccr.2012.02.022] [PMID: 22439926]

[66] Heddleston JM, Li Z, McLendon RE, Hjelmeland AB, Rich JN. The hypoxic microenvironment maintains glioblastoma stem cells and promotes reprogramming towards a cancer stem cell phenotype. Cell Cycle 2009; 8(20): 3274-84.[http://dx.doi.org/10.4161/cc.8.20.9701] [PMID: 19770585]

[67] Méndez O, Zavadil J, Esencay M, *et al.* Knock down of HIF-1α in glioma cells reduces migration *in vitro* and invasion *in vivo* and impairs their ability to form tumor spheres. Mol Cancer 2010; 9(1): 133.[http://dx.doi.org/10.1186/1476-4598-9-133] [PMID: 20515450]

[68] Chung The H, Karkey A, Pham Thanh D, *et al.* A high-resolution genomic analysis of multidrug-resistant hospital outbreaks of Klebsiella pneumoniae. EMBO Mol Med 2015; 7(3): 227-39.[http://dx.doi.org/10.15252/emmm.201404767] [PMID: 25712531]

[69] Subbiah V, Meyer C, Zinner R, *et al.* Phase Ib/II study of the safety and efficacy of combination therapy with

multikinase VEGF inhibitor pazopanib and MEK inhibitor trametinib in advanced soft tissue sarcoma. Clin Cancer Res 2017; 23(15): 4027-34.[http://dx.doi.org/10.1158/1078-0432.CCR-17-0272] [PMID: 28377484]

[70] Cao Z, Scandura JM, Inghirami GG, Shido K, Ding BS, Rafii S. Molecular checkpoint decisions made by subverted vascular niche transform indolent tumor cells into chemoresistant cancer stem cells. Cancer Cell 2017; 31(1): 110-26.[http://dx.doi.org/10.1016/j.ccell.2016.11.010] [PMID: 27989801]

[71] Krishnamurthy S, Warner KA, Dong Z, *et al.* Endothelial interleukin-6 defines the tumorigenic potential of primary human cancer stem cells. Stem Cells 2014; 32(11): 2845-57.[http://dx.doi.org/10.1002/stem.1793] [PMID: 25078284]

[72] Wang Y, Wang Y, Chen H, Liang Q. Endothelial cells promote formation of medulloblastoma stem-like cells *via* Notch pathway activation. J Mol Neurosci 2017; 63(2): 152-8.[http://dx.doi.org/10.1007/s12031-017-0965-2] [PMID: 28856557]

[73] Peñarando J, López-Sánchez LM, Mena R, *et al.* A role for endothelial nitric oxide synthase in intestinal stem cell proliferation and mesenchymal colorectal cancer. BMC Biol 2018; 16(1): 3.[http://dx.doi.org/10.1186/s12915-017-0472-5] [PMID: 29329541]

[74] Ziani L, Chouaib S, Thiery J. Alteration of the antitumor immune response by cancer-associated fibroblasts. Front Immunol 2018; 9: 414.[http://dx.doi.org/10.3389/fimmu.2018.00414] [PMID: 29545811]

[75] Feig C, Jones JO, Kraman M, *et al.* Targeting CXCL12 from FAP-expressing carcinoma-associated fibroblasts synergizes with anti-PD-L1 immunotherapy in pancreatic cancer. Proc Natl Acad Sci USA 2013; 110(50): 20212-7.[http://dx.doi.org/10.1073/pnas.1320318110] [PMID: 24277834]

[76] Vermeulen L, De Sousa E Melo F, van der Heijden M, *et al.* Wnt activity defines colon cancer stem cells and is regulated by the microenvironment. Nat Cell Biol 2010; 12(5): 468-76.[http://dx.doi.org/10.1038/ncb2048] [PMID: 20418870]

[77] Xiong S, Wang R, Chen Q, *et al.* Cancer-associated fibroblasts promote stem cell-like properties of hepatocellular carcinoma cells through IL-6/STAT3/Notch signaling. Am J Cancer Res 2018; 8(2): 302-16.[PMID: 29511600]

[78] Su S. CD10+ GPR77+ cancer-associated fibroblasts promote cancer formation and chemoresistance by sustaining cancer stemness. Cell 2018; 172(4): 841-56.

[79] Cuiffo BG, Karnoub AE. Mesenchymal stem cells in tumor development: emerging roles and concepts. Cell Adhes Migr 2012; 6(3): 220-30.[http://dx.doi.org/10.4161/cam.20875] [PMID: 22863739]

[80] Nishimura K, Semba S, Aoyagi K, Sasaki H, Yokozaki H. Mesenchymal stem cells provide an advantageous tumor microenvironment for the restoration of cancer stem cells. Pathobiology 2012; 79(6): 290-306.[http://dx.doi.org/10.1159/000337296] [PMID: 22688186]

[81] Davis H, Irshad S, Bansal M, *et al.* Aberrant epithelial GREM1 expression initiates colonic tumorigenesis from cells outside the stem cell niche. Nat Med 2015; 21(1): 62-70.[http://dx.doi.org/10.1038/nm.3750] [PMID: 25419707]

[82] Rhodes LV, Antoon JW, Muir SE, Elliott S, Beckman BS, Burow ME. Effects of human mesenchymal stem cells on ER-positive human breast carcinoma cells mediated through ER-SDF-1/CXCR4 crosstalk. Mol Cancer 2010; 9(1): 295.[http://dx.doi.org/10.1186/1476-4598-9-295] [PMID: 21087507]

[83] Halpern JL, Kilbarger A, Lynch CC. Mesenchymal stem cells promote mammary cancer cell migration *in vitro via* the CXCR2 receptor. Cancer Lett 2011; 308(1): 91-9.[http://dx.doi.org/10.1016/j.canlet.2011.04.018] [PMID: 21601983]

[84] Tsai KS, Yang SH, Lei YP, *et al.* Mesenchymal stem cells promote formation of colorectal tumors in mice. Gastroenterology 2011; 141(3): 1046-56.[http://dx.doi.org/10.1053/j.gastro.2011.05.045] [PMID: 21699785]

[85] Liu S, Ginestier C, Ou SJ, *et al.* Breast cancer stem cells are regulated by mesenchymal stem cells through cytokine networks. Cancer Res 2011; 71(2): 614-24.[http://dx.doi.org/10.1158/0008-5472.CAN-10-0538] [PMID: 21224357]

[86] Cabarcas SM, Mathews LA, Farrar WL. The cancer stem cell niche--there goes the neighborhood? Int J Cancer 2011; 129(10): 2315-27.[http://dx.doi.org/10.1002/ijc.26312] [PMID: 21792897]

[87] Yan XL, Fu CJ, Chen L, *et al.* Mesenchymal stem cells from primary breast cancer tissue promote cancer proliferation and enhance mammosphere formation partially *via* EGF/EGFR/Akt pathway. Breast Cancer Res Treat 2012; 132(1): 153-64.[http://dx.doi.org/10.1007/s10549-011-1577-0] [PMID: 21584665]

[88] Nywening TM, Belt BA, Cullinan DR, *et al.* Targeting both tumour-associated CXCR2[+] neutrophils and CCR2[+] macrophages disrupts myeloid recruitment and improves chemotherapeutic responses in pancreatic ductal adenocarcinoma. Gut 2018; 67(6): 1112-23.[http://dx.doi.org/10.1136/gutjnl-2017-313738] [PMID: 29196437]

[89]   Sainz B. Cancer stem cells and macrophages: implications in tumor biology and therapeutic strategies. Mediators of inflammation 2016; 2016

[90]   Castro-Vega LJ, Jouravleva K, Ortiz-Montero P, *et al.* The senescent microenvironment promotes the emergence of heterogeneous cancer stem-like cells. Carcinogenesis 2015; 36(10): 1180-92.[http://dx.doi.org/10.1093/carcin/bgv101] [PMID: 26168819]

[91]   Treps L, Perret R, Edmond S, Ricard D, Gavard J. Glioblastoma stem-like cells secrete the pro-angiogenic VEGF-A factor in extracellular vesicles. J Extracell Vesicles 2017; 6(1)1359479[http://dx.doi.org/10.1080/20013078.2017.1359479] [PMID: 28815003]

[92]   Sun X, Ma X, Wang J, *et al.* Glioma stem cells-derived exosomes promote the angiogenic ability of endothelial cells through miR-21/VEGF signal. Oncotarget 2017; 8(22): 36137-48.[http://dx.doi.org/10.18632/oncotarget.16661] [PMID: 28410224]

[93]   Domenis R, Cesselli D, Toffoletto B, *et al.* Systemic T cells immunosuppression of glioma stem cell-derived exosomes is mediated by monocytic myeloid-derived suppressor cells. PLoS One 2017; 12(1)e0169932[http://dx.doi.org/10.1371/journal.pone.0169932] [PMID: 28107450]

[94]   Nakano I. Extracellular vesicles in the biology of brain tumour stem cells–Implications for inter-cellular communication, therapy and biomarker development. Seminars in cell & developmental biology 2015.[http://dx.doi.org/10.1016/j.semcdb.2015.02.011]

[95]   Rinkenbaugh AL, Baldwin AS. The NF-κB pathway and cancer stem cells. Cells 2016; 5(2): 16.[http://dx.doi.org/10.3390/cells5020016] [PMID: 27058560]

[96]   Dandawate PR. Targeting cancer stem cells and signaling pathways by phytochemicals: Novel approach for breast cancer therapy. Seminars in cancer biology 2016.[http://dx.doi.org/10.1016/j.semcancer.2016.09.001]

[97]   Ye J, Wu D, Wu P, Chen Z, Huang J. The cancer stem cell niche: cross talk between cancer stem cells and their microenvironment. Tumour Biol 2014; 35(5): 3945-51.[http://dx.doi.org/10.1007/s13277-013-1561-x] [PMID: 24420150]

[98]   Shimoda M, Principe S, Jackson HW, *et al.* Loss of the Timp gene family is sufficient for the acquisition of the CAF-like cell state. Nat Cell Biol 2014; 16(9): 889-901.[http://dx.doi.org/10.1038/ncb3021] [PMID: 25150980]

[99]   Lapidot T, Sirard C, Vormoor J, *et al.* A cell initiating human acute myeloid leukaemia after transplantation into SCID mice. Nature 1994; 367(6464): 645-8.[http://dx.doi.org/10.1038/367645a0] [PMID: 7509044]

[100 Bonnet D, Dick JE. Human acute myeloid leukemia is organized as a hierarchy that originates from a
]   primitive hematopoietic cell. Nat Med 1997; 3(7): 730-7.[http://dx.doi.org/10.1038/nm0797-730] [PMID: 9212098]

[101 Guzman ML, Jordan CT. Considerations for targeting malignant stem cells in leukemia. Cancer Contr 2004;
]   11(2): 97-104.[http://dx.doi.org/10.1177/107327480401100216] [PMID: 15024346]

[102 Al-Hajj M, Clarke MF. Self-renewal and solid tumor stem cells. Oncogene 2004; 23(43): 7274-
]   82.[http://dx.doi.org/10.1038/sj.onc.1207947] [PMID: 15378087]

[103 Singh SK, Clarke ID, Terasaki M, *et al.* Identification of a cancer stem cell in human brain tumors. Cancer
]   Res 2003; 63(18): 5821-8.[PMID: 14522905]

[104 Li C, Heidt DG, Dalerba P, *et al.* Identification of pancreatic cancer stem cells. Cancer Res 2007; 67(3):
]   1030-7.[http://dx.doi.org/10.1158/0008-5472.CAN-06-2030] [PMID: 17283135]

[105 Curley MD, Therrien VA, Cummings CL, *et al.* CD133 expression defines a tumor initiating cell population
]   in primary human ovarian cancer. Stem Cells 2009; 27(12): 2875-83.[http://dx.doi.org/10.1002/stem.236] [PMID: 19816957]

[106 Ginestier C, Hur MH, Charafe-Jauffret E, *et al.* ALDH1 is a marker of normal and malignant human
]   mammary stem cells and a predictor of poor clinical outcome. Cell Stem Cell 2007; 1(5): 555-67.[http://dx.doi.org/10.1016/j.stem.2007.08.014] [PMID: 18371393]

[107 Yu Z, Baserga R, Chen L, Wang C, Lisanti MP, Pestell RG. microRNA, cell cycle, and human breast cancer.
]   Am J Pathol 2010; 176(3): 1058-64.[http://dx.doi.org/10.2353/ajpath.2010.090664] [PMID: 20075198]

[108 Phi LTH. Cancer stem cells (CSCs) in drug resistance and their therapeutic implications in cancer treatment.
]   Stem cells international 2018; 2018

[109 Chen K, Huang YH, Chen JL. Understanding and targeting cancer stem cells: therapeutic implications and
]   challenges. Acta Pharmacol Sin 2013; 34(6): 732-40.[http://dx.doi.org/10.1038/aps.2013.27] [PMID: 23685952]

[110 Dragu DL, Necula LG, Bleotu C, Diaconu CC, Chivu-Economescu M. Therapies targeting cancer stem cells:
]   Current trends and future challenges. World J Stem Cells 2015; 7(9): 1185-201.[PMID: 26516409]

[111 Prince ME, Sivanandan R, Kaczorowski A, *et al.* Identification of a subpopulation of cells with cancer stem
] cell properties in head and neck squamous cell carcinoma. Proc Natl Acad Sci USA 2007; 104(3): 973-
8.[http://dx.doi.org/10.1073/pnas.0610117104] [PMID: 17210912]

[112 Katsuno Y, Ehata S, Yashiro M, Yanagihara K, Hirakawa K, Miyazono K. Coordinated expression of REG4
] and aldehyde dehydrogenase 1 regulating tumourigenic capacity of diffuse-type gastric carcinoma-initiating
cells is inhibited by TGF-β. J Pathol 2012; 228(3): 391-404.[http://dx.doi.org/10.1002/path.4020] [PMID:
22430847]

[113 Yamashita T, Wang XW. Cancer stem cells in the development of liver cancer. J Clin Invest 2013; 123(5):
] 1911-8.[http://dx.doi.org/10.1172/JCI66024] [PMID: 23635789]

[114 Yang ZF, Ho DW, Ng MN, *et al.* Significance of CD90+ cancer stem cells in human liver cancer. Cancer
] Cell 2008; 13(2): 153-66.[http://dx.doi.org/10.1016/j.ccr.2008.01.013] [PMID: 18242515]

[115 Hu Y, Fu L. Targeting cancer stem cells: a new therapy to cure cancer patients. Am J Cancer Res 2012; 2(3):
] 340-56.[PMID: 22679565]

[116 Han L. Cancer stem cells: therapeutic implications and perspectives in cancer therapy. Acta Pharm Sin B
] 2013; 3(2): 65-75.[http://dx.doi.org/10.1016/j.apsb.2013.02.006]

[117 Zhang C, Li C, He F, Cai Y, Yang H. Identification of CD44+CD24+ gastric cancer stem cells. J Cancer Res
] Clin Oncol 2011; 137(11): 1679-86.[http://dx.doi.org/10.1007/s00432-011-1038-5] [PMID: 21882047]

[118 Kim CFB, Jackson EL, Woolfenden AE, *et al.* Identification of bronchioalveolar stem cells in normal lung
] and lung cancer. Cell 2005; 121(6): 823-35.[http://dx.doi.org/10.1016/j.cell.2005.03.032] [PMID: 15960971]

[119 Eramo A, Lotti F, Sette G, *et al.* Identification and expansion of the tumorigenic lung cancer stem cell
] population. Cell Death Differ 2008; 15(3): 504-14.[http://dx.doi.org/10.1038/sj.cdd.4402283] [PMID:
18049477]

[120 Du L, Wang H, He L, *et al.* CD44 is of functional importance for colorectal cancer stem cells. Clin Cancer
] Res 2008; 14(21): 6751-60.[http://dx.doi.org/10.1158/1078-0432.CCR-08-1034] [PMID: 18980968]

[121 Hermann PC, Huber SL, Herrler T, *et al.* Distinct populations of cancer stem cells determine tumor growth
] and metastatic activity in human pancreatic cancer. Cell Stem Cell 2007; 1(3): 313-
23.[http://dx.doi.org/10.1016/j.stem.2007.06.002] [PMID: 18371365]

[122 Yu F, Yao H, Zhu P, *et al.* let-7 regulates self renewal and tumorigenicity of breast cancer cells. Cell 2007;
] 131(6): 1109-23.[http://dx.doi.org/10.1016/j.cell.2007.10.054] [PMID: 18083101]

[123 Li L. Antibody against CD44s inhibits pancreatic tumor initiation and postradiation recurrence in mice.
] Gastroenterology 2014; 146(4): 1108-1118. e12.

[124 Boiko AD, Razorenova OV, van de Rijn M, *et al.* Human melanoma-initiating cells express neural crest
] nerve growth factor receptor CD271. Nature 2010; 466(7302): 133-7.[http://dx.doi.org/10.1038/nature09161]
[PMID: 20596026]

[125 Chanmee T, Ontong P, Kimata K, Itano N. Key roles of hyaluronan and its CD44 receptor in the stemness
] and survival of cancer stem cells. Front Oncol 2015; 5: 180.[http://dx.doi.org/10.3389/fonc.2015.00180]
[PMID: 26322272]

[126 Son MJ, Woolard K, Nam DH, Lee J, Fine HA. SSEA-1 is an enrichment marker for tumor-initiating cells in
] human glioblastoma. Cell Stem Cell 2009; 4(5): 440-52.[http://dx.doi.org/10.1016/j.stem.2009.03.003]
[PMID: 19427293]

[127 Singh SK. Identification of human brain tumour initiating cells. Nature 2004; 432(7015): 396-401.
]

[128 Choy W, Nagasawa DT, Trang A, Thill K, Spasic M, Yang I. CD133 as a marker for regulation and potential
] for targeted therapies in glioblastoma multiforme. Neurosurg Clin N Am 2012; 23(3): 391-
405.[http://dx.doi.org/10.1016/j.nec.2012.04.011] [PMID: 22748652]

[129 Kim W-T, Ryu CJ. Cancer stem cell surface markers on normal stem cells. BMB Rep 2017; 50(6): 285-
] 98.[http://dx.doi.org/10.5483/BMBRep.2017.50.6.039] [PMID: 28270302]

[130 Alamgeer M, Ganju V, Szczepny A, *et al.* The prognostic significance of aldehyde dehydrogenase 1A1
] (ALDH1A1) and CD133 expression in early stage non-small cell lung cancer. Thorax 2013; 68(12): 1095-
104.[http://dx.doi.org/10.1136/thoraxjnl-2012-203021] [PMID: 23878161]

[131 Horst D, Kriegl L, Engel J, Kirchner T, Jung A. Prognostic significance of the cancer stem cell markers
] CD133, CD44, and CD166 in colorectal cancer. Cancer Invest 2009; 27(8): 844-
50.[http://dx.doi.org/10.1080/07357900902744502] [PMID: 19626493]

[132 Ishigami S, Ueno S, Arigami T, *et al.* Prognostic impact of CD133 expression in gastric carcinoma.
] Anticancer Res 2010; 30(6): 2453-7.[PMID: 20651407]

[133 Xia P. *CD133* mRNA may be a suitable prognostic marker for human breast cancer. Stem Cell Investig
]   2017; 4: 87.[http://dx.doi.org/10.21037/sci.2017.10.03] [PMID: 29270413]

[134 Nomura A, Banerjee S, Chugh R, *et al.* CD133 initiates tumors, induces epithelial-mesenchymal transition
]   and   increases   metastasis   in   pancreatic   cancer.   Oncotarget   2015;   6(10):   8313-
      22.[http://dx.doi.org/10.18632/oncotarget.3228] [PMID: 25829252]

[135 Chen Y-S, Wu MJ, Huang CY, *et al.* CD133/Src axis mediates tumor initiating property and epithelial-
]   mesenchymal   transition   of   head   and   neck   cancer.   PLoS   One   2011;
      6(11)e28053[http://dx.doi.org/10.1371/journal.pone.0028053] [PMID: 22140506]

[136 Gong A, Huang S. FoxM1 and Wnt/β-catenin signaling in glioma stem cells. Cancer Res 2012; 72(22): 5658-
]   62.[http://dx.doi.org/10.1158/0008-5472.CAN-12-0953] [PMID: 23139209]

[137 Luu HH, Zhang R, Haydon RC, *et al.* Wnt/β-catenin signaling pathway as a novel cancer drug target. Curr
]   Cancer Drug Targets 2004; 4(8): 653-71.[http://dx.doi.org/10.2174/1568009043332709] [PMID: 15578921]

[138 Soner BC, Aktug H, Acikgoz E, *et al.* Induced growth inhibition, cell cycle arrest and apoptosis in
]   CD133+/CD44+ prostate cancer stem cells by flavopiridol. Int J Mol Med 2014; 34(5): 1249-
      56.[http://dx.doi.org/10.3892/ijmm.2014.1930] [PMID: 25216351]

[139 Schmalz PG, Shen MJ, Park JK. Treatment resistance mechanisms of malignant glioma tumor stem cells.
]   Cancers (Basel) 2011; 3(1): 621-35.[http://dx.doi.org/10.3390/cancers3010621] [PMID: 24212632]

[140 Schömig K, Busch G, Steppich B, *et al.* Interleukin-8 is associated with circulating CD133+ progenitor cells
]   in acute myocardial infarction. Eur Heart J 2006; 27(9): 1032-7.[http://dx.doi.org/10.1093/eurheartj/ehi761]
      [PMID: 16455670]

[141 Grosse-Gehling P, Fargeas CA, Dittfeld C, *et al.* CD133 as a biomarker for putative cancer stem cells in solid
]   tumours: limitations,   problems   and   challenges.   J   Pathol   2013;   229(3):   355-
      78.[http://dx.doi.org/10.1002/path.4086] [PMID: 22899341]

[142 Lee HJ, Choe G, Jheon S, Sung SW, Lee CT, Chung JH. CD24, a novel cancer biomarker, predicting disease-
]   free survival of non-small cell lung carcinomas: a retrospective study of prognostic factor analysis from the
      viewpoint of forthcoming (seventh) new TNM classification. J Thorac Oncol 2010; 5(5): 649-
      57.[http://dx.doi.org/10.1097/JTO.0b013e3181d5e554] [PMID: 20354454]

[143 Zheng J, Li Y, Yang J, *et al.* NDRG2 inhibits hepatocellular carcinoma adhesion, migration and invasion by
]   regulating CD24 expression. BMC Cancer 2011; 11(1): 251-, 1-9.[http://dx.doi.org/10.1186/1471-2407-11-
      251] [PMID: 21676268]

[144 Lim SC. CD24 and human carcinoma: tumor biological aspects. Biomed Pharmacother 2005; 59 (Suppl. 2):
]   S351-4.[http://dx.doi.org/10.1016/S0753-3322(05)80076-9] [PMID: 16507407]

[145 Kristiansen G, Winzer KJ, Mayordomo E, *et al.* CD24 expression is a new prognostic marker in breast
]   cancer. Clin Cancer Res 2003; 9(13): 4906-13.[PMID: 14581365]

[146 Kristiansen G, Pilarsky C, Pervan J, *et al.* CD24 expression is a significant predictor of PSA relapse and poor
]   prognosis   in   low   grade   or   organ   confined   prostate   cancer.   Prostate   2004;   58(2):   183-
      92.[http://dx.doi.org/10.1002/pros.10324] [PMID: 14716744]

[147 Kristiansen G, Denkert C, Schlüns K, Dahl E, Pilarsky C, Hauptmann S. CD24 is expressed in ovarian cancer
]   and is a new independent prognostic marker of patient survival. Am J Pathol 2002; 161(4): 1215-
      21.[http://dx.doi.org/10.1016/S0002-9440(10)64398-2] [PMID: 12368195]

[148 Baumann P, Thiele W, Cremers N, *et al.* CD24 interacts with and promotes the activity of c-src within lipid
]   rafts in breast cancer cells, thereby increasing integrin-dependent adhesion. Cell Mol Life Sci 2012; 69(3):
      435-48.[http://dx.doi.org/10.1007/s00018-011-0756-9] [PMID: 21710320]

[149 Kristiansen G, Sammar M, Altevogt P. Tumour biological aspects of CD24, a mucin-like adhesion molecule.
]   J   Mol   Histol   2004;   35(3):   255-62.[http://dx.doi.org/10.1023/B:HIJO.0000032357.16261.c5]   [PMID:
      15339045]

[150 Baumann P, Cremers N, Kroese F, *et al.* CD24 expression causes the acquisition of multiple cellular
]   properties   associated   with   tumor   growth   and   metastasis.   Cancer   Res   2005;   65(23):   10783-
      93.[http://dx.doi.org/10.1158/0008-5472.CAN-05-0619] [PMID: 16322224]

[151 Friederichs J, Zeller Y, Hafezi-Moghadam A, Gröne HJ, Ley K, Altevogt P. The CD24/P-selectin binding
]   pathway initiates lung arrest of human A125 adenocarcinoma cells. Cancer Res 2000; 60(23): 6714-
      22.[PMID: 11118057]

[152 Aigner S, Ramos CL, Hafezi-Moghadam A, *et al.* CD24 mediates rolling of breast carcinoma cells on P-
]   selectin. FASEB J 1998; 12(12): 1241-51.[http://dx.doi.org/10.1096/fasebj.12.12.1241] [PMID: 9737727]

[153 Athanassiadou P, Grapsa D, Gonidi M, Athanassiadou AM, Tsipis A, Patsouris E. CD24 expression has a
]   prognostic   impact   in   breast   carcinoma.   Pathol   Res   Pract   2009;   205(8):   524-

33.[http://dx.doi.org/10.1016/j.prp.2009.01.008] [PMID: 19243896]

[154 Kristiansen G, Schlüns K, Yongwei Y, Denkert C, Dietel M, Petersen I. CD24 is an independent prognostic
] marker of survival in nonsmall cell lung cancer patients. Br J Cancer 2003; 88(2): 231-6.[http://dx.doi.org/10.1038/sj.bjc.6600702] [PMID: 12610508]

[155 Smith SC, Oxford G, Wu Z, *et al.* The metastasis-associated gene CD24 is regulated by Ral GTPase and is a
] mediator of cell proliferation and survival in human cancer. Cancer Res 2006; 66(4): 1917-22.[http://dx.doi.org/10.1158/0008-5472.CAN-05-3855] [PMID: 16488989]

[156 Sagiv E, Kazanov D, Arber N. CD24 plays an important role in the carcinogenesis process of the pancreas.
] Biomed Pharmacother 2006; 60(6): 280-4.[http://dx.doi.org/10.1016/j.biopha.2006.06.006] [PMID: 16824727]

[157 Li D, Zheng L, Jin L, *et al.* CD24 polymorphisms affect risk and progression of chronic hepatitis B virus
] infection. Hepatology 2009; 50(3): 735-42.[http://dx.doi.org/10.1002/hep.23047] [PMID: 19610054]

[158 Yan Y, Zuo X, Wei D. Concise review: emerging role of CD44 in cancer stem cells: a promising biomarker
] and therapeutic target. Stem Cells Transl Med 2015; 4(9): 1033-43.[http://dx.doi.org/10.5966/sctm.2015-0048] [PMID: 26136504]

[159 Takaishi S, Okumura T, Tu S, *et al.* Identification of gastric cancer stem cells using the cell surface marker
] CD44. Stem Cells 2009; 27(5): 1006-20.[http://dx.doi.org/10.1002/stem.30] [PMID: 19415765]

[160 Pietras A, Katz AM, Ekström EJ, *et al.* Osteopontin-CD44 signaling in the glioma perivascular niche
] enhances cancer stem cell phenotypes and promotes aggressive tumor growth. Cell Stem Cell 2014; 14(3): 357-69.[http://dx.doi.org/10.1016/j.stem.2014.01.005] [PMID: 24607407]

[161 Bourguignon LY, Spevak CC, Wong G, Xia W, Gilad E. Hyaluronan-CD44 interaction with protein kinase
] C(ε) promotes oncogenic signaling by the stem cell marker Nanog and the Production of microRNA-21, leading to down-regulation of the tumor suppressor protein PDCD4, anti-apoptosis, and chemotherapy resistance in breast tumor cells. J Biol Chem 2009; 284(39): 26533-46.[http://dx.doi.org/10.1074/jbc.M109.027466] [PMID: 19633292]

[162 Ju S-Y, Chiou S-H, Su Y. Maintenance of the stemness in CD44(+) HCT-15 and HCT-116 human colon
] cancer cells requires miR-203 suppression. Stem Cell Res (Amst) 2014; 12(1): 86-100.[http://dx.doi.org/10.1016/j.scr.2013.09.011] [PMID: 24145190]

[163 Kaufmann M, Heider KH, Sinn HP, von Minckwitz G, Ponta H, Herrlich P. CD44 variant exon epitopes in
] primary breast cancer and length of survival. Lancet 1995; 345(8950): 615-9.[http://dx.doi.org/10.1016/S0140-6736(95)90521-9] [PMID: 7534855]

[164 Thapa R, Wilson GD. The importance of CD44 as a stem cell biomarker and therapeutic target in cancer.
] Stem cells international 2016; 2016[http://dx.doi.org/10.1155/2016/2087204]

[165 Bendall LJ, Gottlieb DJ. CD44 and adhesion of normal and leukemic CD34+ cells to bone marrow stroma.
] Leuk Lymphoma 1999; 32(5-6): 427-39.[http://dx.doi.org/10.3109/10428199909058400] [PMID: 10048415]

[166 Aso T, Matsuo M, Kiyohara H, *et al.* Induction of CD44 variant 9-expressing cancer stem cells might
] attenuate the efficacy of chemoradioselection and Worsens the prognosis of patients with advanced head and neck cancer. PLoS One 2015; 10(3)e0116596[http://dx.doi.org/10.1371/journal.ponc.0116596] [PMID: 25751671]

[167 Uchino M, Kojima H, Wada K, *et al.* Nuclear β-catenin and CD44 upregulation characterize invasive cell
] populations in non-aggressive MCF-7 breast cancer cells. BMC Cancer 2010; 10(1): 414.[http://dx.doi.org/10.1186/1471-2407-10-414] [PMID: 20696077]

[168 Jackson B, Brocker C, Thompson DC, *et al.* Update on the aldehyde dehydrogenase gene (ALDH)
] superfamily. Hum Genomics 2011; 5(4): 283-303.[http://dx.doi.org/10.1186/1479-7364-5-4-283] [PMID: 21712190]

[169 Li T, Su Y, Mei Y, *et al.* ALDH1A1 is a marker for malignant prostate stem cells and predictor of prostate
] cancer patients' outcome. Lab Invest 2010; 90(2): 234-44.[http://dx.doi.org/10.1038/labinvest.2009.127] [PMID: 20010854]

[170 Tulake W, Yuemaier R, Sheng L, Ru M, Lidifu D, Abudula A. Upregulation of stem cell markers ALDH1A1
] and OCT4 as potential biomarkers for the early detection of cervical carcinoma. Oncol Lett 2018; 16(5): 5525-34.[http://dx.doi.org/10.3892/ol.2018.9381] [PMID: 30344706]

[171 Mori Y, Yamawaki K, Ishiguro T, *et al.* ALDH-dependent glycolytic activation mediates stemness and
] paclitaxel resistance in patient-derived spheroid models of uterine endometrial cancer. Stem Cell Reports 2019; 13(4): 730-46.[http://dx.doi.org/10.1016/j.stemcr.2019.08.015] [PMID: 31564647]

[172 Kawasoe M. Acquired resistance of leukemic cells to AraC is associated with the upregulation of aldehyde
] dehydrogenase 1 family member A2. Experimental hematology 2013; 41(7): 597-603. e2.

[173 Prasmickaite L, Engesaeter BØ, Skrbo N, *et al.* Aldehyde dehydrogenase (ALDH) activity does not select for
]   cells with enhanced aggressive properties in malignant melanoma. PLoS One 2010;
     5(5)e10731[http://dx.doi.org/10.1371/journal.pone.0010731] [PMID: 20505780]

[174 Yang L, Wu D, Wang X, Cederbaum AI. Cytochrome P4502E1, oxidative stress, JNK, and autophagy in
]   acute alcohol-induced fatty liver. Free Radic Biol Med 2012; 53(5): 1170-
     80.[http://dx.doi.org/10.1016/j.freeradbiomed.2012.06.029] [PMID: 22749809]

[175 Zhou B-BS, Zhang H, Damelin M, Geles KG, Grindley JC, Dirks PB. Tumour-initiating cells: challenges and
]   opportunities for anticancer drug discovery. Nat Rev Drug Discov 2009; 8(10): 806-
     23.[http://dx.doi.org/10.1038/nrd2137] [PMID: 19794444]

[176 Boumahdi S, Driessens G, Lapouge G, *et al.* SOX2 controls tumour initiation and cancer stem-cell functions
]   in squamous-cell carcinoma. Nature 2014; 511(7508): 246-50.[http://dx.doi.org/10.1038/nature13305]
     [PMID: 24909994]

[177 Ma N, Thanan R, Kobayashi H, *et al.* Nitrative DNA damage and Oct3/4 expression in urinary bladder
]   cancer with Schistosoma haematobium infection. Biochem Biophys Res Commun 2011; 414(2): 344-
     9.[http://dx.doi.org/10.1016/j.bbrc.2011.09.073] [PMID: 21951846]

[178 Thanan R, Pairojkul C, Pinlaor S, *et al.* Inflammation-related DNA damage and expression of CD133 and
]   Oct3/4 in cholangiocarcinoma patients with poor prognosis. Free Radic Biol Med 2013; 65: 1464-
     72.[http://dx.doi.org/10.1016/j.freeradbiomed.2013.07.034] [PMID: 23917144]

[179 Kitamura T, Qian BZ, Soong D, *et al.* CCL2-induced chemokine cascade promotes breast cancer metastasis
]   by enhancing retention of metastasis-associated macrophages. J Exp Med 2015; 212(7): 1043-
     59.[http://dx.doi.org/10.1084/jem.20141836] [PMID: 26056232]

[180 Anido J, Sáez-Borderías A, Gonzàlez-Juncà A, *et al.* TGF-β receptor inhibitors target the CD44high/Id1high
]   glioma-initiating cell population in human glioblastoma. Cancer Cell 2010; 18(6): 655-
     68.[http://dx.doi.org/10.1016/j.ccr.2010.10.023] [PMID: 21156287]

[181 Li T, Zhang C, Ding Y, *et al.* Umbilical cord-derived mesenchymal stem cells promote proliferation and
]   migration in MCF-7 and MDA-MB-231 breast cancer cells through activation of the ERK pathway. Oncol
     Rep 2015; 34(3): 1469-77.[http://dx.doi.org/10.3892/or.2015.4109] [PMID: 26151310]

[182 Wang W, Zhong W, Yuan J, *et al.* Involvement of Wnt/β-catenin signaling in the mesenchymal stem cells
]   promote metastatic growth and chemoresistance of cholangiocarcinoma. Oncotarget 2015; 6(39): 42276-
     89.[http://dx.doi.org/10.18632/oncotarget.5514] [PMID: 26474277]

[183 Lu J, Ye X, Fan F, *et al.* Endothelial cells promote the colorectal cancer stem cell phenotype through a
]   soluble form of Jagged-1. Cancer Cell 2013; 23(2): 171-85.[http://dx.doi.org/10.1016/j.ccr.2012.12.021]
     [PMID: 23375636]

[184 Xu J, Zhang C, He Y, *et al.* Lymphatic endothelial cell-secreted CXCL1 stimulates lymphangiogenesis and
]   metastasis of gastric cancer. Int J Cancer 2012; 130(4): 787-97.[http://dx.doi.org/10.1002/ijc.26035] [PMID:
     21387301]

[185 Johnson LA, Jackson DG. Inflammation-induced secretion of CCL21 in lymphatic endothelium is a key
]   regulator of integrin-mediated dendritic cell transmigration. Int Immunol 2010; 22(10): 839-
     49.[http://dx.doi.org/10.1093/intimm/dxq435] [PMID: 20739459]

[186 Chiquet-Ehrismann R, Orend G, Chiquet M, Tucker RP, Midwood KS. Tenascins in stem cell niches. Matrix
]   Biol 2014; 37: 112-23.[http://dx.doi.org/10.1016/j.matbio.2014.01.007] [PMID: 24472737]

[187 Mani SA, Guo W, Liao MJ, *et al.* The epithelial-mesenchymal transition generates cells with properties of
]   stem cells. Cell 2008; 133(4): 704-15.[http://dx.doi.org/10.1016/j.cell.2008.03.027] [PMID: 18485877]

[188 Morel A-P, Lièvre M, Thomas C, Hinkal G, Ansieau S, Puisieux A. Generation of breast cancer stem cells
]   through epithelial-mesenchymal transition. PLoS One 2008;
     3(8)e2888[http://dx.doi.org/10.1371/journal.pone.0002888] [PMID: 18682804]

[189 Selby C, Yacko LR, Glode AE. Gemtuzumab ozogamicin: Back again. J Adv Pract Oncol 2019; 10(1): 68-
]   82.[PMID: 31308990]

[190 Egan PC, Reagan JL. The return of gemtuzumab ozogamicin: a humanized anti-CD33 monoclonal antibody-
]   drug conjugate for the treatment of newly diagnosed acute myeloid leukemia. OncoTargets Ther 2018; 11:
     8265-72.[http://dx.doi.org/10.2147/OTT.S150807] [PMID: 30538495]

[191 Bennett G, Brown A, Mudd G, *et al.* MMAE delivery using the Bicycle toxin conjugate BT5528. Mol Cancer
]   Ther 2020; 19(7): 1385-94.[http://dx.doi.org/10.1158/1535-7163.MCT-19-1092] [PMID: 32398269]

[192 Jin L, Lee EM, Ramshaw HS, *et al.* Monoclonal antibody-mediated targeting of CD123, IL-3 receptor α
]   chain, eliminates human acute myeloid leukemic stem cells. Cell Stem Cell 2009; 5(1): 31-
     42.[http://dx.doi.org/10.1016/j.stem.2009.04.018] [PMID: 19570512]

[193
]	Jin L, Hope KJ, Zhai Q, Smadja-Joffe F, Dick JE. Targeting of CD44 eradicates human acute myeloid leukemic stem cells. Nat Med 2006; 12(10): 1167-74.[http://dx.doi.org/10.1038/nm1483] [PMID: 16998484]

[194
]	Chandrakesan P, Yao J, Qu D, et al. Dclk1, a tumor stem cell marker, regulates pro-survival signaling and self-renewal of intestinal tumor cells. Mol Cancer 2017; 16(1): 30.[http://dx.doi.org/10.1186/s12943-017-0594-y] [PMID: 28148261]

[195
]	Nakanishi Y, Seno H, Fukuoka A, et al. Dclk1 distinguishes between tumor and normal stem cells in the intestine. Nat Genet 2013; 45(1): 98-103.[http://dx.doi.org/10.1038/ng.2481] [PMID: 23202126]

[196
]	Alkilany AM, Thompson LB, Boulos SP, Sisco PN, Murphy CJ. Gold nanorods: their potential for photothermal therapeutics and drug delivery, tempered by the complexity of their biological interactions. Adv Drug Deliv Rev 2012; 64(2): 190-9.[http://dx.doi.org/10.1016/j.addr.2011.03.005] [PMID: 21397647]

[197
]	Rupp U, Schoendorf-Holland E, Eichbaum M, et al. Safety and pharmacokinetics of bivatuzumab mertansine in patients with CD44v6-positive metastatic breast cancer: final results of a phase I study. Anticancer Drugs 2007; 18(4): 477-85.[http://dx.doi.org/10.1097/CAD.0b013e32801403f4] [PMID: 17351401]

[198
]	Birzele F, Voss E, Nopora A, et al. CD44 isoform status predicts response to treatment with anti-CD44 antibody in cancer patients. Clin Cancer Res 2015; 21(12): 2753-62.[http://dx.doi.org/10.1158/1078-0432.CCR-14-2141] [PMID: 25762343]

[199
]	Perez A. Targeting CD44 in head and neck squamous cell carcinoma (HNSCC) with a new humanized antibody RO5429083 2012.

[200
]	Bidlingmaier S, Zhu X, Liu B. The utility and limitations of glycosylated human CD133 epitopes in defining cancer stem cells. J Mol Med (Berl) 2008; 86(9): 1025-32.[http://dx.doi.org/10.1007/s00109-008-0357-8] [PMID: 18535813]

[201
]	Zhao L, Yang Y, Zhou P, et al. Targeting CD133high colorectal cancer cells in vitro and in vivo with an asymmetric bispecific antibody. J Immunother 2015; 38(6): 217-28.[http://dx.doi.org/10.1097/CJI.0000000000000086] [PMID: 26049545]

[202
]	Druker BJ, Talpaz M, Resta DJ, et al. Efficacy and safety of a specific inhibitor of the BCR-ABL tyrosine kinase in chronic myeloid leukemia. N Engl J Med 2001; 344(14): 1031-7.[http://dx.doi.org/10.1056/NEJM200104053441401] [PMID: 11287972]

[203
]	Han M-E, Jeon TY, Hwang SH, et al. Cancer spheres from gastric cancer patients provide an ideal model system for cancer stem cell research. Cell Mol Life Sci 2011; 68(21): 3589-605.[http://dx.doi.org/10.1007/s00018-011-0672-z] [PMID: 21448722]

[204
]	Alberts DS, Liu PY, Wilczynski SP, et al. Phase II trial of imatinib mesylate in recurrent, biomarker positive, ovarian cancer (Southwest Oncology Group Protocol S0211). Int J Gynecol Cancer 2007; 17(4): 784-8.[http://dx.doi.org/10.1111/j.1525-1438.2007.00882.x] [PMID: 17343607]

[205
]	Cristofanilli M, Morandi P, Krishnamurthy S, et al. Imatinib mesylate (Gleevec) in advanced breast cancer-expressing C-Kit or PDGFR-β: clinical activity and biological correlations. Ann Oncol 2008; 19(10): 1713-9.[http://dx.doi.org/10.1093/annonc/mdn352] [PMID: 18515258]

[206
]	Levina V, Marrangoni A, Wang T, et al. Elimination of human lung cancer stem cells through targeting of the stem cell factor-c-kit autocrine signaling loop. Cancer Res 2010; 70(1): 338-46.[http://dx.doi.org/10.1158/0008-5472.CAN-09-1102] [PMID: 20028869]

[207
]	Pan Q, Li Q, Liu S, et al. Concise review: targeting cancer stem cells using immunologic approaches. Stem Cells 2015; 33(7): 2085-92.[http://dx.doi.org/10.1002/stem.2039] [PMID: 25873269]

[208
]	Bonnet D, Warren EH, Greenberg PD, Dick JE, Riddell SR. CD8(+) minor histocompatibility antigen-specific cytotoxic T lymphocyte clones eliminate human acute myeloid leukemia stem cells. Proc Natl Acad Sci USA 1999; 96(15): 8639-44.[http://dx.doi.org/10.1073/pnas.96.15.8639] [PMID: 10411928]

[209
]	Visus C, Ito D, Amoscato A, et al. Identification of human aldehyde dehydrogenase 1 family member A1 as a novel CD8+ T-cell-defined tumor antigen in squamous cell carcinoma of the head and neck. Cancer Res 2007; 67(21): 10538-45.[http://dx.doi.org/10.1158/0008-5472.CAN-07-1346] [PMID: 17974998]

[210
]	Visus C, Wang Y, Lozano-Leon A, et al. Targeting ALDH(bright) human carcinoma-initiating cells with ALDH1A1-specific CD8[+] T cells. Clin Cancer Res 2011; 17(19): 6174-84.[http://dx.doi.org/10.1158/1078-0432.CCR-11-1111] [PMID: 21856769]

[211
]	Volonté A, Di Tomaso T, Spinelli M, et al. Cancer-initiating cells from colorectal cancer patients escape from T cell-mediated immunosurveillance in vitro through membrane-bound IL-4. J Immunol 2014; 192(1): 523-32.[http://dx.doi.org/10.4049/jimmunol.1301342] [PMID: 24277698]

[212
]	Ning N, Pan Q, Zheng F, et al. Cancer stem cell vaccination confers significant antitumor immunity. Cancer Res 2012; 72(7): 1853-64.[http://dx.doi.org/10.1158/0008-5472.CAN-11-1400] [PMID: 22473314]

[213 Lu L, Tao H, Chang AE, *et al.* Cancer stem cell vaccine inhibits metastases of primary tumors and induces
]   humoral   immune   responses   against   cancer   stem   cells.   OncoImmunology   2015;
     4(3)e990767[http://dx.doi.org/10.4161/2162402X.2014.990767] [PMID: 25949905]

[214 Palucka K, Banchereau J. Cancer immunotherapy *via* dendritic cells. Nat Rev Cancer 2012; 12(4): 265-
]   77.[http://dx.doi.org/10.1038/nrc3258] [PMID: 22437871]

[215 Facucho-Oliveira JM, St John JC. The relationship between pluripotency and mitochondrial DNA
]   proliferation during early embryo development and embryonic stem cell differentiation. Stem Cell Rev Rep
     2009; 5(2): 140-58.[http://dx.doi.org/10.1007/s12015-009-9058-0] [PMID: 19521804]

[216 Panopoulos AD, Yanes O, Ruiz S, *et al.* The metabolome of induced pluripotent stem cells reveals metabolic
]   changes   occurring   in   somatic   cell   reprogramming.   Cell   Res   2012;   22(1):   168-
     77.[http://dx.doi.org/10.1038/cr.2011.177] [PMID: 22064701]

[217 Liu PP, Liao J, Tang ZJ, *et al.* Metabolic regulation of cancer cell side population by glucose through
]   activation   of   the   Akt   pathway.   Cell   Death   Differ   2014;   21(1):   124-
     35.[http://dx.doi.org/10.1038/cdd.2013.131] [PMID: 24096870]

[218 Ciavardelli D, Rossi C, Barcaroli D, *et al.* Breast cancer stem cells rely on fermentative glycolysis and are
]   sensitive   to   2-deoxyglucose   treatment.   Cell   Death   Dis   2014;   5(7):   e1336-
     6.[http://dx.doi.org/10.1038/cddis.2014.285] [PMID: 25032859]

[219 Liao J, Qian F, Tchabo N, *et al.* Ovarian cancer spheroid cells with stem cell-like properties contribute to
]   tumor generation, metastasis and chemotherapy resistance through hypoxia-resistant metabolism. PLoS One
     2014; 9(1)e84941[http://dx.doi.org/10.1371/journal.pone.0084941] [PMID: 24409314]

[220 Zhou Y, Zhou Y, Shingu T, *et al.* Metabolic alterations in highly tumorigenic glioblastoma cells: preference
]   for   hypoxia   and   high   dependency   on   glycolysis.   J   Biol   Chem   2011;   286(37):   32843-
     53.[http://dx.doi.org/10.1074/jbc.M111.260935] [PMID: 21795717]

[221 Janiszewska M, Suvà ML, Riggi N, *et al.* Imp2 controls oxidative phosphorylation and is crucial for
]   preserving   glioblastoma   cancer   stem   cells.   Genes   Dev   2012;   26(17):   1926-
     44.[http://dx.doi.org/10.1101/gad.188292.112] [PMID: 22899010]

[222 Lagadinou ED, Sach A, Callahan K, *et al.* BCL-2 inhibition targets oxidative phosphorylation and selectively
]   eradicates   quiescent   human   leukemia   stem   cells.   Cell   Stem   Cell   2013;   12(3):   329-
     41.[http://dx.doi.org/10.1016/j.stem.2012.12.013] [PMID: 23333149]

[223 Sancho P, Burgos-Ramos E, Tavera A, *et al.* MYC/PGC-1α balance determines the metabolic phenotype and
]   plasticity   of   pancreatic   cancer   stem   cells.   Cell   Metab   2015;   22(4):   590-
     605.[http://dx.doi.org/10.1016/j.cmet.2015.08.015] [PMID: 26365176]

[224 Pandya K, Meeke K, Clementz AG, *et al.* Targeting both Notch and ErbB-2 signalling pathways is required
]   for   prevention   of   ErbB-2-positive   breast   tumour   recurrence.   Br   J   Cancer   2011;   105(6):   796-
     806.[http://dx.doi.org/10.1038/bjc.2011.321] [PMID: 21847123]

[225 Messersmith WA, Shapiro GI, Cleary JM, *et al.* A Phase I, dose-finding study in patients with advanced solid
]   malignancies   of   the   oral   γ-secretase   inhibitor   PF-03084014.   Clin   Cancer   Res   2015;   21(1):   60-
     7.[http://dx.doi.org/10.1158/1078-0432.CCR-14-0607] [PMID: 25231399]

[226 Gavai AV, Quesnelle C, Norris D, *et al.* Discovery of clinical candidate BMS-906024: a potent pan-notch
]   inhibitor   for   the   treatment   of   leukemia   and   solid   tumors.   ACS   Med   Chem   Lett   2015;   6(5):   523-
     7.[http://dx.doi.org/10.1021/acsmedchemlett.5b00001] [PMID: 26005526]

[227 Ahmadzadeh M, Rosenberg SA. TGF-β 1 attenuates the acquisition and expression of effector function by
]   tumor   antigen-specific   human   memory   CD8   T   cells.   J   Immunol   2005;   174(9):   5215-
     23.[http://dx.doi.org/10.4049/jimmunol.174.9.5215] [PMID: 15843517]

[228 Yen W-C, Fischer MM, Axelrod F, *et al.* Targeting Notch signaling with a Notch2/Notch3 antagonist
]   (tarextumab) inhibits tumor growth and decreases tumor-initiating cell frequency. Clin Cancer Res 2015;
     21(9): 2084-95.[http://dx.doi.org/10.1158/1078-0432.CCR-14-2808] [PMID: 25934888]

[229 Crane AM, Kramer P, Bui JH, *et al.* Targeted correction and restored function of the CFTR gene in cystic
]   fibrosis   induced   pluripotent   stem   cells.   Stem   Cell   Reports   2015;   4(4):   569-
     77.[http://dx.doi.org/10.1016/j.stemcr.2015.02.005] [PMID: 25772471]

[230 Stechishin OD, Luchman HA, Ruan Y, *et al.* On-target JAK2/STAT3 inhibition slows disease progression in
]   orthotopic   xenografts   of   human   glioblastoma   brain   tumor   stem   cells.   Neuro-oncol   2013;   15(2):   198-
     207.[http://dx.doi.org/10.1093/neuonc/nos302] [PMID: 23262510]

[231 Wang-Gillam A. Phase I study of defactinib combined with pembrolizumab and gemcitabine in patients with
]   advanced cancer. American Society of Clinical Oncology 2018.